BEST MEDICINE

Asthma

Dr George Kassianos
Professor Fan Chung
Dr Kevin Gruffydd-Jones
Dr Mike Thomas
Professor David Price

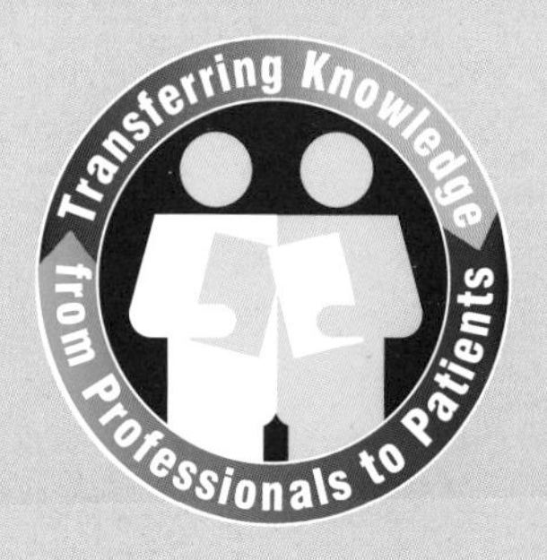

Foreword by Claire Rayner
President of the Patients Association

Managing Editor: Dr Scott Chambers
Medical Writers: Dr Eleanor Bull, Dr Rebecca Fox-Spencer, Dr Anna Palmer, Dr Susan Chambers
Editorial Controller: Emma Catherall
Operations Manager: Julia Potterton
Designer: Chris Matthews
Typesetter: Julie Smith
Indexer: Laurence Errington
Director – Online Business: Peter Llewellyn
Publishing Director: Julian Grover
Publisher: Stephen I'Anson

1 Bankside
Lodge Road
Long Hanborough
Oxfordshire
OX29 8LJ, UK
Tel: +44 (0)1993 885370
Fax: +44 (0)1993 881868
Email: *enquiries@bestmedicine.com*

www.bestmedicine.com
www.csfmedical.com

You are strongly urged to consult your doctor before taking, stopping or changing any of the products reviewed or referred to in *BESTMEDICINE* or any other medication that has been prescribed or recommended by your doctor.

A catalogue record for this book is available from the British Library.

ISBN: 1-905064-94-2

Typeset by Creative, Langbank, Scotland.
Printed and bound in Wales.
Distributed by NBN International, Plymouth, Devon.

Contents

Foreword

Claire Rayner
President of The Patients Association

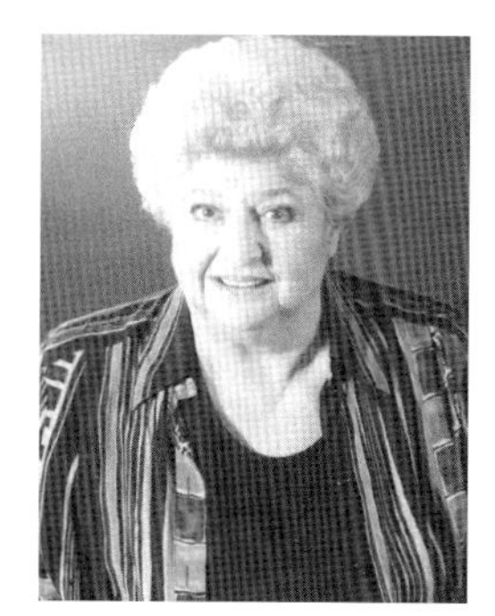

Photograph courtesy of Amanda Rayner

Patients and their families are rightly entitled to have access to good-quality, independent and reliable information concerning a diverse range of conditions and a wide variety of medications that are available to treat them. Indeed, there is a growing recognition amongst the majority of healthcare professionals that well-informed patients are more likely to adopt a more active role in the management of their illness and will therefore feel more satisfied with the care that they receive. Such an effect has the potential not only to directly benefit the patient and their families, but can also maximise limited healthcare resources within an already over-stretched NHS. However, at present access to this kind of information is limited, despite the fact that as many as one-in-four adults (12 million people in the UK alone) want ready access to this knowledge prior to visiting their doctor.

The importance of patient self-management is a key component of current NHS strategy. Indeed, this has been widely acknowledged in an NHS-led campaign called the Expert Patient Programme (*www.expertpatient.nhs.uk*). This is a self-management course which aims to give people the confidence, skills and knowledge to manage their condition better and take more control of their lives. The Expert Patient Programme defines an Expert Patient as one who has had the condition for long enough to have learnt the language doctors use.

BESTMEDICINE aims to meet the information and educational needs of both patients and healthcare professionals alike. The information found in the *BESTMEDICINE* series will assist patients and their families to obtain the level of information they now need to understand and manage their medical condition in partnership with their doctor. However, as *BESTMEDICINE* draws much of its content from medical publications written by doctors for doctors, some readers may find these books rather challenging when they first approach them. Despite this, I strongly believe that the effort that you invest in reading this book will be fully repaid by the increased knowledge they you will gain about this condition. Indeed, the extensive glossary of terms that can be found within each book certainly makes understanding the text a great deal easier, and the Patient Notes section is also very informative and reassuringly written by a doctor for the less scientifically minded reader. *BESTMEDICINE* represents the world's first source of independent, unabridged medical information that will appeal to patients and their families as well as healthcare professionals. This development should be welcomed and applauded, and I would commend these books to you.

Claire Rayner, November 2004

Claire Rayner has been involved with the Patients Association for many years and has considerable expertise and experience from a professional background in nursing and journalism and her personal experience as a patient and carer. She is well known as a leading 'Agony Aunt' and as a medical correspondent for many popular magazines. Claire has also published articles in a number of professional journals, as well as over forty medical, nursing and patient advice books.

An introduction to *BESTMEDICINE*

The source: information for healthcare professionals

Over the years, it has become increasingly apparent that there is a dearth of drug-related information that is independently compiled and robustly reviewed, and which also acknowledges the challenges faced by healthcare professionals when applying evidence-based medicine whilst practising at the 'front line' of patient care. As such, many healthcare professionals feel a certain ambivalence towards the numerous drug review publications that are currently on offer and, indeed, many do not have confidence in the information that can be found within their pages. In response to the need for a more impartial information resource – one that is independent of the pharmaceutical industry and the health service – we developed a novel publication, which was launched to meet this perceived lack of independent information. This peer-reviewed publication is called *Drugs in Context* and was launched in May 2003 and is the source of much of what you will find in this edition of *BESTMEDICINE*.

Uniquely independent

Drugs in Context is unique in that it reviews the significant clinical and pharmacological evidence underpinning the use of a single drug, in the disease area(s) where it is used and the practice setting where it is most commonly prescribed. Over 50 issues are published each year covering numerous diseases and conditions. The principal goal of *Drugs in Context* is to become the definitive drug and disease management resource for all healthcare professionals. As such, over the coming years, the publication plans to review all of the significant drugs that are currently used in clinical practice.

Reliable and impartial information for patients too

In addition to the lack of impartial information for the healthcare professional, we also firmly believe that there is a significant and growing number of patients who are not served well in this regard either. Indeed, it is becoming apparent to us that many patients would welcome access to the same sources of information on drugs and diseases that their doctors and other healthcare professionals have access to.

There are numerous sources of information currently available to patients – ranging from leaflets and books to websites and other electronic media. However, despite their best intentions, the rigour and accuracy of many of these resources cannot be relied upon due to significant variation in the quality of the material. Perhaps the major problem facing a patient or a loved one who is hunting for specific information relating to a disease or the drug that has been prescribed by their doctor is that there is simply too much material available, making sifting through it to find a relevant fact akin to looking for a needle in a haystack! More importantly, many of these resources can often (albeit unintentionally) patronise the reader who has made every effort to actively seek out information that can serve to reassure themselves about the concerned illness and about the medication(s) prescribed for it.

Can knowledge be the '*BESTMEDICINE*'?

We firmly believe as healthcare professionals, that an informed patient is more likely to take an active role in the management of their disease or condition and, therefore, will be more likely to benefit from any course of treatment. This means that everyone will benefit – the patient, their family and friends, the healthcare professionals involved in their care, and the NHS and the country as a whole! Indeed, such is the importance of patient education, that the NHS has launched an initiative emphasising the need for patients to assume a more active role in the management of their condition via the acquisition of knowledge and skills related specifically to their disease. This initiative is called the Expert Patients Programme (*www.expertpatients.nhs.uk*).

Filling the need for quality information

Many of our observations about the lack of quality education have underpinned the principles behind the launch of *BESTMEDICINE*, much of the content of which is drawn directly from the pages of *Drugs in Context*, as written by and for healthcare professionals. *BESTMEDICINE* aims to appeal primarily to the patient, loved-one or carer who wants to improve their knowledge of the disease in question, the evidence for and against the drugs available to treat the disease and the practical challenges faced by healthcare professionals in managing it.

A whole new language!

We fully acknowledge that a lot of medical terminology used in order to expedite communication amongst the medical community will be new to many of you, some terms may be difficult to pronounce and sometimes surplus to requirements. However, rather than significantly abridge the content and risk excluding something of importance to the reader, we have instead provided you with a comprehensive glossary of terms and what we hope will be helpful additional GP discussion pieces at the end of each section to aid understanding further. We have also provided you with an introduction to the processes underlying drug development and the key concepts in disease management which we hope you will also find informative and which we strongly recommend that you read before tackling the rest of this edition of *BESTMEDICINE*.

No secrets

By providing the same information to patients and their families as healthcare professionals we believe that *BESTMEDICINE* will help to foster better relationships between patients, their families and doctors and other healthcare professionals and ultimately may even improve treatment outcomes.

This edition is one of a number of unique collections of disease summaries and drug reviews that we will be making widely available over the coming months. You will find details about each issue as it is published at *www.bestmedicine.com*.

We do hope that you find this edition of *BESTMEDICINE* illuminating.

Dr George Kassianos, GP, Bracknell; Editor-in-Chief – *Drugs in Context*; Editor – *BESTMEDICINE*
Dr Jonathan Morrell, GP, Hastings; Medical Editor (Primary Care) – *Drugs in Context*
Dr Michael Schachter, Consultant Physician, St Mary's Hospital Paddington; Clinical Pharmacology Editor – *Drugs in Context*

Reader's guide

We acknowledge that some of the medical and scientific terminology used throughout *BESTMEDICINE* will be new to you and will address sometimes challenging concepts. However, rather than abridge the content and risk excluding important information, we have included this Reader's Guide to dissect and explain the contents of *BESTMEDICINE* in order to make it more digestible to the less scientifically minded reader. We recommend that you familiarise yourself with the drug development process, summarised below, before embarking on the Drug Reviews. This brief synopsis clarifies and contextualises many of the specialist terms encountered in the Drug Reviews.

Following this Reader's Guide, you will find that *BESTMEDICINE* is made up of two main sections – a Disease Overview and the Drug Reviews – both of which are evidence-based and as such have been highly referenced. All references are listed at the end of a section. Importantly, the manuscript has been 'peer-reviewed', which means that it has undergone rigorous checks for accuracy both by a practising doctor and a specialist in drug pharmacology. The Disease Overview and Drug Reviews are sandwiched between two opinion pieces, an Editorial, written by a recognised expert in the field, and an Improving Practice article, written by a practising GP with a specialist interest in the disease area. It is important to bear in mind that these authors are addressing their professional colleagues, rather than a 'lay' reader, providing you with a fascinating and unique insight into many of the challenges faced by doctors in the day-to-day practice of medicine.

The Disease Overview, Drug Reviews and Improving Practice sections are all followed by a short commentary by Dr Mike Thomas and Professor David Price entitled Patient Notes. In these sections, Dr Thomas and Professor Price reiterate some of the key issues raised in rather more 'user-friendly' language.

As mentioned previously, much of the content of *BESTMEDICINE* has been taken directly from *Drugs in Context,* which is written by and for healthcare professionals. Consequently, some of the language used may be difficult for the less scientifically minded reader. To help with this, in addition to the Patient Notes, we have included a comprehensive glossary of those terms underlined in the text. Terms will not be underlined in tables or figures, but the more difficult words will be defined in the Glossary.

Disease overview

The disease overview provides a brief synopsis of the disease, its symptoms, diagnosis and a critique of the currently available treatment options.

- The epidemiology, or incidence and distribution of the disease within a population, is discussed, with particular emphasis on UK-specific data.

- The aetiology section describes the specific causes or origins of the disease, which are usually a result of both genetic and environmental factors. Multifactorial diseases result from more than one causative element. If an individual has a genetic predisposition, they are more susceptible to developing the disease as a result of their genetic make-up.
- The functional changes that accompany a particular syndrome or disease constitute its pathophysiology.
- The management of a disease may be influenced by treatment guidelines, specific directives published by government agencies, professional societies, or by the convening of expert panels. The National Institute for Clinical Excellence (NICE), an independent sector of the NHS comprised of experts in the field of treatment, is one such body.
- The social and economic factors that characterise the influence of the disease, describe its socioeconomic impact. Such factors include the cost to the healthcare provider to treat the disease – in terms of GP consultations, drug costs and the subsequent burden on hospital resources – or the cost to the patient or employer with respect to the number of work days lost as a consequence of ill health.

Drug reviews

The pharmacokinetics of a drug are of interest to healthcare professionals because it is important for them to understand the action of a drug on the body over a period of time.

The drug reviews are not intended to address every available treatment for a particular disease. Rather, we focus on the major drugs currently available in the UK for the treatment of the featured disease and evaluate their performance in clinical trials and their safety in clinical practice. The basic pharmacology of the drug – the branch of science that deals with the origin, nature, chemistry, effects and uses of drugs – is discussed initially. This includes a description of the mechanism of action of the drug, the manner in which it exerts its therapeutic effects, and its pharmacokinetics (or the activity of the drug within the body over a period of time). Pharmacokinetics encompasses the absorption of the drug into or across the tissues of the body, its distribution to specific functional areas, its metabolism – the process by which it is broken down within the body into by-products (metabolites) – and ultimately, its removal or excretion from the body. The most frequently used pharmacokinetic terms that are used in the drug review sections of this issue of *BESTMEDICINE* are explained in Table 1.

Whilst the basic pharmacology of a drug is clearly important, the main focus of the drug review is to summarise the drug's performance in controlled clinical trials. Clinical trials examine the effectiveness, or clinical efficacy, of the drug against the disease or condition it was developed to treat, as well as its safety and tolerability – the side-effects associated with the drug and the likelihood that the patient will tolerate treatment. Adherence to drug treatment, or patient compliance, reflects the tendency of patients to comply with the terms of their treatment regimen. Compliance may be affected by treatment-related side-effects or the convenience of drug treatment. The safety of the drug also

Table 1. Key terms.

Term	Definition
Agonist	A drug/substance that has affinity for specific cell receptors thereby triggering a biological response.
Antagonist	A drug/substance that blocks the action of another by binding to a specific cell receptor without eliciting a biological response.
AUC (area under curve)	A plot of the concentration of a drug against the time since initial administration. It is a means of analysing the bioavailability of a drug.
Binding affinity	An attractive force between substances that causes them to enter into and remain in chemical contact.
Bioavailability	The degree and rate at which a drug is absorbed into a living system or is made available at the site of physiological activity.
Clearance	The rate at which the drug is removed from the blood by excretion into the urine through the kidneys.
C_{max}	The maximum concentration of the drug recorded in the blood plasma.
Cytochrome P450 (CYP) system	A group of enzymes responsible for the metabolism of a number of different drugs and substances within the body.
Dose dependency	In which the effect of the drug is proportional to the concentration of drug administered.
Enzyme	A protein produced in the body that catalyses chemical reactions without itself being destroyed or altered. The suffix 'ase' is used when designating an enzyme.
Excretion	The elimination of a waste product (in faeces or urine) from the body.
Half-life ($t_{1/2}$)	The time required for half the original amount of a drug to be eliminated from the body by natural processes.
Inhibitor	A substance that reduces the activity of another substance.
Ligand	Any substance that binds to another and brings about a biological response.
Potency	A measure of the power of a drug to produce the desired effects.
Protein binding	The extent to which a drug attaches to proteins, peptides or enzymes within the body.
Receptor	A molecular structure, usually (but not always) situated on the cell membrane, which mediates the biological response that is associated with a particular drug/substance.
Synergism	A phenomenon in which the combined effects of two drugs are more powerful than when either drug is administered alone.
t_{max}	The time taken to reach C_{max}.
Volume of distribution (V_D)	The total amount of drug in the body divided by its concentration in the blood plasma. Used as a measure of the dispersal of the drug within the body once it has been absorbed.

encompasses its contra-indications, conditions under which the drug should never be prescribed. This may mean avoiding use in special patient populations (e.g. young or elderly patients, or those with co-existing or comorbid conditions, such as liver or kidney disease) or avoiding co-administration with certain other medications.

A brief synopsis of the drug development process is outlined below, in order to clarify and put into context many of the specialist terms encountered throughout the drug reviews.

The drug development process

Launching a new drug is an extremely costly and time-consuming venture. The entire process can cost an estimated £500 million and can take between 10 and 15 years from the initial identification of a potentially useful therapeutic compound in the laboratory to launching the finished product as a treatment for a particular disease (Figure 1). Much of this time is spent fulfilling strict guidelines set out by regulatory authorities, in order to ensure the safety and quality of the end product. As a consequence of this, a drug can fail at any stage of the development process and its development abandoned. Once identified and registered, the new drug can be protected by a patent for 20 years, after which time other companies are free to manufacture and market identical drugs, called generics. Thus, the pharmaceutical company has a finite period of time before patent expiry to recoup the cost of drug development (of both successful drugs and those drugs that do not make it to the marketplace) and return a profit to their shareholders.

Figure 1. The drug development process.

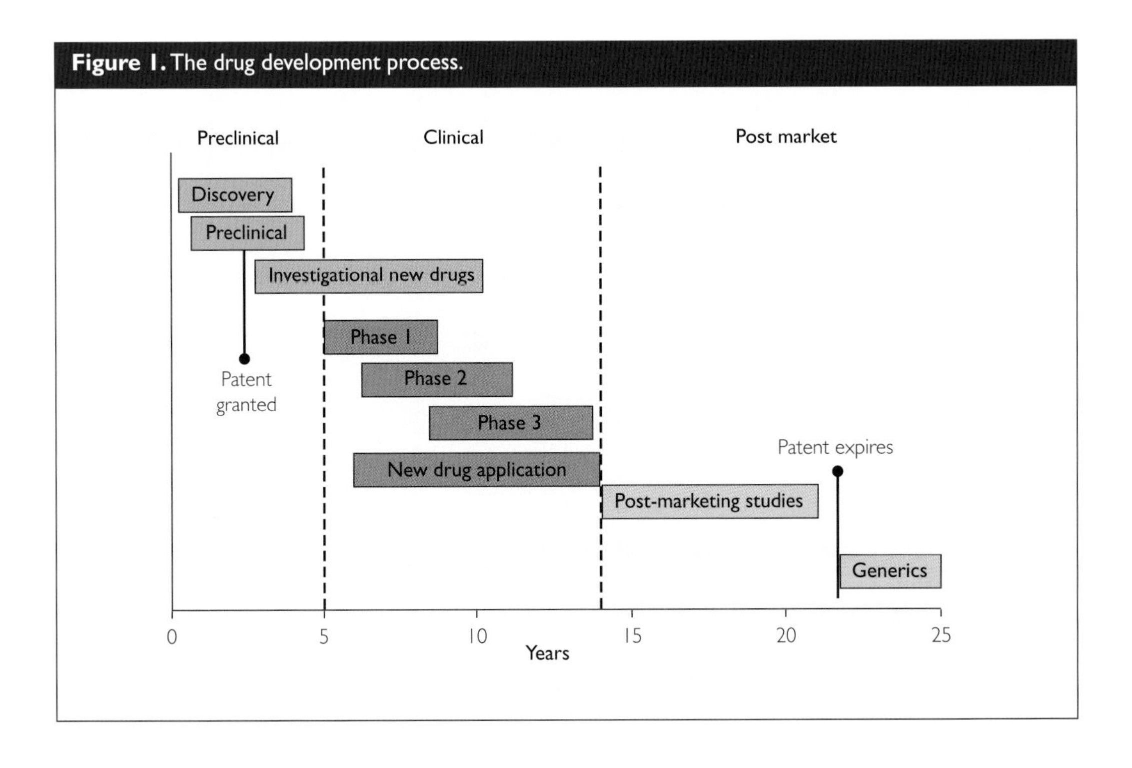

Potential new drugs are identified by the research and development (R&D) department of the pharmaceutical company. After a candidate drug has been selected for development, it enters a rigorous testing procedure with five distinct phases – preclinical, which takes place in the laboratory, and phases 1, 2, 3 and 4, which involve testing in humans. Approval from the regulatory body is essential before the drug can be marketed and is dependent on the satisfactory completion of all phases of testing. In the UK, the Medicines and Healthcare Products Agency (MHRA) and the European Medicines Evaluation Agency (EMEA) regulate the development process and companies must apply to these organisations for marketing authorisation. Within Europe, the Mutual Recognition Procedure means that the approval of a drug in one country (the Reference Member State), forms the basis for its subsequent approval in other European Union member states. This can make the approval process more efficient and may lead to approval being granted in several European countries at once. Once approval has been granted, the drug will be given a licence detailing the specific disease or conditions it is indicated to treat and the patient groups it may be used in. The drug will be assigned either prescription-only medicine (POM) or over-the counter (OTC) status. POMs can only be obtained following consultation with a doctor, who will actively supervise their use.

Preclinical testing

Preclinical testing is essential before a drug can progress to human clinical trials. It is estimated that only one of every 1000 compounds that enter the preclinical stage continue into human testing (phases 1–4). Preclinical testing, or screening, is for the main-part performed in animals, and every effort is made to use as few animals as possible and to ensure their humane and proper care. Generally, two or more species (one rodent, one non-rodent) are tested, since a drug may affect one species differently from another.

Although a drug will never act in exactly the same way in animals as in humans, animal models are designed to mimic a human disease condition as closely as possible and provide information essential to drug development. *In vitro* experiments – literally meaning 'in glass' – are performed outside the living system in a laboratory setting. *In vivo* experiments are performed in the living cell or organism.

It is during the preclinical phase that the pharmacodynamics of the drug will first be examined. These include its mechanism of action, or the way in which it exerts its therapeutic effects. The drug's pharmacokinetics, toxicology (potentially hazardous or poisonous effects) and the formulation of the drug – the manner in which it is taken (e.g. tablet, injection, liquid) – are also assessed at this point in development.

Phase I

Phase 1 trials are usually conducted in a small group of 10–80 healthy volunteers and further evaluate the biochemical and physiological effects of the drug – its chemical and biological impact within the body. An appropriate dosage range will be established at this point – the maximum and minimum therapeutic concentrations of the drug which are associated with a tolerable number of side-effects (secondary and usually adverse events unrelated to the beneficial effects of the drug). The mechanism of action and pharmacokinetic effects of the drugs are also further explored in this, the first group of human subjects to receive the drug.

Phase 2

If no major problems are revealed during phase 1 development, the drug can progress to phase 2 screening which takes place in 100–300 patients diagnosed with the disease or condition that the drug is designed to treat. At this stage it is important to determine the effectiveness, or efficacy, of the drug. If the drug is no better than placebo then it will not be granted a licence. The side-effect or adverse event profile of the drug is re-examined at this stage, and is particularly pertinent in these patients, who may react more severely to the drug than healthy volunteers. The likelihood and severity of drug interactions is also of great importance in this patient group. Drug interactions – in which the action of one drug interferes with the action of another – can occur if the patient is taking more than one form of medication for the treatment of a comorbid disease or condition. If multiple drugs are administered together, or concomitantly, then the risk of drug interactions is increased.

Phase 3

Phase 3 clinical trials involve between 1000 and 3000 patients diagnosed with the relevant disease or condition. The recruitment of patients and the co-ordination and analysis of the trials is costly, so the pharmaceutical company will not embark on this stage unless they are sufficiently convinced of the therapeutic benefits of their drug. Essentially, phase 3 trials are replications of phase 2 trials but on a larger scale. The duration of the trial depends on the type of drug and the length of time required in order to determine the efficacy of the drug. For example, an antibiotic trial will have a shorter duration than the trial of a drug intended to treat long-term conditions, such as Alzheimer's disease. Acute treatment describes a short-term schedule given over a period of days or weeks, and chronic treatment refers to longer-term treatment schedules, lasting over periods of months or years.

Clinical trials may compare the new drug with an existing drug – a comparative trial – or may simply compare the new drug with no active drug treatment at all – a placebo-controlled trial. The participants who receive a comparator treatment or placebo are termed controls. In placebo-controlled trials, patients are given a placebo – an inert substance with no specific pharmacological activity – in place of the active drug. Patients will be unaware that the substance they are taking is placebo, which will be visually identical to the active treatment. This approach rules out any psychological effects of drug treatment – a patient may perceive that their condition has improved simply through the action of taking a tablet. In order to be considered clinically effective, the experimental drug must produce better results than the placebo.

The clinical trial should be designed in such a way as to limit the degree of bias it carries. The blinding of the trial is one means of eliminating bias. Double-blind trials, in which neither the doctor nor the patient knows which is the real drug and which is the placebo or comparator drug, are the most informative. In single-blind trials, only the patient is unaware of what they are taking, and in open-label trials, all participants are aware of treatment allocation. Conducting the trial across a number of clinics or hospitals, either abroad or in the same country (multicentre trials), further eliminates bias, as does randomisation, the random allocation of patients to treatment groups. At the start of the study, the baseline characteristics of the study population are recorded and are used as a starting point for all subsequent comparisons.

☛ Someone is always aware of who is taking what in a clinical trial. Whilst neither a doctor nor a patient may be aware of their treatment in a double-blind trial, there is a secure coding system, known only to the investigator, which contains the various treatment allocations.

Efficacy is commonly measured by means of primary and secondary endpoints. Endpoints mark a recognised stage in the disease process and are used to compare the outcome in different treatment arms of clinical trials. The endpoint of one trial may be a marker of improvement or recovery whereas another trial may use the deterioration of the patient (morbidity) or death (mortality) to signify the end of the trial. Either way, endpoints represent valid criteria by which to compare treatments. On a similar note, surrogate markers are laboratory measurements of biological activity within the body that provide an indirect measure of the effect of treatment on disease state (e.g. blood pressure and cholesterol levels).

Statistical analysis allows the investigator to draw rational conclusions from clinical trials regarding the effectiveness of their drug. If the patient data generated during the course of a clinical trial are statistically significant, then there is a high probability that the given result, be it an improvement or a decline in the health of the patient, is due to a specific effect of drug treatment, rather than a chance occurrence. The data are put through a number of mathematical procedures that ultimately produce a *p*-value. This value reflects the probability that the result occurred by chance. For example, if the *p*-value is less than or equal to 0.05, the result is usually considered to be statistically significant. Such a *p*-value indicates that there is a 95% probability that the result did not occur by chance. The smaller the *p*-value, the more significant the result. When quoting clinical findings, the *p*-value is often given in brackets in order to emphasise the importance of the finding.

Once a drug has progressed through the key stages of development and demonstrated clear efficacy with an acceptable safety profile, the data are collated and the pharmaceutical company will then submit a licence application to the regulatory authorities – a new drug application (NDA).

Phase 4 (Post-marketing studies)

Phase 4 testing takes place after the drug has been marketed and involves large numbers of patients, sometimes including those groups that may have previously been excluded from clinical trials (e.g. pregnant women and elderly or young patients). These trials are usually open-label, so the patient is aware of what they are taking, without control groups. They provide valuable information regarding the tolerability of the drug, and may reveal any long-term adverse events associated with treatment. Post-marketing surveillance continues throughout the life-span of the drug, and constantly monitors the safety, usage and performance. Doctors are advised to inform the MHRA and the Committee on Safety of Medicines (CSM) of any adverse events they encounter.

Editorial

Professor K Fan Chung
Royal Brompton Hospital and National Heart and Lung Institute
Imperial College, London

Asthma continues to be a major clinical burden with a significant economic impact. The World Health Organization (WHO) estimates that up to 150 million people suffer from asthma worldwide, with more than 3 million of these in the UK. An increase in its prevalence has occurred over the last three decades, whilst asthma accounted for 1521 deaths in the UK in 1999.

Remember that the author of this Editorial is addressing his healthcare professional colleagues rather than the 'lay' reader. This provides a fascinating insight into many of the challenges faced by doctors in the day-to-day practice of medicine (see Reader's Guide).

Over the last 10 years, important advances have been made in the management of the condition, and these have now been embodied within the recently published Global Initiative for Asthma (GINA) and the British Asthma Guidelines. It is not the introduction of new asthma drugs such as the leukotriene receptor antagonist that have made the most important impact, but the consolidation of inhaled corticosteroids and the discovery of the additive effects of combining inhaled corticosteroids with long-acting β_2-agonists. The benefits of early treatment of mild asthma with low-dose inhaled corticosteroid therapy are now well defined and include prevention of severe exacerbations and improvement of asthma control. The dose–response of inhaled corticosteroids has been evaluated and most of their beneficial effects are seen within the low-to-middle range of licensed doses. At the more severe end, additive effects on asthma control and on the reduction of severe exacerbations are obtained when long-acting β_2-agonists are taken together with inhaled corticosteroid therapy. This additive benefit does not appear to be as marked in patients with mild asthma. Therefore, combination therapy of inhaled corticosteroids and long-acting β_2-agonists has become the mainstay in moderate-to-severe asthma. When compared with low-dose inhaled corticosteroids in mild-to-moderate asthma, leukotriene receptor antagonists are not as effective, but are a useful alternative to long-acting β_2-agonists in combination with inhaled corticosteroids.

Given the availability of such effective agents, has the control of asthma improved in the community? The answer to this question remains unclear. One clear trend over the past few years has been the steady decrease in the number of hospitalisations for acute severe asthma, which has mirrored the increase in inhaled corticosteroid therapy. There has also been a small but steady decline in asthma deaths, again coinciding with the increase in prescriptions for inhaled corticosteroids. On the other hand, telephone or postal surveys indicate that significant asthma-related morbidity persists in the community. One example of this paradox is the persistence of uncontrolled asthma (including regular exacerbations) in some patients despite their continuance on high levels of treatments. Lack of adherence and inadequate (sometimes inappropriate) treatment may be the main reasons for this. However, little attention is given to patient education and the establishment of self-management programmes. In addition, asthma drugs may be less effective when used in the clinical field than under controlled trial conditions. Furthermore, a small proportion (1–5%) of the asthmatic population derive less beneficial response to currently available drugs (including β-adrenergic bronchodilators and corticosteroids), and this is reflected by persistent asthma despite adequate therapy. One likely and preventable cause of this treatment resistance is cigarette smoking.

We must also recognise the limitations of current therapies. The search for new agents continues, with the first antibody-based therapy (anti-immunoglobulin E monoclonal antibody) now available in the US for treating severe asthma, which provides an improvement when added to other therapies. In seeking out new medications, and ultimately a cure, a greater understanding of airway abnormalities is required through the application of genetics, molecular biology and proteomics. The inflammatory process and structural changes are at the root of asthma control and increasing numbers of 'targets' are being identified. As such, even more effective treatments can be expected within the next two or three decades. However, in the meantime it is important that we implement the recent management guidelines in the community, provide the right level and type of treatment according to disease severity, and teach as well as encourage our asthmatics to manage their disease and pre-empt exacerbations.

1. Disease overview – Asthma

Dr Eleanor Bull
CSF Medical Communications Ltd

Summary

Asthma is a chronic inflammatory disorder of the airways associated with airway hyper-responsiveness, reversible airflow limitation and other respiratory problems. Characteristically, the symptoms of asthma are variable in nature and worsen at night or following exposure to recognised triggers. In this manner, asthma is distinguished from other respiratory disorders. Asthma is one of the most common chronic diseases worldwide, affecting between 100 and 150 million people – thus it imposes a substantial economic burden on healthcare resources. For the individual, asthma can impact greatly on quality of life through the periodic limitation of everyday activities. The causes of asthma are multifactorial and many relate to an inherited predisposition. Environmental factors, including animal allergens, tobacco smoke and air pollution, may aggravate the condition. There is no current cure for asthma, and once established, no intervention can prevent the natural course of disease development, although steroidal agents may slow the rate of progression. In general, available treatments provide symptomatic relief of varying degrees and may reduce the frequency of exacerbations, but do not address the underlying cause of disease.

Introduction

Asthma is characterised by widespread but variable airflow obstruction that is mostly reversible, either spontaneously or with treatment. A dynamic condition, the severity of asthma varies with time such that episodic worsening of airflow is a major feature of the disease. Exacerbations of asthma (attacks or worsening of symptoms and lung function) can be rapid in onset or occur gradually. Severe exacerbations can be fatal if not treated appropriately, although the mortality rate for asthma has decreased to some extent, thanks largely to improved treatment options and patient education.

Asthma is characterised by widespread but variable airflow obstruction that is mostly reversible, either spontaneously or with treatment.

Symptoms

The main symptoms of asthma are shared with other respiratory disorders, including chronic obstructive pulmonary disease (COPD), bronchiectasis, cystic fibrosis and obliterative bronchiolitis. What differentiates asthma from these other diseases is the frequency of occurrence and aetiology of the symptoms. In addition, there will commonly be a personal or family history of asthma or other atopic conditions (e.g. allergic rhinitis and atopic eczema), in which abnormal amounts of IgE antibodies are produced in response to common environmental allergens. The principal, non-specific symptoms of asthma include:

- wheeze
- cough
- shortness of breath
- chest tightness.

When these symptoms are related specifically to asthma, they tend to be:

- variable in severity
- intermittent
- worse at night
- provoked by triggers including exercise and allergen exposure in susceptible individuals.

Epidemiology

It has been estimated that asthma affects between 100 and 150 million people worldwide, and its prevalence is on the increase (Figure 1).[1,2] There are insufficient data to determine the likely causes of this growth, although factors associated with a western lifestyle are thought to contribute. The socioeconomic status of an individual is a recognised factor that contributes strongly to disease severity. Inner-city living is associated with a greater prevalence of asthma, which may be related to higher levels of environmental pollution, dampness and poor ventilation.[3,4] Alternatively, in westernised countries the surrounding environment is more sterile and infants' immune systems may fail to develop appropriately as a result of reduced microbial exposure in early life, thereby increasing susceptibility to atopic disease development, a concept known as the 'hygiene hypothesis'.[5,6]

In the UK, over 5 million people are currently receiving treatment and 8 million people have been diagnosed as having asthma at some point in their lives.

An International Study of Asthma and Allergies in Childhood (ISAAC) survey reported that in children aged 13–14 years, the UK has the fifth highest prevalence of asthma (20.7% [Table 1]) out of 56 countries worldwide.[7] In the UK, out of a population of 59 million, over 5 million people are currently receiving treatment and 8 million people have been diagnosed as having asthma at some point in their lives. Furthermore, in 2000, over 18,000 first or new episodes of asthma presented every week to GPs in the UK.[8] Although mortality rates are decreasing, around 1500 people still die from asthma each year in the UK. The majority of these deaths are in the elderly, but in 1999, 25 children and over 500 adults under the age of 65 years died as a result of asthma.[8]

Figure 1. The global prevalence of asthma.[2]

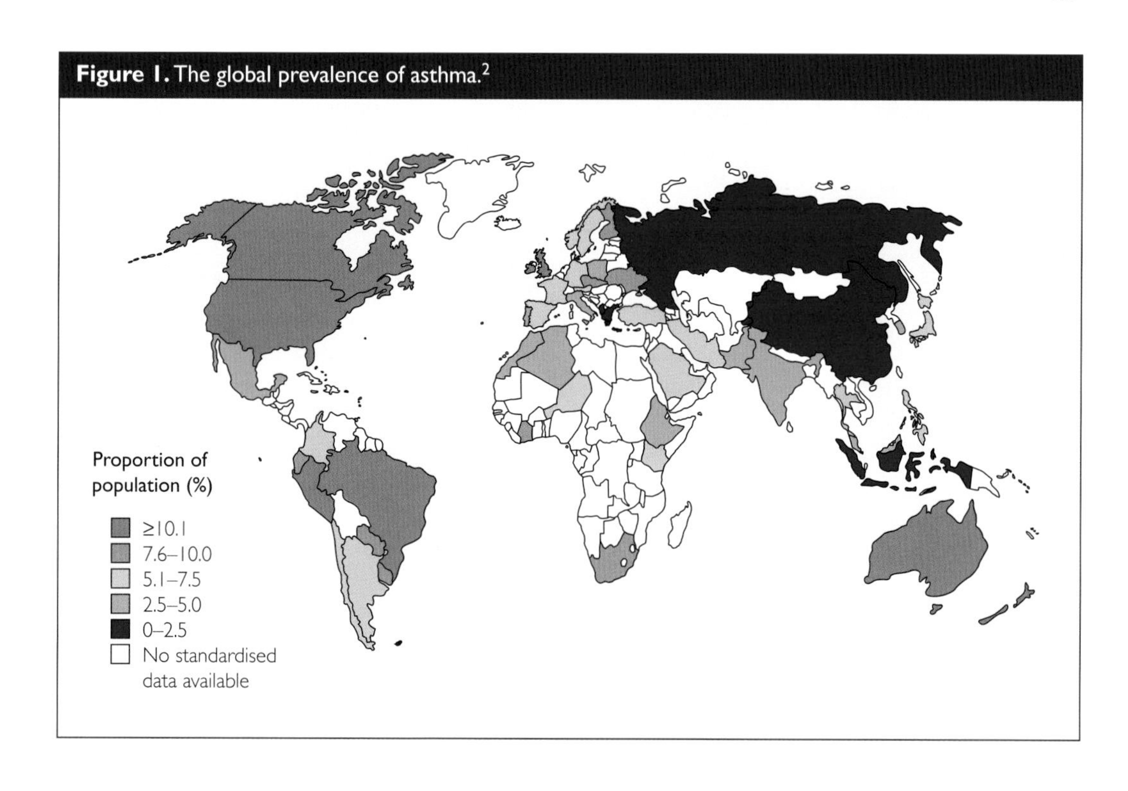

Table 1. International comparison of asthma prevalence in children aged 13–14 years – a selection of countries with the highest and lowest prevalence.[7]

Country	Percentage of population diagnosed with asthma
Australia	28.2
Peru	28.0
New Zealand	24.4
Singapore	20.9
UK	20.7
South Korea	2.4
Russia	2.4
Uzbekistan	1.7
Indonesia	1.6
Albania	1.6

Pathophysiology

Asthma is a chronic inflammatory disorder of the airways in which many cells and mediators play a role (Table 2). The pathophysiological features of the asthmatic response are illustrated in Figure 2.

Table 2. Summary of the inflammatory cells and mediators involved in asthma.

Inflammatory cell type	Role in asthma
Eosinophils	Induce airway epithelial damage through release of basic proteins and oxygen-derived free radicals
Mast cells	Acute response to allergens Multiple roles: histamine release, airway remodelling
Neutrophils	Induce airway obstruction and epithelial damage through release of lipid mediators and oxygen-derived free radicals
T lymphocytes	Release IgE antibodies and cytokines, resulting in recruitment and maintenance of eosinophils
Macrophages	Release cytokines
Inflammatory mediator	
Histamine, prostaglandins, leukotrienes	Contract airway smooth muscle, increase microvasculature leakage, mucus secretion and chemotaxis of inflammatory cells
Platelet-activating factor	Increases vascular permeability, chemotaxis of inflammatory cells
Substance P, neurokinin A, calcitonin gene-related peptide	Inflammatory neurotransmitters: increase and extend inflammatory response
Cytokines	Chronic inflammation, multiple roles
Endothelins	Vasoconstriction, bronchoconstriction, airway smooth muscle proliferation, fibrosis

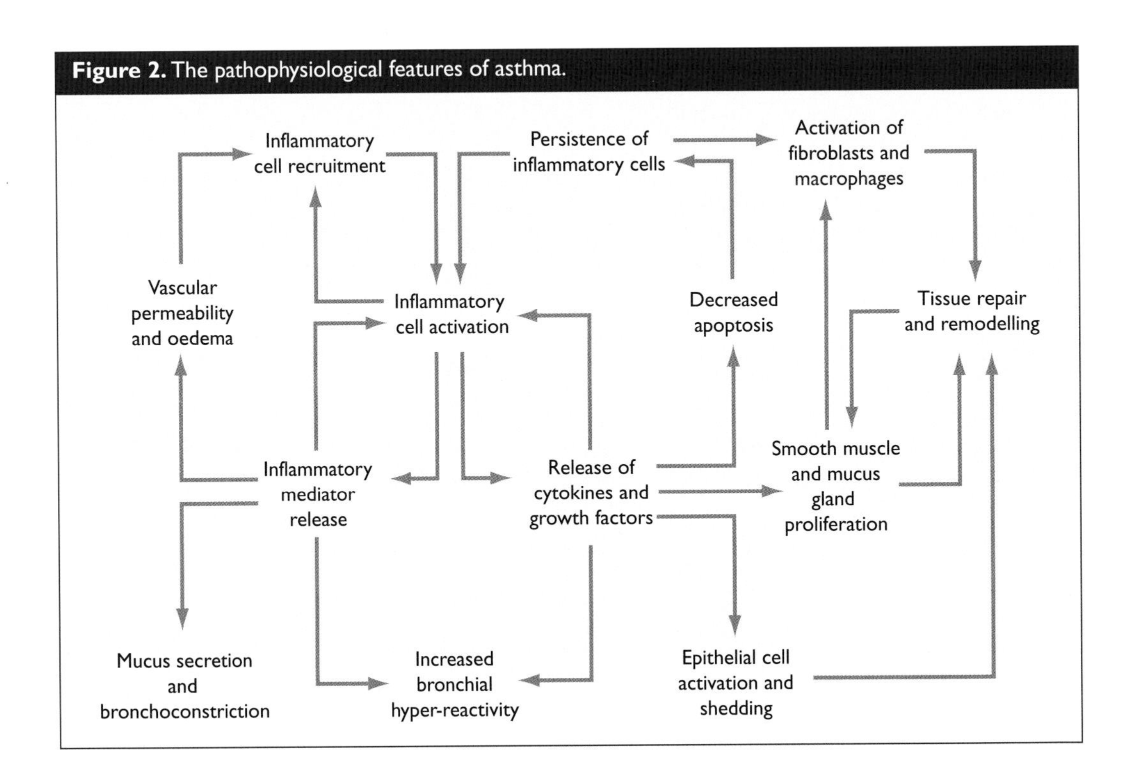

Figure 2. The pathophysiological features of asthma.

Airway hyper-responsiveness

In patients with asthma, the smooth muscle of the airway is hyper-reactive to various spasmogens, resulting in the exaggerated narrowing of the airways in response to normally non-inflammatory stimuli. Ultimately, this leads to an increased variation in airway calibre and increased basal airway tone. Airway hyper-responsiveness can be elicited by the infiltration and accumulation of activated inflammatory cells, including eosinophils, T lymphocytes, mast cells and macrophages. These cells produce chemical mediators (leukotrienes, cytokines, histamine), which perpetuate airway hyper-responsiveness and exacerbate tissue damage.[9]

Airway hyper-responsiveness can be elicited by the infiltration and accumulation of activated inflammatory cells, including eosinophils, T lymphocytes, mast cells and macrophages.

T lymphocytes are differentiated into Th1 and Th2 phenotypes. An imbalance of these cells in favour of the Th2 phenotype commonly occurs in patients with allergic asthma.[10] Following exposure to an allergen, Th2 cells stimulate the secretion of IgE antibodies from B-lymphocytes and produce a distinct profile of cytokines (specifically interleukins 4, 5 and 13) that are strongly associated with the pathophysiology of asthma and other atopic diseases.[11] Interleukin 5 in particular is responsible for the recruitment and activation of eosinophils. Eosinophil infiltration into the airways is considered to be a defining feature of asthma, and the mediators released following eosinophil activation – major basic protein and eosinophilic cationic protein – are thought to be integral to the epithelial damage that is characteristic of asthma pathophysiology.

Airway epithelial shedding

Damage to, or loss of, the cells forming the bronchial epithelium further contributes to airway hyper-responsiveness. Many factors can initiate epithelial shedding including chemical sensitisers, viral infection, allergen exposure and inflammatory mediators released from inflammatory cells, in particular, eosinophils.[12] As a consequence, clumps of epithelial cells aggregate in the lumen of the airways of asthmatics, where they may obstruct airflow. Furthermore, epithelial damage also results in the loss of enzymes, relaxant properties and protective barrier functions attributed to the bronchial epithelium.

Occlusion of airways by mucus plugs

In patients with asthma, the epithelial goblet cells responsible for mucus production in the airways proliferate rapidly, causing mucus hypersecretion. Excess mucus may form obstructive plugs in the airways and accumulates cellular debris from necrotic epithelial cells. Increased microvascular leakage can be evoked by many of the inflammatory mediators implicated in asthma and may also lead to mucosal oedema of the airway wall and increased airway secretions.[13]

Activation of airway sensory nerve endings

The exposure of sensory nerves as a result of epithelial damage may elicit reflex neural effects in asthmatics, including cough and chest tightness. In addition, the release of the inflammatory neuropeptides – substance P, neurokinin A and calcitonin gene-related peptide – from sensitised inflammatory nerves in the airways further impacts on the overall inflammatory response.[14]

Airway wall remodelling

Patients with chronic asthma may undergo long-term structural changes in their airways caused by the accumulation of collagen in subepithelial tissue (subepithelial fibrosis).[15] Airway integrity is further modified by smooth muscle hypertrophy and hyperplasia, leading to an overall increase in airway smooth muscle.[16] Both of these factors result in an exaggerated degree of airway wall narrowing, which profoundly reduces air supply to the patient, particularly in instances of airway smooth muscle contraction.

Airway smooth muscle contraction

Patients with asthma exhibit increased shortening in measurements of isotonic contraction of airway smooth muscle.[17,18] The enhanced contractility observed in asthma seems to be associated with an increased velocity of shortening.[19] It is thought that the reorganisation of contractile filaments and the plasticity of smooth muscle cells may underlie chronic airway hyper-responsiveness.[20]

Aetiology

Asthma is a heritable condition and in the majority of cases the individual is predisposed to disease development as a result of pre-existing, innate characteristics.

The causes of asthma are multifactorial and differ according to individual patients. Asthma is a heritable condition and in the majority of cases the individual is predisposed to disease development as a result of pre-existing, innate characteristics.[21,22] Environmental factors contribute to the manifestation of disease symptoms in a predisposed individual.

A number of host factors influence the likelihood of predisposing a patient to asthma. These factors include:

- atopy
- airway hyper-responsiveness
- gender
- race/ethnicity.

Environmental factors influence the susceptibility of a predisposed individual to develop asthma. Such factors include:

- indoor allergens (house-dust mites, animal allergens, fungi, moulds, yeast)
- outdoor allergens (pollens, fungi, moulds, yeast)
- occupational sensitisers (requiring special assessment)

- tobacco smoke
- air pollution
- respiratory infection
- parasitic infection
- socioeconomic status
- diet
- drugs
- obesity
- an increasingly sterile environment with reduced microbial exposure: the 'hygiene hypothesis'.

Furthermore, a number of environmental factors precipitate asthma exacerbations, and include:

- indoor and outdoor allergens
- indoor and outdoor air pollutants
- respiratory and viral infections
- exercise
- weather changes
- sulphur dioxide
- foods, additives, drugs (e.g. aspirin, non-steroidal anti-inflammatory drugs, paracetamol)
- extreme emotional suppression
- tobacco smoke (inhaled passively or actively).

The onset of asthma may occur at any stage of life, although the factors that influence onset may differ between individuals. In infants, asthma is primarily related to atopy, which predisposes the airways to sensitisation by allergens, and, is characterised by a predominance of Th2 lymphocytes. There is evidence to suggest that children living in affluent societies may be exposed to lower levels of pathogens and that, as a result, their immune systems may polarise towards a Th2 rather than Th1 phenotype and hence increase the chances of developing allergic disease.[6] Exposure to pathogens in early life may confer protection against allergic diseases through the suppression of Th2-mediated immunity. In older children, allergy is the predominant feature associated with asthma. In adults, asthma can result from the occupational sensitisation of the airways and from the development of atopy in later life.

The onset of asthma may occur at any stage of life, although the factors that influence onset may differ between individuals.

Diagnosis

Asthma is under-diagnosed throughout the world and as a consequence it is under-treated. The principal underlying reason behind this is that many patients tolerate intermittent respiratory symptoms before seeking medical advice. Diagnosis can be made on the basis of presenting symptoms; however, measurements of lung function greatly enhance diagnostic accuracy.

Lung function tests measure the peak expiratory flow (PEF) rate, forced vital capacity (FVC) and forced expiratory volume in 1 second (FEV_1). These measurements depend on airflow limitation relating directly to the luminal size of airways and the elastic properties of the surrounding lung tissue, and will be markedly decreased in asthmatic patients, with a pronounced variability of function. Lung function tests should be conducted in both the presence and absence of symptoms. If function is normal in the presence of symptoms, a diagnosis of asthma is unlikely. Considering the diurnal variation of symptoms in asthma, patient self-monitoring is particularly important. Patients are encouraged to maintain a diary card of their PEF and to record any reduction in peak flow following exposure to a recognised trigger (including exercise).

In short, a diagnosis of asthma should be considered if there is a:

- history of classic symptoms (e.g. cough, wheeze, shortness of breath, tightness, exercise-induced symptoms)
- 15–20% or greater variability in lung function between morning and evening as measured by changes in PEF, FVC and FEV_1
- response to asthma treatment (i.e. an increase in lung function after inhalation of a short-acting β_2-agonist or after a trial of corticosteroid tablets)
- a decrease in lung function after 6 minutes of exercise (e.g. running).

The severity of asthma can be judged on the basis of the severity and frequency of symptoms and the level of medication required for their adequate control, as well as the degree to which the patient's lifestyle is limited. The aetiology and the pattern of airflow limitation are also useful indicators of the severity of the disease. Figure 3 illustrates the asthma classification scheme developed by the Global Initiative for Asthma (GINA).[23]

Outcome measures in clinical trials

In order to understand how to optimise asthma treatment, it is important to be able to evaluate with some accuracy, the effectiveness of potential drug therapies. This can be achieved through the careful design of clinical trials and the selection of appropriate outcome measures. The duration of an asthma trial should be tailored towards the nature of the

Figure 3. The asthma classification scheme developed by the Global Initiative for Asthma (GINA).[23]
Severe exacerbations can affect patients at any level of severity.
FEV_1, forced expiratory volume in 1 second; PEF, peak expiratory flow.
[a]Predicted values based on age, gender and height.
[b]Variability between morning and evening FEV_1.

	Asthma severity	Lung function		Symptom frequency	Nocturnal symptoms	Exacerbations
		PEF or FEV_1[a]	PEF variability[b]			
	Severe	≤60%	>30%	Continual	Frequent	Frequent
Persistent	Moderate	>60–80%	>30%	Daily	>1/week	Affect activity
	Mild	≥80%	20–30%	>2/week<1/day	>2/month	May affect activity
Intermittent	Mild	≥80%	<20%	≤2/week	≤2/month	Are brief

drug being tested. An acute trial of a short-acting β_2-agonist need only last a few days, whereas controller therapies may require at least 3 months for long-lasting treatment effects to emerge.

When assessing the effectiveness of drug therapy in asthma, no outcome measure should be used in isolation. Asthma is a complex disease and more than one parameter is necessary to determine the level of asthma control. Healthcare professionals and patients may have different expectations of asthma therapy and different ideas of what constitutes asthma control, and all viewpoints should be taken into account before making an overall judgement.

When assessing the effectiveness of drug therapy in asthma, no outcome measure should be used in isolation.

Outcome measures commonly used to assess drug efficacy in asthma clinical trials are outlined in detail below.

- Symptoms – including cough, wheeze, chest tightness and dyspnoea, which are usually self-reported by the patient using diary cards.
- Lung function – assessed using the spirometry measures described previously, including FEV_1, PEF and FVC. These measures correlate well with improved asthma symptoms, are highly repeatable, standardised and relatively easy to perform.[24]
- Changes in concomitant medication – this usually confirms an improvement in lung function and symptoms. Often this measure refers to the use of short-acting β_2-agonist rescue medication, but can also refer to the dose of an inhaled or an oral corticosteroid.[24]
- Exacerbations – this combines symptoms, airflow and additional medication needs. All aspects of an exacerbation, including frequency, duration and severity should be recorded.[24]
- Quality of life – specifically tailored questionnaires are available to evaluate the impact of asthma symptoms and treatment on the quality of life of adults, adolescents and children.[24]
- Measurements of inflammation – including exhaled nitric oxide (NO) and levels of eosinophils in the sputum.[24]

Objective measures

Objective measures of airflow and lung function (e.g. FEV_1, PEF, FVC) have become the standard means of evaluating drug efficacy, both in clinical practice and in randomised controlled trials, and provide an accurate snapshot of asthma severity.[24] In general, these parameters are easy to perform, robust, highly repeatable and accurately reflect airway calibre.[24] However, they are not without their disadvantages. For example, neither FEV_1 nor PEF are sensitive enough to detect obstruction in the lung periphery. Furthermore, patient self-measurement of PEF over extended periods of time, whilst helpful on one level, may also introduce unnecessary errors into the investigation. In addition, the use of mean lung function data (e.g. mean FEV_1) often disguises the variability of the response; patients do not always fall into distinct responder and non-responder groups and mean values do not take this into account.[25]

Objective measures of airflow and lung function (e.g. FEV_1, PEF, FVC) have become the standard means of evaluating drug efficacy and provide an accurate snapshot of asthma severity.

Bronchoprovocation tests, which measure bronchial hyper-responsiveness by the inhalation of bronchoprovocators such as methacholine, histamine, bradykinin or adenosine monophosphate

(AMP), provide an effective means of examining airway function. However, such studies may be time-consuming and are not definitive – it is possible to be hyper-responsive and not to have asthma, for example.[25] Surrogate markers of inflammation, including sputum eosinophil counts, exhaled NO, bronchoalveolar lavage and bronchial biopsy, whilst useful, are not without their difficulties. Sputum measurement is difficult to perform and interpret and some patients cannot produce sufficient sputum to allow assessment. In contrast, recording exhaled NO levels is technically simple, non-invasive and correlates well with several clinical parameters.[25]

Outcome measures in childhood asthma

Outcome measurements that work well in adult populations may not always be appropriate for paediatric patient populations. Symptom reporting and lung function parameters often prove unreliable or are impractical in very young children and, consequently, physicians are often forced to rely on information from parents and caregivers.[26] The accuracy of such information is questionable, particularly concerning nocturnal awakenings, cough and wheezing. For example, if the symptom is not severe enough to awaken the parent, it will go unreported.[26] Days without asthma symptoms and quality of life assessments are more useful when assessing childhood asthma, since these take into account the impact of asthma on routine daily activities. In addition, given the variability in responses, recording discrete measurements of FEV_1 may be more meaningful than just presenting the mean values, whilst specific airway resistance (sRAW) measured using a plethysmograph may be a more appropriate measurement of airway function in younger age groups.[26]

Evaluating the effects of early intervention on asthma progression in children requires years of outcome monitoring, and should involve an evaluation of the effects of treatment on airway remodelling, growth, peak bone mineral density, physical impairment and psychosocial development.[26,27] To be informative, such studies should extend for several years in duration.

Treatment of asthma

The main aims of asthma treatment are the control of symptoms, the prevention of exacerbations and achievement of best possible pulmonary function with minimal side-effects. Although pharmacological interventions are effective in controlling symptoms and improving quality of life in the majority of patients, the prevention of asthma exacerbations by non-pharmacological means is of great importance in the management of the disease. By limiting exposure to risk factors such as allergens and environmental pollutants, the likelihood of asthma exacerbations can be greatly reduced. Additional lifestyle changes should also be implemented.

By limiting exposure to risk factors such as allergens and environmental pollutants, the likelihood of asthma exacerbations can be greatly reduced.

Prophylactic lifestyle changes that reduce the impact of asthma include:

- dietary manipulations
- weight reduction
- smoking cessation
- self-management plans
- breathing retraining in patients with symptoms suggestive of dysfunctional breathing.

Pharmacological treatment

Pharmacological intervention should be selected on the basis of disease severity in the individual patient and in accordance with clearly defined treatment guidelines. These guidelines advocate a stepwise approach, in which treatment is started at the step most appropriate for the individual patient. Treatment guidelines issued jointly by the Scottish Intercollegiate Guidelines Network (SIGN) and the British Thoracic Society (BTS) for the treatment of asthma in adults, children aged 5–12 years and in pre-school children are shown in Figures 4, 5 and 6, respectively.[28] Many patients can be treated adequately with inhaled corticosteroids but an important number require additional therapy. Representative large-scale surveys in the UK have revealed that one-in-ten people living with asthma have severe or moderately severe asthma that is not effectively controlled.[29] Newly developed therapies should aim to improve symptom control in severe cases, minimise side-effects and improve patient compliance. The current treatments of choice are described in the following sections.

Treatment guidelines advocate a stepwise approach, in which treatment is started at the step most appropriate for the individual patient.

Medications for asthma are usually administered by inhalation, the advantage of this being that drugs are delivered directly to the airways where they are needed at high concentrations and the onset of action is accelerated. However, inhaler devices can be associated with reduced compliance and localised side-effects (see Inhaler Devices, below).

When treating paediatric patients, the basic treatment principles remain the same as those for adults. However, in children under 3 years of age, the only recommended controller medications are the inhaled corticosteroids.

Short-acting β_2-agonists

β_2-agonists (e.g. salbutamol and terbutaline) are effective bronchodilators and as such are commonly prescribed for the relief of the acute asthmatic response, with maximum effects achieved within 30 minutes and maintained for 4–6 hours. They relax airway smooth muscle, increase mucociliary clearance, inhibit mediator release from mast cells and decrease vascular permeability. Side-effects are limited but can include tremor, palpitations and tachycardia at high doses. Tolerance, associated with a loss of bronchodilator activity, may also occur.[30]

β_2-agonists are effective bronchodilators and as such are commonly prescribed for the relief of the acute asthmatic response.

Figure 4. The stepwise pharmacological management of adults with asthma.[28]

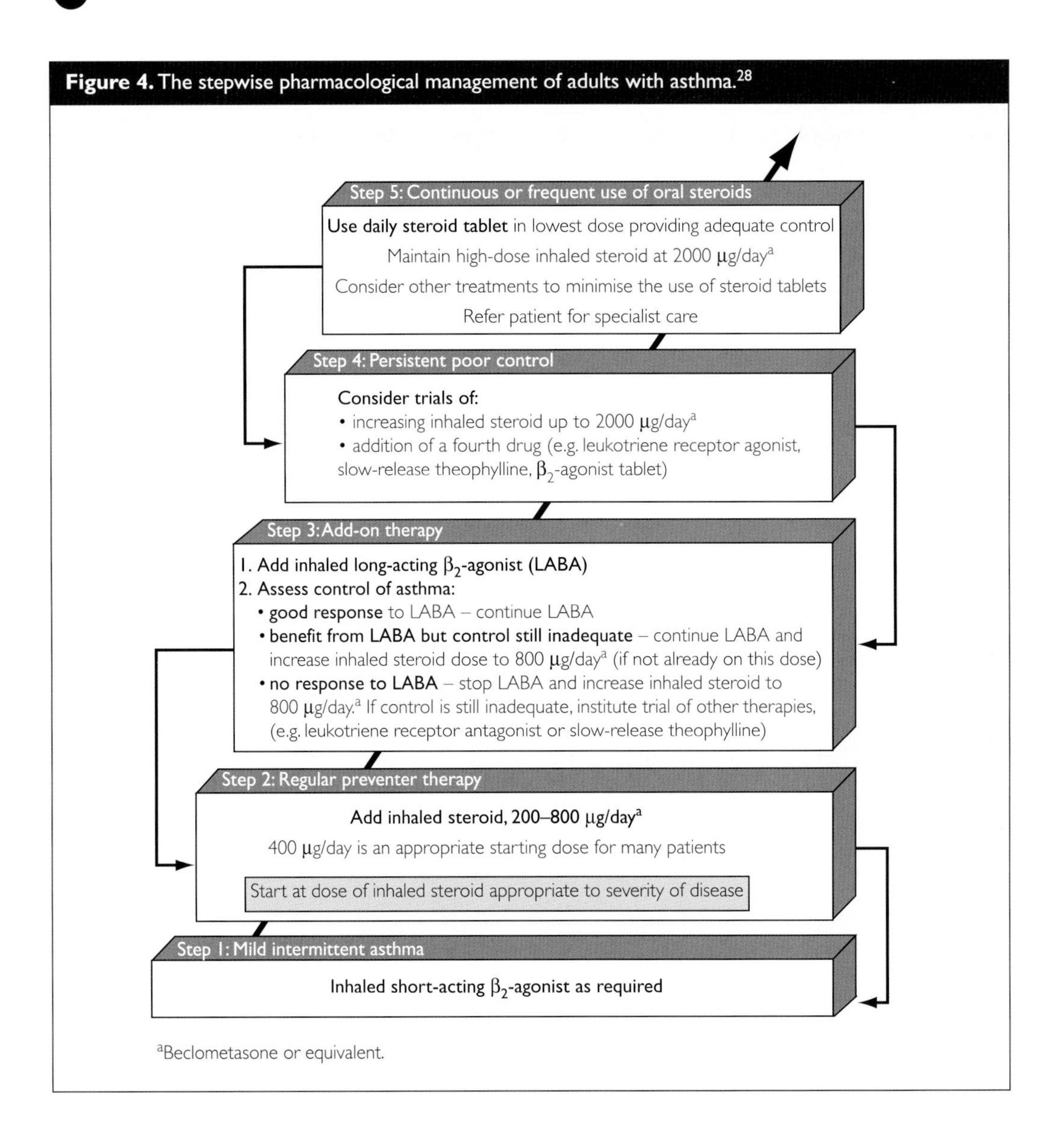

[a]Beclometasone or equivalent.

Long-acting β_2-agonists

Compounds in this class (e.g. salmeterol, formoterol) act in the same manner as the short-acting β_2-agonists but efficacy is sustained for up to 12 hours. This extended duration of action warrants their use in the treatment of moderate persistent asthma as a means of improving asthma control and reducing exacerbations, rather than the immediate symptomatic relief of the acute asthma response. Inhaled steroids are the recommended first-line intervention for both adults and children for the effective control of asthma.

Figure 5. The stepwise pharmacological management of children aged 5–12 years with asthma.[28]

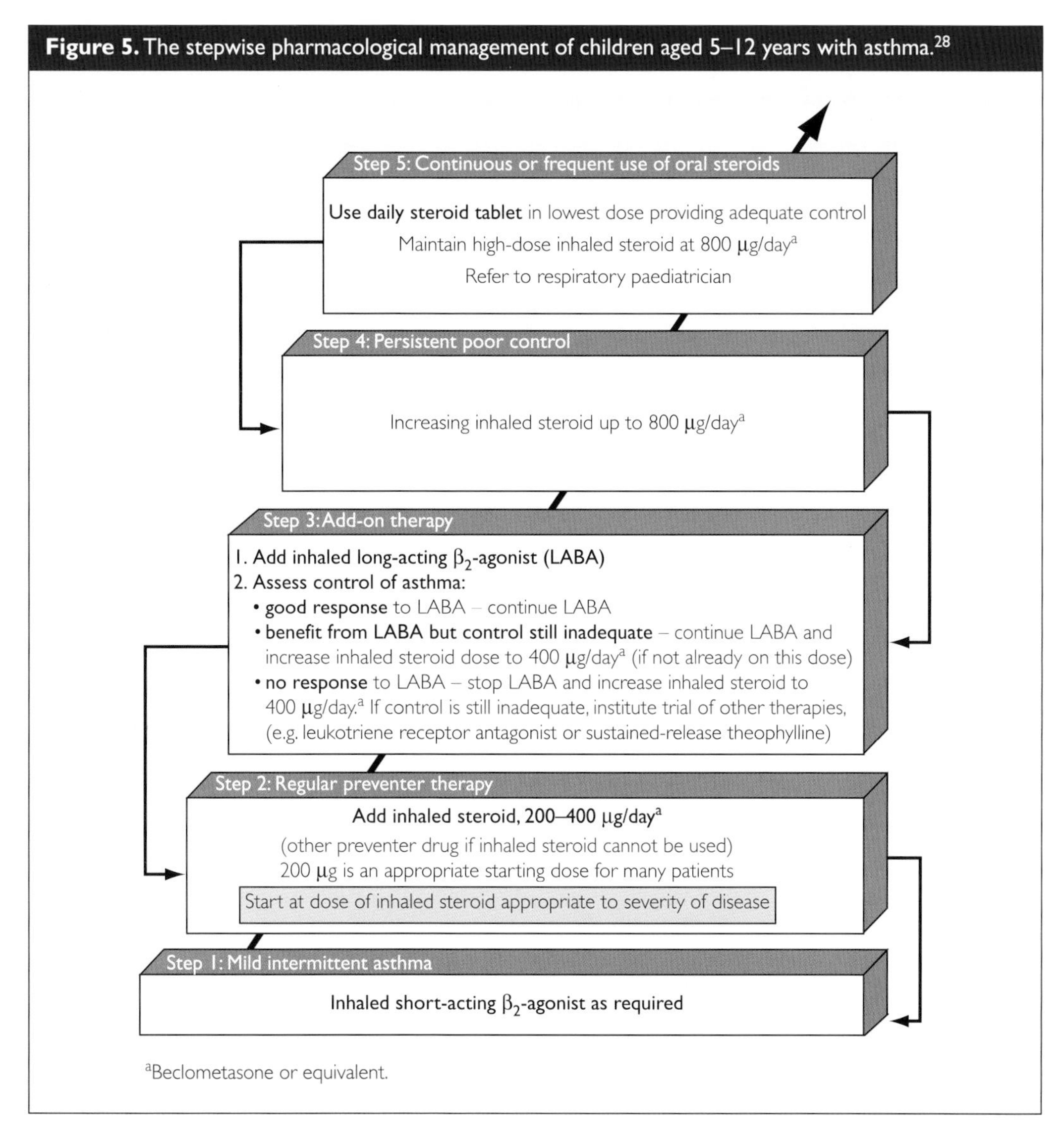

[a]Beclometasone or equivalent.

Low-dose inhaled corticosteroids

Corticosteroids (e.g. beclometasone, fluticasone, mometasone and budenoside) are currently the most effective anti-inflammatory medications available for asthma at all levels of severity. They act by directly inhibiting a range of inflammatory cells, particularly eosinophils, and by activating glucocorticoid receptors leading to the altered regulation of transcription of target genes.[31] This leads to dramatic improvements in airway hyper-responsiveness, lung function and a reduction in the frequency of exacerbations. In the short term, side-effects commonly include dysphonia

> Corticosteroids act by directly inhibiting a range of inflammatory cells and by activating glucocorticoid receptors leading to the altered regulation of transcription of target genes.

Figure 6. The stepwise pharmacological management of pre-school children (under the age of 5 years with asthma).[28]

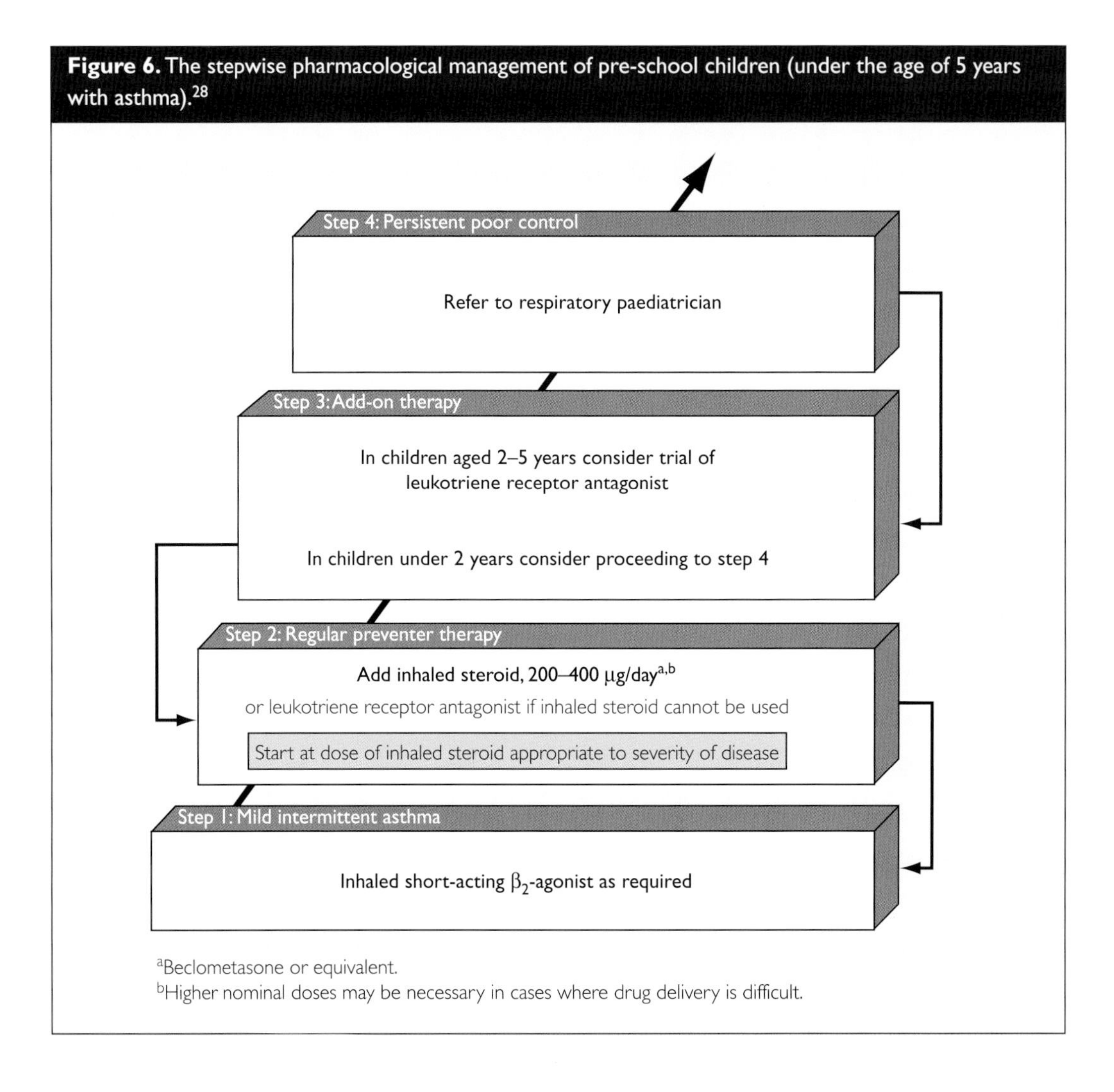

[a]Beclometasone or equivalent.
[b]Higher nominal doses may be necessary in cases where drug delivery is difficult.

and oral candidiasis, although this may be prevented by the use of spacer devices and the 'gargling' of water following drug administration. However, it is the long-term systemic consequences of exposure that are of most concern, with bruising, reduced bone mineral density and suppression of the adrenocortical axis reported, albeit rarely, in both paediatric and adult patients, and usually in those receiving high doses.[32,33]

Inhaler devices:

The use of inhaled bronchodilator and anti-inflammatory therapy is the mainstay of current asthma treatment and thus, effective delivery to the lungs is a critical factor in disease management. Three types of inhaler are currently available:

- metered dose inhaler (MDI)
- breath actuated inhalers (BAI)
- dry powder inhalers (DPI).

The most commonly prescribed inhaler is the MDI (also sometimes referred to as pressurised metered dose inhaler or pMDI). These devices require the patient to activate the device simultaneously with inspiration in order to deliver an aerosolised metered dose of drug to the lungs.[34] However, co-ordinating inspiration and actuation can be problematic in certain patient groups, particularly the very young or those with the most severe breathing difficulties. This problem has been overcome, to some extent, by the use of a spacer device (a tube attached to a mouthpiece or mask to simplify actuation) or more recently, by the development of the BAI group of inhalers. Release of a dose of drug by a BAI device is triggered by slow inspiration and, as such, this represents a far simpler inhaler option.[34] As a consequence of environmental concerns, the traditional use of chlorofluorocarbon (CFC) as the propellant molecule in both MDI and BAI devices is currently being phased out, with hydrofluoroalkane (HFA) now the favoured propellant of choice, as it is considered to be a non-greenhouse gas and is therefore a more environmentally friendly option. Finally, DPI devices are also activated by a deep breath and were developed to provide a simple alternative to the classical MDIs. In general, the bulk of current research suggests that there are no significant differences in treatment outcomes between these different inhaler delivery systems.[35–38]

Cromones

Cromones (e.g. sodium cromoglycate and nedocromil sodium) are occasionally used in conjunction with corticosteroids. Although their mechanism of action is not fully understood, it is thought to involve the suppression of the IgE-mediated inflammatory response.[39] Side-effects are minimal although an inconvenient dosing regimen and a lack of effectiveness in adults limit the widespread use of these agents.

Leukotriene receptor antagonists

The leukotriene receptor antagonists (e.g. montelukast and zafirlukast) act by blocking the inflammatory effects of leukotrienes. In this way they remain active over a wide spectrum of asthma severity and exhibit both anti-inflammatory and bronchodilator activity.[40] Initial findings indicate that these drugs are not as effective as the corticosteroids, although they are well tolerated, with few side-effects reported. As such they are commonly employed as add-on therapy to an existing inhaled corticosteroid treatment regimen.

Methylxanthines

Theophylline is a bronchodilator with possible anti-inflammatory activity, employed as preventer therapy and as an adjunct to corticosteroids. However, it has a very low therapeutic index and its use is limited by side-effects including gastrointestinal upset, nausea and vomiting, tachycardia, arrhythmia and tremor.[41]

Socioeconomic impact

The treatment of asthma exerts a particularly high burden on the primary healthcare system, with almost 4 million consultations for asthma each year in the UK and estimated annual healthcare costs of over £850 million.[8,42,43]

In the UK, asthma is a major cause of work and school absence, with consequent repercussions in professional and educational attainment.

The morbidity associated with asthma is such that a high proportion of patients are hospitalised for treatment. In the UK in 1999 there were 80,000 admissions to hospital due to asthma, with over 30,000 of these accounted for by children.[7] Over 18 million working days are lost due to asthma each year.[32] In the UK, asthma is a major cause of work and school absence, with consequent repercussions in professional and educational attainment. Recent findings suggest that the perception of the severity of asthma-related lifestyle restrictions differs between paediatric patients and healthcare professionals such that lifestyle limitation is underestimated by the latter group (Figure 7).[44] Measures should be taken to address this discrepancy in order to improve patient outcomes.

Clearly, reducing the number and severity of attacks will improve both patients' quality of life and the efficiency of the healthcare system.

Figure 7. Asthma symptom prevalence of at least once a month: a comparison of statements of children and parents with the views of healthcare professionals.[44]

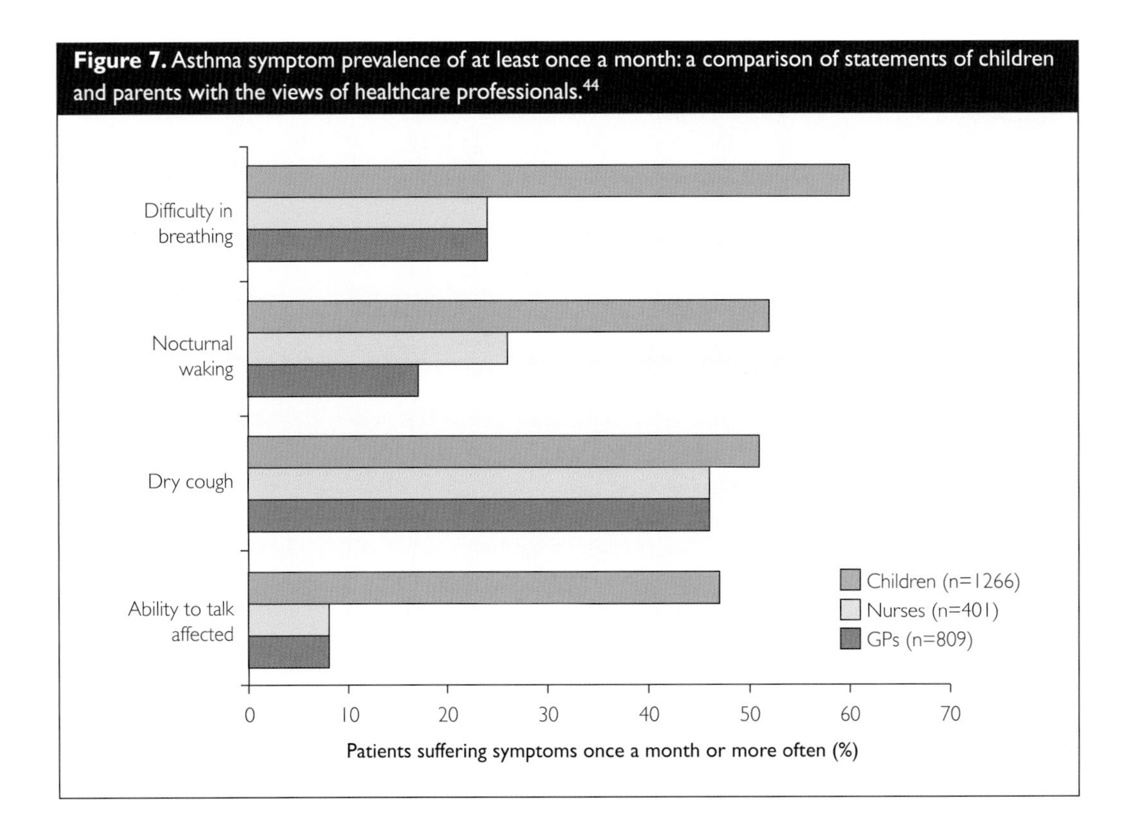

Key points

- Asthma is a chronic inflammatory disorder of the airways with recurrent exacerbations.
- The increasing worldwide incidence of asthma exerts significant pressure on healthcare resources.
- The main symptoms are wheeze, cough, shortness of breath and chest tightness; these are intermittent, worsen at night and are provoked by recognised triggers.
- Asthma is characterised by airway hyper-responsiveness, airway obstruction, epithelial damage and long-term structural remodelling of the airways.
- Asthma diagnosis should be made on the basis of presenting symptoms and measurements of lung function (e.g. FEV_1, PEF and FVC).
- The causes of asthma are multifactorial with genetic and environmental contributions, including tobacco smoke, air pollution and animal allergens.
- Current asthma therapy is directed at treating chronic inflammation and improving lung function through bronchodilation, although non-pharmacological preventative measures should be taken where possible to avoid exacerbations.
- The treatment of asthma should be tailored to the individual patient and revised regularly in line with current treatment recommendations.
- Inhaled corticosteroids remain the cornerstone of treatment, with the addition of add-on therapy if symptoms persist.
- The major financial costs associated with asthma management are principally related to the medical cost of hospitalisation, emergency care and drug therapy. Indirectly, asthma also accounts for costs attributed to the loss of school or work days.

References

A list of the published evidence which has been reviewed in compiling the preceding section of *BESTMEDICINE.*

1. World Health Organization. WHO Factsheet No. 206: Bronchial Asthma. 2000.
2. Masoli M, Fabian D, Holt S, Beasley R. Global Burden of Asthma. Global Initiative for Asthma, 2003.
3. Shapiro G, Stout J. Childhood asthma in the United States: urban issues. *Pediatr Pulmonol* 2002; **33**: 47–55.
4. Cesaroni G, Farchi S, Davoli M, Forastiere F, Perucci C. Individual and area-based indicators of socioeconomic status and childhood asthma. *Eur Respir J* 2003; **22**: 619–24.
5. Strachan D. Hay fever, hygiene, and household size. *BMJ* 1989; **299**: 1259–60.
6. Strachan D. Family size, infection and atopy: the first decade of the "hygiene hypothesis". *Thorax* 2000; **55**: S2–10.
7. Worldwide variations in the prevalence of asthma symptoms: the International Study of Asthma and Allergies in Childhood (ISAAC). *Eur Respir J* 1998; **12**: 315–35.
8. National Asthma Campaign. Out in the open: a true picture of asthma in the United Kingdom today. *The Asthma Journal* 2001; **6**: 1–14.
9. Fireman P. Understanding asthma pathophysiology. *Allergy Asthma Proc* 2003; **24**: 79–83.
10. Umetsu D, DeKruyff R. TH1 and TH2 CD4+ cells in human allergic diseases. *J Allergy Clin Immunol* 1997; **10**: 1–6.
11. Tattersfield A, Knox A, Britton J, Hall I. Asthma. *Lancet* 2002; **360**: 1313–22.
12. Barnes P. Pathophysiology of asthma. *Br J Clin Pharmacol* 1996; **42**: 3–10.
13. Barnes P, Chung K, Page C. Inflammatory mediators and asthma. *Pharmacol Rev* 1988; **40**: 49–84.
14. Barnes P. Sensory nerves, neuropeptides, and asthma. *Ann N Y Acad Sci* 1991; **629**: 359–70.
15. Djukanovic R, Roche W, Wilson J *et al.* Mucosal inflammation in asthma. *Am Rev Respir Dis* 1990; **142**: 434–57.
16. Ebina M, Yaegashi H, Chiba R, Takahashi T, Motomiya M, Tanemura M. Hyperreactive site in the airway tree of asthmatic patients revealed by thickening of bronchial muscles. A morphometric study. *Am Rev Respir Dis* 1990; **141**: 1327–32.
17. Bai T. Abnormalities in airway smooth muscle in fatal asthma. *Am Rev Respir Dis* 1990; **141**: 552–7.
18. Thomson R, Bramley A, Schellenberg R. Airway muscle stereology: implications for increased shortening in asthma. *Am J Respir Crit Care Med* 1996; **154**: 749–57.
19. Mitchell R, Ruhlmann E, Magnussen H, Leff A, Rabe K. Passive sensitization of human bronchi augments smooth muscle shortening velocity and capacity. *Am J Physiol* 1994; **267**: L218–22.
20. Gunst S, Tang D. The contractile apparatus and mechanical properties of airway smooth muscle. *Eur Respir J* 2000; **15**: 600–16.
21. Holgate S. Genetic and environmental interaction in allergy and asthma. *J Allergy Clin Immunol* 1999; **104**: 1139–46.
22. Palmer L, Burton P, James A, Musk A, Cookson W. Familial aggregation and heritability of asthma-associated quantitative traits in a population-based sample of nuclear families. *Eur J Hum Genet* 2000; **8**: 853–60.
23. National Heart Lung and Blood Institute. Global strategy for asthma management and prevention. NHLBI /WHO Workshop Report. National Institute of Health, 1995.
24. Holgate S, Bousquet J, Chung K *et al.* Summary of recommendations for the design of clinical trials and the registration of drugs used in the treatment of asthma. *Respir Med* 2004; **98**: 479–87.
25. Spahn J. Clinical trial efficacy: what does it really tell you? *J Allergy Clin Immunol* 2003; **112**: S102–6.
26. Skoner D. Outcome measures in childhood asthma. *Pediatrics* 2002; **109**: 393–8.
27. Pedersen S. Long-term outcomes in paediatric asthma. *Allergy* 2002; **57**: 58–74.
28. Scottish Intercollegiate Guidelines Network and the British Thoracic Society. British Guideline on the Management of Asthma, 2004. *www.sign.ac.uk*
29. National Asthma Campaign. Greater expectations? Findings from the National Asthma Campaign's representative study of the Needs of People with Asthma (NOPWA) in the UK. *The Asthma Journal* 2000; **5**(3).
30. O'Connor B, Aikman S, Barnes P. Tolerance to the nonbronchodilator effects of inhaled beta 2-agonists in asthma. *N Engl J Med* 1992; **327**: 1204–8.
31. Green R, Brightling C, Pavord I, Wardlaw A. Management of asthma in adults: current therapy and future directions. *Postgrad Med J* 2003; **79**: 259–67.
32. Clark D, Lipworth B. Adrenal suppression with chronic dosing of fluticasone propionate compared with budesonide in adult asthmatic patients. *Thorax* 1997; **52**: 55–8.
33. Israel E, Banerjee T, Fitzmaurice G, Kotlov T, LaHive K, LeBoff M. Effects of inhaled glucocorticoids on bone density in premenopausal women. *N Engl J Med* 2001; **345**: 941–7.
34. Price D, Thomas M, Mitchell G, Niziol C, Featherstone R. Improvement of asthma control with a breath-actuated pressurised metred dose inhaler (BAI): a prescribing claims study of 5556 patients using a traditional pressurised metred dose inhaler (MDI) or a breath-actuated device. *Respir Med* 2003; **97**: 12–19.

35 Wolfe J, Kreitzer S, Chervinsky P *et al.* Comparison of powder and aerosol formulations of salmeterol in the treatment of asthma. *Ann Allergy Asthma Immunol* 2000; **84**: 334–40.

36 Campbell LM, Anderson TJ, Parashchak MR *et al.* A comparison of the efficacy of long-acting beta 2-agonists: eformoterol via Turbohaler and salmeterol via pressurized metered dose inhaler or Accuhaler, in mild to moderate asthmatics. Force Research Group. *Respir Med* 1999; **93**: 236–44.

37 Barry PW, O'Callaghan C. The influence of inhaler selection on efficacy of asthma therapies. *Adv Drug Deliv Rev* 2003; **55**: 879–923.

38 Lundback B, Alexander M, Day J *et al.* Evaluation of fluticasone propionate (500 micrograms day-1) administered either as dry powder via a Diskhaler inhaler or pressurized inhaler and compared with beclomethasone dipropionate (1000 micrograms day-1) administered by pressurized inhaler. *Respir Med* 1993; **87**: 609–20.

39 Diaz P, Galleguillos F, Gonzalez M, Pantin C, Kay A. Bronchoalveolar lavage in asthma: the effect of disodium cromoglycate (cromolyn) on leukocyte counts, immunoglobulins, and complement. *J Allergy Clin Immunol* 1984; **74**: 41–8.

40 Lipworth B. Leukotriene-receptor antagonists. *Lancet* 1999; **353**: 57–62.

41 Pollard S, Spector S, Yancey S, Cox F, Emmett A. Salmeterol versus theophylline in the treatment of asthma. *Ann Allergy Asthma Immunol* 1997; **78**: 457–64.

42 National Asthma Campaign. National Asthma Audit: Direct Publishing Solutions Ltd, 1999/2000.

43 Hoskins G, McCowan C, Neville R, Thomas G, Smith B, Silverman S. Risk factors and costs associated with an asthma attack. *Thorax* 2000; **55**: 19–24.

44 Price D, Ryan D, Pearce L *et al.* The burden of paediatric asthma is higher than health professionals think: results from the Asthma in Real Life (AIR) study. *Prim Care Respir J* 2002; **11**: 30–3.

Acknowledgements

Figure 1 is adapted from Masoli, 2003.[2]
Figure 3 is adapted the National Heart Lung and Blood Institute.[23]
Figures 4–6 are adapted from the Scottish Intercollegiate Guidelines Network (SIGN), 2004.[28]

PATIENT NOTES

Dr Mike Thomas and Professor David Price

Asthma has become one of the most common long-term and persistent illnesses in industrialised and affluent westernised societies.

The global burden of asthma

Asthma has become one of the most common long-term and persistent (chronic) illnesses in industrialised and affluent westernised societies. Despite effective treatment, asthma continues to impact on many patients' lives. Although we do have useful treatments at our disposal, both to prevent attacks and to treat symptoms when they do occur, there is no current 'cure' for asthma. For most people, asthma treatment needs to be long-term, as treatment is only effective whilst it is being used. The preventative treatments currently available are effective and safe, and recent research has shown it is possible to control most patients' asthma for most of the time, enabling them to live full and unrestricted lifestyles. International guidelines such as those produced by the World Health Organization aim for very high levels of asthma control (see Box 1).

Surveys in the UK and in other countries, however, have shown that many people continue to suffer significant symptoms from asthma and have a poorer quality of life as a consequence. Many patients avoid participating in pleasurable leisure activities for fear of triggering asthma, many have symptoms affecting their routine daily activities and many have disturbed sleep because of asthma. Therefore, for the majority of patients, asthma control could be greatly improved. Reasons for the persistently poor outcomes from asthma are not fully understood, but it seems that some patients are unaware of how much better their asthma control could be, whilst doctors are sometimes not fully aware of the impact of the condition on their patient. Some patients also have concerns about using long-term 'preventer' medication.

Box 1. Aims of asthma treatment. Adapted from the Global Initiative in Asthma (GINA) Guidelines.

- Minimal symptoms
- No exacerbations (attacks)
- No activity limitation
- No emergency visits
- Minimal need for rescue medication
- Minimal side-effects from medication
- Normal/near-normal lung function
- Minimal diurnal (between morning and night) peak flow variability

Poor asthma control can result in persistent symptoms – particularly wheezing, coughing and breathlessness – and can result in frightening and potentially dangerous asthma attacks. Most attacks will subside after appropriate treatment, but every year many people are hospitalised due to acute severe asthma and potentially avoidable deaths do occur. In the UK, over 1500 deaths occur each year due to asthma. Although this has fallen from approximately 2000 deaths per year in the 1990s, avoidable factors are often found and most deaths could have been prevented by better treatment and education.

Why does asthma occur?

The organ principally affected by asthma is the lungs, though many patients with asthma also have other allergic diseases. The main part of the lung affected is the air-carrying tubes – the larger airways (bronchi) and the smaller airways (bronchioli). These branching tubes are essential for the passage of air into the air sacs (alveoli) and for oxygen to be taken into the body and carbon dioxide removed, and contain mucus-producing glands and a ring of muscle in the wall of the tube. In asthma, the lining of the tubes becomes inflamed. The inflammatory process has a number of consequences. Firstly, the muscles in the bronchi become 'twitchy' (hyper-reactive), and if they come in contact with a precipitating factor (trigger) they may tighten up leading to a narrowing in the airway – a process known as bronchoconstriction. This restricts the passage of air in and out of the lung, and so noisy breathing (wheezing), sensations of chest tightness and breathlessness are common. Triggers include cold air, pollutants (such as tobacco smoke), allergens (particles containing proteins to which the sufferer is allergic, such as house-dust mite, pollen, dog or cat dander) or viruses. Contact with a trigger can result in acute bronchoconstriction and an asthma attack. Inflammation also results in an increase in mucus production and in damage to cells in the lining layer of the tubes, which can result in 'plugs' of mucus and accumulation of damaged cells that block the tubes and disrupt airflow further, and also produce a cough productive of phlegm. The presence of a cough and phlegm in people with asthma does not necessarily imply an infection in the airways ('bronchitis'), but may simply indicate active asthma.

Triggers of asthma include cold air, pollutants allergens or viruses.

The chronic inflammation occurring in the bronchi can result in changes to the structure of the airways ('airway remodelling'), with fibrous (scar) tissue in the walls and thickened membranes. This can result in stiffened and narrowed airways resulting in ongoing symptoms like wheeze, breathlessness and cough particularly when exposed to triggers, and in more severe asthma may lead to a progressive loss in lung function. In acute attacks, bronchoconstriction and mucus plugging may prevent the exchange of gases – the central function of the lungs – and in life-threatening cases increases in carbon dioxide and a fall in oxygen in the blood occurs. In this situation, emergency drugs to open the constricted air tubes ('bronchodilators') and supplementary oxygen can be life-saving. However, the mainstay of modern asthma treatment is the use of anti-inflammatory agents to 'damp down' the inflammatory process and prevent asthma attacks and symptoms occurring. All asthma outcomes have been shown to be improved by regular treatment. Unfortunately, for a variety of reasons, some people do not take their recommended preventive treatment regularly, either through misunderstanding of the need for long-term treatment or because of concerns about the safety of this treatment. Doctors can help allay these fears in many cases.

Why has there been a large increase in asthma cases in recent years?

Asthma has become far more common over the last 30 years. In the UK, approximately one-in-20 people currently receive treatment for asthma. The condition is most common in childhood and adolescence, and in many people it may spontaneously go into remission as they enter adulthood. In some patients, however, it can be a lifelong illness, and in others in whom it remits, it may recur in later life. Less commonly, asthma may start in later life, possibly triggered by occupational exposures. Asthma is often associated with other allergic ('atopic') illnesses like eczema and allergic rhinitis (or 'hay fever' when the triggering allergen is pollen). Asthma also has a strong genetic component, and having an affected parent or sibling greatly increases the chances of a child developing asthma.

Asthma is more common in affluent than in developing societies, and the prevalence of asthma in countries such as the UK, the US and New Zealand may be ten-times higher than in the Third World. Families who move to areas with a high prevalence of asthma adopt the local lifestyle rapidly and begin to show a similar prevalence as the local population. The reasons why this should occur are not fully understood; some have proposed that increased cleanliness and reduced exposure to infections enjoyed in affluent societies, particularly by young children, may adversely affect the maturation of the juvenile immune system, leading to the development of asthma and allergies – the so-called 'hygiene hypothesis'. This theory has been supported by observations that children who grow up in environments with more exposure to infections at an early age have a lower chance of developing asthma. For example, it has been shown that children growing up on farms, children with older siblings and large families under one roof, children with pets in the house and

Increased cleanliness and reduced exposure to infections enjoyed in affluent societies may adversely affect the maturation of the juvenile immune system.

children attending day care with other children all have lower asthma risks – all situations associated with increased exposure to early infections.

What can be done to prevent asthma?

It is possible to reduce house-dust mite populations by using impermeable covers for beds and furniture, special vacuum cleaners and hard flooring.

Unfortunately, at present we do not have a 'cure' for asthma and do not have preventative treatment that would completely stop asthma occurring in a susceptible individual. That said, intensive research is underway in these areas. For example, in the future it may be possible to provide a 'vaccination' for asthma that stimulates the immune system away from the allergic type of inflammation characteristic of asthma. There is also significant interest in 'secondary prevention' – measures to reduce the severity and impact of asthma once it has initially developed. For example, it is possible to reduce house-dust mite populations – the most common causative allergen for asthma, which persists in mattresses, carpets and soft furniture – by using impermeable covers for beds and furniture, special vacuum cleaners and hard flooring. However, as yet these measures have not yet been shown to reduce the severity of asthma in affected individuals, possibly because we can't as yet get the levels low enough to avoid the triggering threshold. Cat and dog dander are also common allergic triggers, and people with such allergies are usually advised not to have pets in the house and to minimise contact with them. Desensitisation injections may be useful in people with a single main allergic trigger, but are rarely performed in the UK because of safety concerns.

Tobacco smoke can be an important trigger for asthma, and can also make the lungs insensitive to the anti-inflammatory effects of inhaled medications. As such, it is particularly important that people with asthma should not smoke. Infection with respiratory viruses (e.g. influenza) is another potential trigger for asthma and may result in a loss of asthma control. As a result, many countries (including the UK) recommend annual influenza vaccination for people with asthma. Although exercise can act as a trigger for some people with asthma, effective treatment exists and it is important that good physical health is maintained by regular exercise. A healthy balanced diet is important, and there is growing evidence that naturally occurring vitamins and 'antioxidants' that are found in fresh fruit and vegetables may protect the lungs.

2. Drug review – Beclometasone (Becotide®)

Dr Rebecca Fox-Spencer
CSF Medical Communications Ltd

You are strongly urged to consult your doctor before taking, stopping or changing any of the products reviewed or referred to in *BESTMEDICINE* or any other medication that has been prescribed or recommended by your doctor.

Summary

Beclometasone is an inhaled corticosteroid used extensively in the prophylactic treatment of persistent asthma. International guidelines are driving the development of drug formulations which do not depend on chlorofluorocarbon (CFC)-based propellants, and a CFC-free formulation of beclometasone is already available in the UK. This is reported to be equally effective and well tolerated as twice the dose of the CFC-based formulation, with an improved pattern of deposition due to the smaller particle size. The CFC-based formulation of beclometasone is less potent than several alternative inhaled corticosteroids, though preliminary evidence suggests that the new formulation may prove to be better ranked in terms of potency among the impending CFC-free generation of inhaled corticosteroids. The one major safety concern with beclometasone treatment, as for other inhaled corticosteroids, is the dose-related risk of reduced growth velocity in children, though further investigation is required into whether this extends to an impairment of final height attainment.

Introduction

Corticosteroids have been used as maintenance therapy for asthma for over 50 years. Although tolerability was generally good for corticosteroids administered orally, concern regarding the systemic side-effect profile, particularly in children, provided an impetus for the development of inhaled formulations. These are now the mainstay of prophylactic treatment for persistent asthma. A new chapter in the use of inhaled corticosteroids in asthma is now commencing following the ruling of the Montreal Protocol that delivery devices dependent on chlorofluorocarbon (CFC) propellants should be phased out.[1] CFC propellants are an inexpensive, reliable and effective option for delivering inhaled corticosteroids, but are now recognised as having deleterious effects on the ozone layer. The most promising alternatives to date appear to be the hydrofluoroalkane (HFA) corticosteroid formulations, though these too will most likely be phased out for environmental reasons at a later date.[2] The differing physical and chemical properties of HFA propellants, however, necessitate new clinical data to support the use of inhaled corticosteroids for asthma. Dry powder inhalers do not use a propellant, and are therefore unaffected by this ruling, but are not suitable for all patients.

Beclometasone dipropionate (referred to hereafter as beclometasone) was the first effective and well-tolerated corticosteroid to be marketed as an inhaled formulation.[3] It was also the first CFC-free inhaled corticosteroid to be made available in the UK. Given the impending changes in practice with respect to the use of CFC-free inhaled corticosteroids, this review highlights recent data concerning the efficacy and safety of new HFA formulations of beclometasone. There is also a strong emphasis on comparative trials of beclometasone and other asthma therapies, as well as those evaluating the relative efficacy of beclometasone delivered by alternative devices.

Beclometasone is no longer patent protected (see Reader's Guide), and a variety of branded and non-proprietary formulations of the drug are now available (Table 1).[4] This range of products offers a choice of alternative doses and different delivery devices. However, the data presented in this review are generally applicable to all of these treatment options.

The chemistry of beclometasone is of essentially academic interest and most healthcare professionals will, like you, skip this section.

Pharmacology

Chemistry

The chemical structure of beclometasone is shown in Figure 1. The high lipophilicity of the beclometasone molecule results in poor solubility in water. This is an ideal property for an inhaled corticosteroid, as it slows

Table 1. Summary of formulations of beclometasone available in the UK.[4]

Name	Manufacturer	Doses available per inhalation/ actuation/blister	Delivery devices available
Beclometasone	Non-proprietary	50, 100, 200, 250, 400 μg	MDI, DPI
Aerobec®	3M Health Care Ltd.	50, 100 μg (Aerobec Forte® 250 μg)	Breath-actuated MDI
Asmabec®	Celltech Pharmaceuticals Ltd.	50, 100, 250 μg	Clickhaler® DPI
Beclazone Easi-Breathe®	IVAX Pharmaceuticals UK Ltd.	50, 100, 250 μg	MDI
Becodisks®	Allen & Hanbury's	100, 200, 400 μg	DPI
Becotide®	Allen & Hanbury's	50, 100, 200 μg	MDI
Qvar®	IVAX Pharmaceuticals UK Ltd.	50, 100 μg	MDI and breath-actuated MDI, (both CFC-free)

CFC, chlorofluorocarbon; DPI, dry powder inhalation; MDI, metered dose inhaler.

Figure 1. The chemical structure of beclometasone dipropionate.

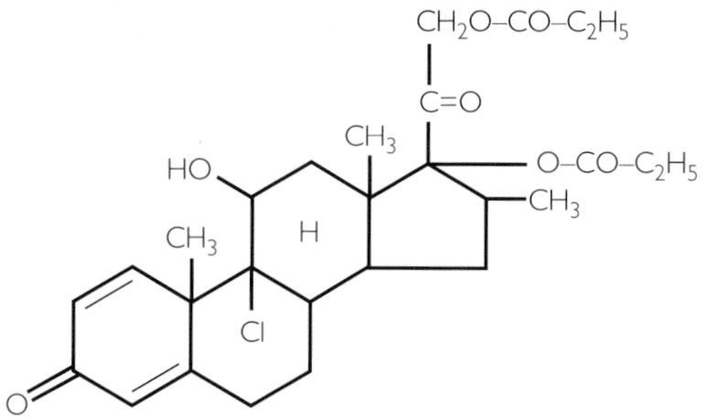

the rate of absorption into the aqueous mucus layer of the bronchial mucosa, thereby increasing the time the active compound spends in contact with the lung surface.[5]

When beclometasone is formulated with a propellant, its physical properties are affected. CFC–beclometasone has a mean particle size of 3.5 μm, compared with only 1.1 μm for HFA–beclometasone. Furthermore, CFC formulations of beclometasone are suspensions, whereas HFA–beclometasone is a solution of beclometasone in an HFA propellant. The HFA aerosol is, as a result of these properties, a warmer, gentler spray than the CFC equivalent.

Mechanism of action

Although the pathology of bronchial hyper-reactivity in asthma is not fully understood, inflammation in the airways is considered a central causative factor.[6] When corticosteroids are inhaled, they are taken up into cells lining the airways, where they bind to cytoplasmically located glucocorticoid receptors.[7] The corticosteroid–receptor complex translocates to the cell nucleus where it modifies the transcription of a wide range of inflammatory mediators (e.g. cytokines, histamine, eicosanoids, leukotrienes) and thereby inhibits the inflammatory component of chronic asthma. Corticosteroids also reduce mucosal oedema, mucus secretion and potentiate β-adrenergic responsiveness. Chronic use of inhaled corticosteroids may reduce the number of mast cells in the airways and the level of immune response to allergens and exercise.[8] These drugs do not, however, appear to have any significant impact on the levels of leukotrienes.[9]

The *in vitro* affinity of beclometasone for corticosteroid receptors is poor when compared with other currently available drugs in the same class.

In vitro *activity*

The potency of inhaled corticosteroids can be estimated by measuring their binding affinity for corticosteroid receptors. The *in vitro* affinity of beclometasone for glucocorticoid receptors is poor when compared with other currently available drugs in this class, as shown in Table 2.[10] It is important to appreciate, however, that the binding affinity of

Table 2. Relative receptor binding affinity and topical potencies of beclometasone and other inhaled corticosteroids. All values, for receptor binding affinity and MacKenzie skin blanching test, are expressed relative to dexamethasone, for which the value is set at 1.0.[10]

	Beclometasone	Budesonide	Flunisolide	Fluticasone	Triamcinolone
Receptor binding affinity	0.4	9.4	1.8	18.0	3.6
MacKenzie skin blanching test	600	980	330	1200	390

beclometasone for corticosteroid receptors *in vitro* may not accurately reflect its behaviour *in vivo*, particularly within specific inflammatory cell types. Furthermore, it is thought that the effectiveness of corticosteroids depends on more complex interactions than basic receptor binding alone.[11]

Although beclometasone compares unfavourably with other currently available inhaled corticosteroids in terms of receptor affinity, it is further activated in the lung by metabolism. The resulting metabolite, 17-beclometasone monopropionate, has a relative receptor affinity for glucocorticoid receptors 1.5-times that of budesonide, which in turn is over 20-times greater than that of beclometasone (Table 2).[5] As a consequence of this metabolic activation, the clinical efficacy of beclometasone may outweigh that otherwise predicted by its poor receptor affinity.

In vivo *activity*

The most common method of assessing corticosteroid potency is the MacKenzie skin blanching test.[10] The extent of skin whitening following several hours of contact with a solution of the drug is reflective of its potency. According to this test, beclometasone has average potency compared with other drugs in the class, as shown in Table 2, where values are indexed against dexamethasone, for which the value is set at 1.0.[10] This vasoconstrictive activity of corticosteroids is, however, of little relevance to their mechanism of action in asthma, and so may not accurately reflect the comparative clinical efficacy of beclometasone when used in this setting.

The pharmacokinetics of a drug are of interest to healthcare professionals because it is important for them to understand the action of a drug on the body over a period of time.

Pharmacokinetics

The pharmacokinetics of inhaled corticosteroids, along with their clinical efficacy and safety, are heavily dependent on the characteristics of the inhaler and the drug formulation selected. The features of the devices used for administering inhaled corticosteroids are summarised in Box 1. The poor solubility of beclometasone in water means that the maximum dose which can be formulated for use in a nebuliser is lower than that for the other inhaled corticosteroids.[5]

Box 1. Devices used to administer inhaled corticosteroids.

Metered dose inhaler (MDI)

- Most widely used device
- Delivers fixed dose each actuation
- Requires a propellant – traditionally CFCs, shortly to be replaced by non-CFCs (e.g. HFA)
- Requires some hand–breath co-ordination, but the use of a spacer can double the amount of drug delivered to the lungs
- Lung deposition is good, though this is dependent on user co-ordination and the size of particles

Breath-actuated aerosol

- Similar to MDIs and delivers a fixed dose per actuation
- An alternative option to an MDI plus spacer when the patient has poor hand–breath coordination, as release of the drug is triggered by inspiration

Dry powder inhaler (DPI)

- Also useful if a patient has poor hand–breath coordination, as it is breath dependent
- Does not require a propellant
- Lung deposition depends on the individual device and inspiratory flow rate

Nebuliser

- Good pulmonary deposition with no hand–breath coordination required
- Despite this, there is no evidence for improved clinical outcomes compared with hand-held inhalers
- Used mainly for young or elderly patients who find other devices difficult to use

CFC, chlorofluorocarbon; HFA, hydrofluoroalkane.

The main pharmacokinetic properties of beclometasone are shown in Table 3.[5,12–14] Depending on the device used, only 10–30% of the inhaled corticosteroid dose is expected to reach the lungs. The HFA formulation of beclometasone is, however, associated with improved lung deposition compared with the CFC formulation. This is most likely a consequence of its considerably smaller particle size and the slower velocity of aerosol emitted from the inhaler, which reduces the dependence on good co-ordination.[15] Whereas CFC–beclometasone only appears to reach the central airways, HFA–beclometasone reaches central, intermediate and peripheral airways.[16] This improved deposition is illustrated in Figure 2.

> The HFA formulation of beclometasone is associated with improved lung deposition over the CFC formulation.

Of the proportion of the drug which is ingested, approximately 70% undergoes first-pass metabolism prior to reaching the systemic circulation. Beclometasone is hydrolysed to the metabolites 17-beclometasone monopropionate and 21-beclometasone monopropionate in the lung, and to a greater extent in the liver, where biotransformation is mediated by the 3A family of cytochrome P450 (CYP) isoenzymes.[17] The 17-beclometasone monopropionate

Table 3. The pharmacokinetic properties of beclometasone.[5,12–14]

Pharmacokinetic parameter	
Oral bioavailability (%)	~30%
t_{max} (hours)	3–5
C_{max} (μg/L)	1.3[a]
Plasma protein binding (%)	87
Steady-state volume of distribution (L)	20
Plasma $t_{1/2}$ (hours)	0.5 (intravenous)/0.1 (inhaled)
Total clearance (L/hour)	150

[a]Following inhaled dose of 2000 μg.
$t_{1/2}$, elimination half-life; t_{max}, time to peak plasma concentrations (C_{max}).

Figure 2. Deposition of beclometasone formulated with a hydrofluoroalkane (HFA) propellant and delivered by a standard metered dose inhaler in an asthmatic patient.[16]

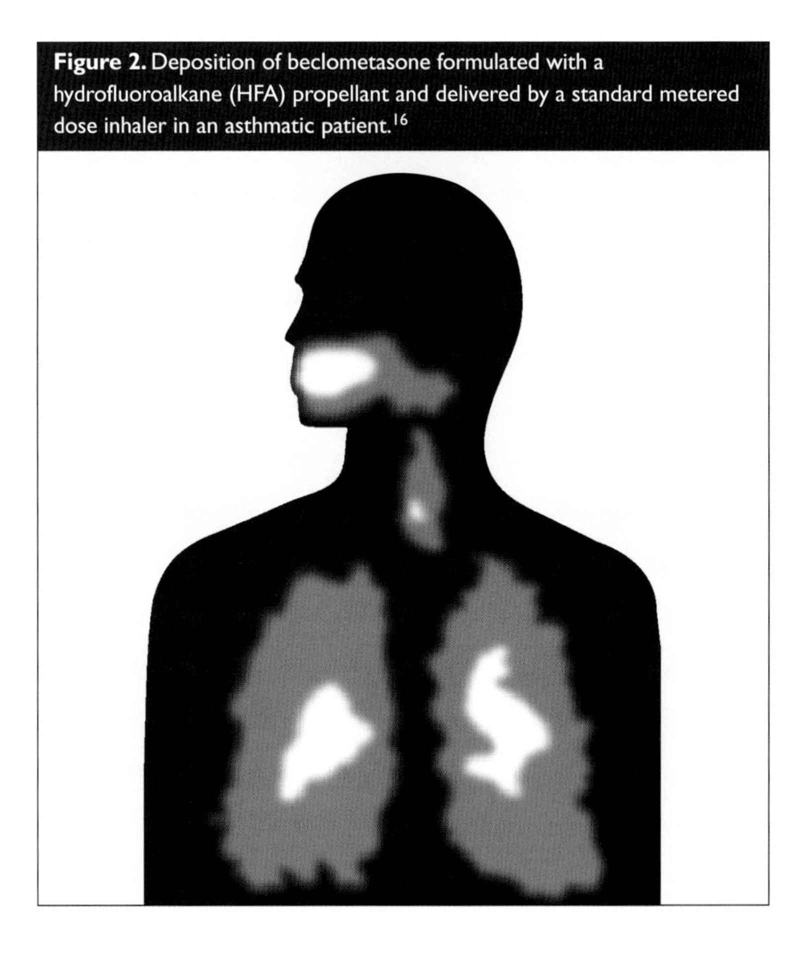

metabolite is highly stable in lung tissue, but may be converted to 21-beclometasone monopropionate in the plasma. In the liver, both 17-beclometasone monopropionate and 21-beclometasone monopropionate may be further metabolised to other, inactive metabolites. The plasma elimination of beclometasone is very rapid following its inhalation, as shown in Table 3, though the elimination of 17-beclometasone monopropionate is considerably slower (6.5 hours following inhalation). Within 96 hours following intravenous administration of beclometasone, it is reported that approximately 60% of the dose is excreted in the faeces (mainly via the bile) and approximately 12% in the urine, in both cases mainly in the form of free and conjugated metabolites.[14,18] Plasma protein binding is relatively high, at approximately 87%.[14]

Clinical efficacy

Placebo-controlled trials

The clinical efficacy of beclometasone has already been well established by placebo-controlled trials. Recent trials reflect the evolution of beclometasone therapy, as they consider means by which the therapy may be further improved, and provide initial evidence of the efficacy of the non-CFC formulations.[19–21] Table 4 summarises three such randomised, blinded, placebo-controlled trials. One of these has evaluated the use of a CFC-propelled MDI with a high dose per actuation,[19] specifically developed to improve compliance, and the remaining two consider various doses of the HFA–beclometasone formulation.[20,21]

Beclometasone delivered by MDI with 84 μg per actuation was clinically equivalent in terms of both safety and its superiority over placebo as an equivalent total daily dose administered by MDI with 42 μg per actuation.[19] A four-fold increase in the total daily dose delivered by the 84 μg per actuation MDI generated additional improvement over placebo.[19] In those trials evaluating the use of HFA–beclometasone, this new formulation was found to be superior to placebo in terms of pulmonary function and asthma symptom suppression, with a good level of tolerability. There was also evidence of a dose–response effect of HFA–beclometasone treatment on pulmonary function, though this was not apparent when considering other parameters such as amelioration of asthma symptoms.[20,21]

Comparative trials of beclometasone

A number of trials have been performed in order to compare different methods of administration or different formulations of beclometasone. Most commonly, these trials did not include placebo groups, though some used placebo devices to create a 'double-dummy' setting (i.e. to generate blinding when two treatments differ significantly in their appearance and function).

Table 4. Summary of randomised, placebo-controlled studies of the efficacy and safety of beclometasone.[19–21]

Study	Asthma severity at baseline	Dose(s) and delivery device	Main outcomes
Nathan *et al.*[19] Double-blind Children and adults (n=423) 28 days	Moderate (baseline FEV_1 50–80% of predicted normal) Increase of ≥15% in FEV_1 in response to short-acting β_2-agonist	336 µg/day (Beclometasone 84: 4 puffs/day) 336 µg/day (Beclometasone 42: 8 puffs/day) 1344 µg/day (Beclometasone 84: 16 puffs/day) All by MDI	• All three active treatment groups demonstrated significant benefits over placebo in mean percentage change from baseline in FEV_1 (+7% in both lower dose groups [$p \leq 0.01$ *vs* placebo], +16% in high-dose group [$p \leq 0.03$ *vs* placebo] and –6% in placebo group). • Similar trends were observed for the effects on $FEF_{25\%-75\%}$, FVC and PEF. The two lower dose groups were not significantly different from each other but were generally superior to placebo. The higher dose demonstrated increased efficacy over placebo at all time points on all of these measures ($p<0.01$ *vs* placebo). • A similar pattern was seen for patient- and physician-rated severity of asthma symptoms. The two lower doses were significantly superior to placebo (generally $p \leq 0.01$) but equivalent to each other, whilst the higher dose generated the greatest improvement. • Use of rescue salbutamol treatment increased in the placebo group and decreased in the three active treatment groups. Only the highest dose group was significantly superior to placebo at all time points ($p<0.01$). • A similar adverse event profile was reported in all groups.

$FEF_{25\%-75\%}$, forced expiratory flow during the middle half of a forced expiratory volume; FEV_1, forced expiratory volume in 1 second; FVC, forced vital capacity; HFA, hydrofluoroalkane; MDI, metered dose inhaler; PEF, peak expiratory flow.

Beclometasone *vs* beclometasone: varying delivery device

One such double-dummy study compared the efficacy and safety of beclometasone administered via a DPI to that administered via a pressurised MDI with a large volume spacer.[22] This 12-week trial of 204 adult patients with mild-to-moderate asthma confirmed that beclometasone administered by these two methods was clinically

Table 4. Continued

Study	Asthma severity at baseline	Dose(s) and delivery device	Main outcomes
Nayak *et al.*[20] Double-blinded Children (n=353) 12 weeks	Moderate (baseline FEV_1 50–80% of predicted normal) Reversibility with short-acting β_2-agonist Use of β_2-agonist therapy at least once a day on at least 50% days in 2-week run-in	80 µg/day HFA–beclometasone 160 µg/day HFA–beclometasone Delivered by breath-actuated MDI	• Both doses were significantly superior to placebo in improving FEV_1 at 12 weeks (mean change from baseline in % predicted FEV_1: +9.2% and +10.0% for the lower and higher dose groups, respectively; both $p \leq 0.01$ *vs* placebo, [+3.9%]). • The percentage of patients demonstrating a clinically relevant improvement in FEV_1 (≥12%) was 48.3% in the 80 µg/day group ($p=0.03$ *vs* placebo), 57.8% in the 160 µg/day group ($p=0.001$ *vs* placebo) and 34.2% in the placebo group). • Active treatment was superior to placebo in improving morning PEF. In the higher dose group, this superiority was significant at all time points ($p \leq 0.01$), whereas in the lower dose group it was significant only at weeks 1–2 ($p \leq 0.05$). • Both active treatment groups were superior to placebo at increasing the percentage of days free from asthma. However, both were significant only in the late stages of the study (160 µg/day, $p \leq 0.05$ from week 7–8 onwards; 80 µg/day, $p \leq 0.05$ during weeks 7–8 and 9–10). • Both active treatment groups reduced β-agonist use, though only the higher dose group was significantly superior ($p \leq 0.05$). • There was no significant difference in the incidence or nature of adverse events or plasma cortisol levels, between active and placebo groups. • Severe adverse events were reported by 5.8, 2.6 and 7.8% of the lower and higher dose groups, and placebo, respectively.

$FEF_{25\%-75\%}$, forced expiratory flow during the middle half of a forced expiratory volume; FEV_1, forced expiratory volume in 1 second; FVC, forced vital capacity; HFA, hydrofluoroalkane; MDI, metered dose inhaler; PEF, peak expiratory flow.

equivalent in terms of pulmonary function and day- and night-time asthma symptom scores. Beclometasone administered by DPI and MDI generated improvements in morning PEF of +3.5 and +3.0 L/minute, respectively, and in evening PEF of +1.7 and +1.4 L/minute. The mean

Table 4. Continued

Study	Asthma severity at baseline	Dose(s) and delivery device	Main outcomes
Hampel *et al.*[21] Blinded Adults (n=270) 6 weeks	Mild-to-moderate (baseline FEV_1 65–85% of predicted normal) Increase of ≥15% in FEV_1 in response to short-acting β_2-agonist Use of β_2-agonist therapy at least 12 times during a 2-week run-in.	100 μg/day HFA–beclometasone 200 μg/day HFA–beclometasone Delivered by breath-actuated MDI	• Both doses were significantly superior to placebo in improving FEV_1 (mean change from baseline in % of predicted normal: 6.7, 8.6 and 0.4% for the lower and higher doses, and placebo, respectively; $p \le 0.01$ for both doses *vs* placebo). • Active treatments were also significantly superior to placebo in terms of morning PEF ($p \le 0.01$), evening PEF ($p \le 0.05$), $FEF_{25\%-75\%}$ ($p \le 0.01$) and nights without sleep disturbance (100 μg/day, $p \le 0.05$; 200 μg/day, $p \le 0.01$). • Only the lower dose of beclometasone was significantly superior to placebo in reducing wheeze and cough ($p \le 0.05$), whilst only the higher dose reduced shortness of breath ($p \le 0.05$). No significant benefit of active treatment was observed in reducing chest tightness. • Only the lower dose significantly reduced daily β-agonist use ($p \le 0.05$). • Both doses were well tolerated, and demonstrated similar adverse event profiles.

$FEF_{25\%-75\%}$, forced expiratory flow during the middle half of a forced expiratory volume; FEV_1, forced expiratory volume in 1 second; FVC, forced vital capacity; HFA, hydrofluoroalkane; MDI, metered dose inhaler; PEF, peak expiratory flow.

improvements in daytime symptom scores were –0.11 and –0.18 symptom score units, respectively. For night-time symptom scores, the mean improvements were –0.02 and –0.14. None of these relationships demonstrated a significant superiority of one device over the other. The mean daily doses used (837 and 867 μg/day, respectively) and the duration of treatment (83 and 82 days) were also similar in both groups. The limited benefits afforded by treatment in this study probably reflect the fact that patients were selected on the basis of stability on beclometasone following a 4-week run-in period.

Equivalence between delivery devices was further indicated by data from two further studies which used double-dummy strategies to compare beclometasone administered by MDI and by a nebuliser.[23,24] One trial of 124 adult patients with moderate-to-severe asthma evaluated 12 weeks of treatment with beclometasone, 3000–4000 μg/day, given via a nebuliser compared with beclometasone, 1500–2000 μg/day, given via an MDI with a spacer.[23] Both the nebuliser and MDI groups demonstrated significant improvements in terms of morning PEF (10.5 and 7.8 L/minute, respectively), evening PEF (13.7 and 13.1 L/minute), FEV_1 (0.4 and 0.3 L) and FVC (0.4 and 0.2 L) compared with the run-in period, during which time they were already inhaling high-dose corticosteroids. There were no significant differences between the two treatment groups in any of these measures of pulmonary function, nor in terms of symptom scores or patient evaluation of drug effectiveness. Tolerability was also reported to be good, and was comparable in the two treatment groups. The second study compared the use of beclometasone, 1600 μg/day, delivered by a nebuliser and an 800 μg/day dose given by an MDI plus spacer in 51 children with moderate-to-severe asthma.[24] Statistically equivalent and significant benefits were reported after 4 weeks' treatment in both the nebuliser and MDI groups with respect to morning PEF (mean change from baseline 88.1 and 92 L/minute, respectively), evening PEF (89.1 and 85.9 L/minute), FEV (0.6 L for both), FVC (0.5 and 0.6 L), rescue salbutamol use (–2.1 and –1.1 puffs/day), together with patient- and investigator-assessment of effectiveness. The two treatments were also equally well tolerated.

When considering these data, it should be borne in mind that the clinical trial setting may be subject to a bias towards better outcomes with MDIs than would be observed in the general population. This is because trials often exclude patients who cannot use MDIs correctly, thus skewing the outcomes in MDI groups towards more favourable outcomes.[25] This effect will be less pronounced in groups using devices which are less dependent on the user's co-ordination and skill.

Beclometasone *vs* beclometasone: varying dose

A trial carried out in Scotland assessed the clinical implications of reducing the dose of beclometasone, with the premise that this would improve its side-effect profile.[26] Prior to enrolment into this study, the participants were already receiving inhaled beclometasone (≥800 μg/day; or an equivalent dose of budesonide or fluticasone propionate), following a diagnosis of asthma at least 1 year previously. Data from the 212 adult patients who completed the study indicated that the dose of beclometasone can be reduced by an average of 25% without any significant loss of efficacy. It should be considered that participation in the study may have led patients to adhere more strictly to their treatment regimen than in a non-trial setting, thus facilitating this dose reduction. It is also of note that the study did not itself demonstrate any reduction in side-effects at the reduced dosage.

Beclometasone *vs* beclometasone: varying formulation

Two further double-dummy trials without a placebo arm evaluated the relative effect of beclometasone in CFC and HFA formulations. The first of these studies compared equal doses (100, 400 and 800 μg/day) of CFC–beclometasone and HFA–beclometasone in 323 adult asthma patients with baseline FEV_1 50–75% of the predicted value and at least

12% reversibility in response to an inhaled β_2-agonist.[27] This 6-week study demonstrated that the reformulation of beclometasone in HFA enables effective control of asthma at lower doses than the CFC formulation. It was reported that 2.6-times the dose of CFC–beclometasone as HFA–beclometasone was required to mediate the same improvement in FEV_1. This multiple was increased to 3.2 for improvements in $FEF_{25\%-75\%}$. For certain other outcomes – specifically days free of wheeze, chest tightness and daily inhaled β-agonist use – there was a significant dose–response effect in both the CFC and HFA groups. Tolerability was reported to be good in all treatment groups evaluated with the exception of the group of patients receiving the lowest dose of CFC–beclometasone, in whom asthma symptoms remained considerable. The only significant safety concern associated with the HFA–beclometasone formulation was the relatively high number of reports of pharyngitis in the highest dosage group (27 *vs* 17% in the 800 μg/day CFC–beclometasone group). However, few of these reports of pharyngitis were attributed to study treatment by the investigators.

The second report comparing the CFC and HFA formulations of beclometasone recognised that lower doses of the latter were necessary to elicit equivalent responses and, therefore, employed doses of 1500 and 800 μg/day, respectively.[28] In this 6-month study, patients (n=141) were over the age of 14 years and were diagnosed with moderate-to-severe asthma, which was controlled with CFC–beclometasone, 1000–2000 μg/day, prior to entry into the study. There were no significant differences between the two treatment groups in terms of mean change from baseline in either FEV_1 or $FEF_{25\%-75\%}$, nor in morning or evening PEF values, at all of the time points on which these parameters were assessed. Asthma symptom and sleep disturbance scores were occasionally superior in the HFA group, but more commonly the two treatment groups were statistically equivalent. The adverse event profile was similar in both groups, and there was no evidence of any difference in adrenal suppression. This study indicates, therefore, that a near halving in the dose of beclometasone when switching from a CFC to an HFA formulation results in at least as effective control of pulmonary function and asthma symptoms, with a comparable safety profile.

A near halving in the dose of beclometasone when switching from a CFC to an HFA formulation results in at least as effective asthma control.

A placebo-controlled trial has also been performed to compare the effects of HFA–beclometasone and CFC–beclometasone on asthma-related quality of life, as assessed by the Asthma Quality of Life questionnaire (AQLQ).[29] However, this 12-week trial was not blinded and different canisters were used for the two active treatments. Patients and investigators were, however, unaware of whether the patient was receiving active treatment or placebo. Following 7–12 days of treatment with oral prednisone to confirm steroid responsiveness, 347 adults with moderate asthma were randomised to HFA–beclometasone at 400 μg/day, CFC–beclometasone at 800 μg/day, or placebo. At these doses, HFA–beclometasone was at least as effective as CFC–beclometasone in terms of improvement in quality of life scores. Thus, 2.4 patients needed to be treated with HFA–beclometasone to generate significant quality of life benefit in one patient, compared with 3.0 in the CFC group. There was a trend in favour of HFA–beclometasone in terms of AQLQ score, but this was not statistically significant compared with the CFC–beclometasone group.

A number of trials have compared CFC–beclometasone with HFA-beclometasone, but used a 'non-extra fine' HFA formulation.[3] By bringing the particle size as close as possible to that of the CFC formulation, it is suggested that disruption to prescribers and patients during the transition to non-CFC propellants, in terms of the need to re-establish the maintenance dose, will be minimised. Indeed, these trials have demonstrated that equivalent efficacy and safety profiles are still obtained with equivalent doses of CFC–beclometasone and non-extra fine HFA–beclometasone.[3] Although this new formulation should eliminate the need to re-establish the optimal maintenance dose, it would appear to contradict other efforts to reduce the long-term dose intake of inhaled corticosteroids.[26] The equivalence of non-extra fine HFA–beclometasone and CFC–beclometasone suggests that the increased potency of the conventional HFA–beclometasone formulation is directly related to the smaller particle size and thus improved airway deposition. However, the beneficial effect of smaller particle size in other CFC-free formulations does not appear to be common to all inhaled corticosteroids. Indeed, a CFC-free formulation of fluticasone propionate and an alternative CFC-free beclometasone formulation demonstrated only equivalent efficacy as the corresponding CFC formulations.[12] It would appear sensible, therefore, to exploit the improved drug delivery observed with the conventional HFA–beclometasone formulation, and this may ultimately result in its recommendation over other drugs in the class once CFC propellants have been phased out.

Comparative trials of beclometasone and other asthma therapies

There is a wealth of data available which highlights the relative efficacy and tolerability of beclometasone and alternative inhaled corticosteroids, as well as other anti-asthmatic drugs with alternative mechanisms of action. Comparative trials of beclometasone have generally used the CFC formulations, and therefore, further trials are now warranted which evaluate the relative strengths and weaknesses of these drugs with non-CFC formulations of each agent.

Beclometasone *vs* mometasone furoate

Beclometasone has been compared in clinical trials with the most recently introduced inhaled corticosteroid, mometasone furoate (hereafter referred to as mometasone).[30,31] One study compared two doses of mometasone (100 μg twice daily and 200 μg twice daily), administered by a DPI, with a single dose of beclometasone (168 μg twice daily), administered via an MDI, and also included a placebo group.[30] The study population comprised 227 patients, aged between 13 and 75 years, who were previously maintained on inhaled triamcinolone, beclometasone, fluticasone or flunisolide. Each of these patients demonstrated an FEV_1 of between 60 and 90% of the predicted normal prior to randomisation. Reversibility was indicated by an increase of at least 12% in FEV_1 and an absolute volume increase of at least 200 mL within 30 minutes of two inhalations of salbutamol. This 12-week trial reported that all active treatments were significantly superior to placebo in terms of improving wheezing ($p<0.01$) and breathing difficulty scores ($p\leq0.02$), as well as in reducing the use of rescue β-agonist medication ($p<0.01$) and increasing the estimated time until worsening of asthma symptoms ($p<0.01$). In terms of pulmonary function, there was no significant difference between active treatments in the effects on FVC, $FEF_{25\%-75\%}$ or PEF. The higher dose of mometasone was more effective in reducing FEV_1 than the other two active treatment groups, but this superiority was not statistically significant. The investigators emphasised that the study was not powered to detect differences between mometasone and beclometasone; the latter was included only as an active control to benchmark the effects of mometasone and complement the placebo-controlled trial. Indeed, the different delivery devices used in this trial may well have influenced the comparative data obtained.

A study of similar design compared three doses of mometasone (56, 200 or 500 μg twice daily) with one beclometasone dose (168 μg twice daily[a]) and a placebo arm.[31] In this double-dummy, 4-week trial, both drugs were administered by an MDI. The 395 study participants were between the ages of 18 and 65 years, with FEV_1 between 50 and 90% of the predicted value, with reversibility of at least 15% in response to inhaled β_2-agonist (or at least 20% if the baseline FEV_1 was 86–90% of the predicted normal). All active treatment groups were significantly superior to placebo in terms of FEV_1, FVC, $FEF_{25\%-75\%}$ and PEF. The two higher doses of mometasone had significantly greater effects on FEV_1 ($p<0.01$), FVC ($p<0.01$) and $FEF_{25\%-75\%}$ than beclometasone (all $p<0.05$). The lowest mometasone dose was comparable in efficacy to the beclometasone group. All three doses of mometasone were significantly superior to beclometasone in terms of morning PEF (two higher doses, $p<0.01$; lowest dose, $p=0.04$). All active treatments were well tolerated, with headache and pharyngitis the most common adverse events reported. The only dose-related effect in terms of the safety profile was an increased rate of oral candidiasis in the highest dose mometasone group (5 *vs* 0% in both the placebo and beclometasone groups).

Beclometasone, 168 μg twice daily, is closest in clinical efficacy to mometasone, 56 μg twice daily.

Thus, this 4-week study indicated that beclometasone, 168 μg twice daily, is closest in clinical efficacy to mometasone, 56 μg twice daily. Mometasone is recognised to be a particularly potent corticosteroid, and these data indicate that it is as effective at lower doses as beclometasone, which may make it more favourable in terms of the risk of local side-effects, such as those of the mouth and throat. Mometasone has now been reformulated with HFA-227, however, and future non-CFC

[a]This non-standard dose describes the fixed dose delivered per MDI actuation, as opposed to the metered dose released ex-valve (200 μg).

comparative trials will be needed to determine any differences in relative performance with this new formulation.

Beclometasone *vs* fluticasone propionate

The relative efficacy and safety profiles of beclometasone and fluticasone propionate (hereafter referred to as fluticasone) administered by a nebuliser, have been compared in a study of 205 adult patients with moderate, persistent asthma.[32] Fluticasone is an inhaled corticosteroid, more recently introduced than beclometasone. The 12-week trial compared beclometasone, 2400 μg/day, with fluticasone, 2000 μg/day, and demonstrated that these treatments are equally effective and well tolerated. Both treatments generated comparable improvements in terms of pulmonary function (PEF, FEV_1 and FVC) and asthma symptoms (i.e. number reporting 'excellent' symptom scores, number of symptom-free days and nights, and use of rescue medication). Adverse events and drug reactions were rare and there were no significant differences in terms of laboratory evaluations of safety. Two patients in the beclometasone group and four in the fluticasone group reported adverse drug reactions. Only one, who was in the beclometasone group, discontinued the study due to treatment-related adverse events.

It is much more common in clinical practice for inhaled corticosteroids to be administered via an MDI than by a nebuliser, and comparative studies of beclometasone and fluticasone using MDIs have demonstrated an efficacy relationship more in favour of fluticasone. For example, a study of 398 paediatric patients, aged between 4 and 19 years, with mild-to-moderate asthma randomised participants to fluticasone, 200 μg/day, or beclometasone, 400 μg/day, and showed that these doses were equivalent on most measurements of efficacy.[33] At certain time points, fluticasone was shown to be superior in terms of per cent predicted PEF, per cent of days with symptom-free exercise and per cent of days without rescue medication. The only significant difference with regards to safety was a higher incidence of sore throat in the fluticasone group ($p<0.001$). The investigators concluded that fluticasone was at least as effective and well tolerated as twice the dose of beclometasone. It should be considered, however, that the increased potency observed with the HFA formulation of beclometasone is a trend which does not appear to be mirrored with the HFA formulation of fluticasone. It would appear that fluticasone is one of the most promising inhaled corticosteroids to be introduced in clinical practice, hence it will be important that further comparative trials between these two drugs are carried out once CFC-free formulations of both agents are better established.

Fluticasone is at least as effective and well tolerated as twice the dose of beclometasone.

Beclometasone *vs* budesonide

The efficacy and safety of nebulised beclometasone and budesonide have been compared in 127 children, aged between 6 and 14 years, with mild-to-moderate persistent asthma.[34] Patients were treated for 4 weeks with beclometasone, 800 μg/day, or budesonide, 1000 μg/day. Both

Beclometasone and budesonide are clinically equivalent and equally well tolerated in children with mild-to-moderate persistent asthma.

beclometasone and budesonide generated significant and comparable benefits in PEFR, FEV_1, use of rescue medication, asthma symptom score and number of nocturnal awakenings ($p<0.001$ *vs* baseline in all cases, no significant difference between groups). Both treatments were also well tolerated, with mostly mild-to-moderate adverse events, none of which caused any patient to discontinue treatment. At these high doses, and given the consistent good drug delivery afforded by nebulisation, beclometasone and budesonide are, therefore, clinically equivalent and equally well tolerated in children with mild-to-moderate persistent asthma.

Beclometasone *vs* montelukast

A number of trials have compared the efficacy and safety of beclometasone to that of montelukast, an orally active, potent and specific cysteinyl leukotriene receptor antagonist.[35–41] One such study, of 730 asthmatic patients, aged 15–65 years with FEV_1 50–85% of the predicted value with at least 15% reversibility in response to an inhaled β_2-agonist, examined the degree of overlap of patient responses to 6 weeks of beclometasone or montelukast therapy.[35] The drugs were dosed at 200 μg twice daily and 10 mg once daily, respectively. There was a high degree of overlap between the two groups; 96% for distribution of responses in terms of FEV_1 and 89% for proportion of asthma control days, a combined measure of the extent of β-agonist use, nocturnal awakenings, use of oral corticosteroid rescue therapy and need for unscheduled asthma-related medical care. A placebo group was also included in this trial, and both drugs were shown to be significantly superior in both FEV_1 ($p<0.05$) and proportion of asthma control days ($p<0.05$) relative to placebo. In terms of the latter outcome, beclometasone was significantly more effective than montelukast ($p<0.05$). The same was true according to the patient's global evaluation ($p<0.05$), though there was no significant difference in global evaluation by the physician.

Similar findings were reported in a 6-week, placebo-controlled trial of 782 asthmatic patients over the age of 15 years, with FEV_1 between 50 and 85% of the predicted value, and FEV_1 reversibility of at least 15% in response to an inhaled β_2-agonist.[36] Beclometasone was administered at 200 μg twice daily and montelukast at 10 mg once daily. In this trial, there was a 98% overlap in patients' clinical response, using the measure of percentage days of asthma control. Both drugs were superior to placebo in all efficacy outcomes, and beclometasone generated a statistically better response with regard to the FEV_1 than montelukast ($p<0.001$). According to more clinically relevant outcomes (i.e. frequency of asthma attacks, asthma flare-ups and use of rescue corticosteroid therapy), montelukast was at least as effective as beclometasone. The most common adverse events reported were infections of the upper respiratory tract, headache, sinusitis and asthma exacerbations, and these did not differ between the treatment groups.

The lack of consensus over whether either of these drugs is clinically superior was further fuelled by a 12-week trial of 895 patients with mild-to-moderate asthma (FEV_1 between 50 and 85% of the predicted value).[37] Beclometasone was administered at 200 μg twice daily and montelukast at 10 mg once daily. In these patients, who were between the ages of 15 and 85 years, both drugs generated significant benefits over placebo in terms of their effects on FEV_1, daytime asthma symptom scores, PEF, quality of life scores, nocturnal awakenings, asthma attacks, asthma control days and days with asthma exacerbations ($p<0.001$ *vs* placebo for each parameter). In this trial, however, beclometasone was significantly superior to montelukast on all of these measures ($p<0.01$ in each case). Montelukast, in contrast, was more effective than beclometasone in terms of speed of onset of action, and the extent of the initial effect.

In a slight deviation from this standard comparative protocol, one study has evaluated the benefits of administering montelukast as an add-on therapy for those patients whose asthma was incompletely controlled with beclometasone, 200 μg twice daily.[38] This double-dummy trial of 642 patients included a placebo group and also enabled a direct comparison between montelukast and beclometasone when used independently of each other. Patients had a history of at least 1 year of intermittent or persistent asthma symptoms, and had been treated with inhaled corticosteroids for at least 6 weeks prior to the study. Supplemental treatment with montelukast, 10 mg once daily, in these patients afforded significant additional benefit over continued treatment with beclometasone alone in terms of improvements in the FEV_1 ($p<0.001$), daytime asthma symptom score ($p=0.041$), nocturnal awakenings ($p=0.027$), morning PEF ($p=0.004$) and physician's global evaluation ($p=0.001$). Complete substitution of beclometasone for montelukast resulted in worse outcomes than in those patients who continued on beclometasone alone, though montelukast monotherapy was still superior to placebo. The investigators concluded that montelukast generates additional benefit to those patients inadequately controlled by beclometasone alone, but when used in isolation, beclometasone is the superior of the two drugs, as shown in Figure 3.

Montelukast generates additional benefit to those patients inadequately controlled by beclometasone alone.

It has been reported that patient adherence to treatment is higher for oral montelukast than for inhaled beclometasone, particularly amongst children.[39,40] The data from the 12-week trial described above suggest that, although montelukast has a more rapid onset of action, beclometasone appears to be more effective in the long term.[37] Open-label comparative studies of beclometasone and montelukast have, however, suggested otherwise, indicating that, in clinical practice, the poorer levels of patient adherence associated with inhaled treatment may limit the overall efficacy of beclometasone.[41] It is important that future comparative trials, including those using CFC-free formulations, are of sufficient duration to consider the influence of treatment concordance. In general, the currently available data are consistent with current prescribing trends and guidelines, with inhaled corticosteroids considered to be the initial controller therapy, with oral antileukotriene agents as an alternative or add-on controller therapy option.[35] A 2-year, single-blind, randomised controlled trial is currently being undertaken

Figure 3. Mean percentage change from baseline in forced expiratory volume in 1 second (FEV_1) with montelukast (10 mg/day) and beclometasone (200 μg twice daily), alone and in combination, and placebo.[38]

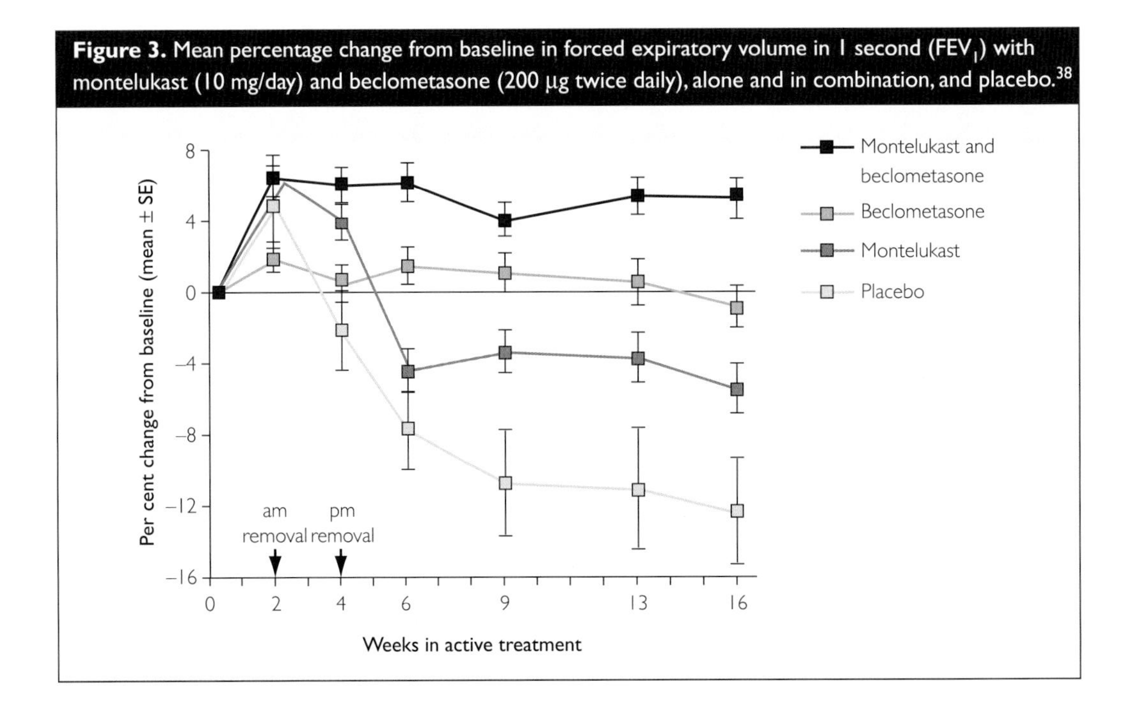

in the UK to assess the relative value of antileukotriene agents and other therapies, including corticosteroids, for improving asthma-related quality of life and other clinically relevant asthma outcomes.[42]

Beclometasone *vs* theophylline

The bronchodilator theophylline is now considered a second-line agent for the treatment of patients with moderate-to-severe asthma, though it is still used by some as a first-line option.[43] Studies comparing beclometasone with theophylline are consistently supportive of the former as the better choice, at least in adult patients. A year-long randomised, double-blind, placebo-controlled study has compared the efficacy and safety of the two drugs when administered twice daily at their optimum doses.[43] The study population comprised of 747 patients between the ages of 6 and 65 years who were considered by their physicians to be candidates for continuous treatment, and had FEV_1 greater than 50% of the predicted value prior to treatment randomisation, with at least 15% reversibility in response to an inhaled β_2-agonist. Both treatments promptly reduced symptoms, levels of absence from work or school and the requirement for emergency treatment. In terms of pulmonary function, both had similar beneficial effects on PEF and FEV_1. There was no evidence in support of the investigators' hypothesis that theophylline would have a faster onset of action. Theophylline was not found to be superior to beclometasone in any measures of efficacy. Beclometasone, in contrast, was significantly more effective at certain time points in terms of symptom control, supplemental bronchodilator and systemic corticosteroid use,

There was no evidence that theophylline had a faster onset of action than beclometasone.

methacholine sensitivity (which is an indicator of bronchial hyperreactivity and inflammation), physician's global assessment and eosinophil count. More of the patients receiving theophylline reported headaches and other adverse events associated with the central nervous system, along with gastrointestinal problems. The beclometasone group, in contrast, reported more oropharyngeal candidiasis, voice disturbance, hoarseness and pharyngitis. The incidence of upper respiratory tract infections was similar in the two groups.

Beclometasone and theophylline have also been compared in a trial focusing on childhood asthma. Although theophylline was recommended as a maintenance therapy for adults and children for many years, this is no longer the case as there is increasing concern over its side-effect profile, particularly in children. A randomised, double-blind, placebo-controlled trial investigated the use of beclometasone and theophylline in 195 patients, with mild-to-moderate asthma, aged between 6 and 16 years.[44] The dose of beclometasone was set at 84 μg four-times daily, whereas theophylline was administered at a dose established by the physician to offer optimal clinical asthma control with minimal side-effects. The target theophylline blood level was 8–15 μg/mL, 12 hours after dose administration. The two drugs demonstrated comparable symptom control, but beclometasone was associated with less use of rescue bronchodilator therapy and systemic steroids. There was no significant difference between the two groups in FEV_1, response to methacholine challenge, medical consultations for asthma or global evaluation by the physician. As in the previous study, there was no evidence that theophylline exerted a therapeutic effect more rapidly that beclometasone. Adverse events were more common in the theophylline group. The only major concern in terms of the safety of beclometasone in this patient group was its effect on growth. Although there was no significant difference between measurements of absolute height in the two treatment groups, beclometasone therapy was reported to reduce growth velocity. The effect appeared to be biased towards boys, though there was insufficient evidence to conclude that only males are subject to retarded growth velocity in response to beclometasone. The investigators concluded that in terms of disease control, there is a clear preference for beclometasone over theophylline. The concern over the effect on growth rate, however, may prove to be an important global consideration for the use of inhaled corticosteroids in children.

Adverse events were more common in the theophylline than the beclometasone group.

Beclometasone *vs* salmeterol

Although the long-acting β_2-agonist salmeterol is not advised to be used in place of a corticosteroid, it has been compared with beclometasone in a placebo-controlled study of 241 children with asthma.[4,45] This 12-month study reported that beclometasone significantly reduced airway responsiveness (assessed by sensitivity to methacholine challenge) relative to placebo or salmeterol, which had similar effects on this parameter. Both drugs generated similar benefits over placebo in most parameters of pulmonary function (i.e. FEV_1, $FEF_{25\%-75\%}$, $FEF_{25\%}$,

$FEF_{50\%}$, $FEF_{75\%}$ and PEF), though neither afforded significant benefits with regard to FVC. Treatment with beclometasone, 200 µg twice daily, was superior to salmeterol, 50 µg twice daily, in controlling asthma symptoms (the percentage of days and nights when β-agonist use was not required was significantly lower than placebo in the beclometasone group [$p<0.001$] but not in the salmeterol group) and reducing the eosinophil count ($p<0.001$ *vs* salmeterol). The adverse event profile was similar in both treatment groups, though height increase over the course of 12 months was significantly less in the beclometasone-treated children than those receiving salmeterol ($p=0.004$) or placebo ($p=0.018$).

Efficacy in exercise-induced asthma

In most cases, exercise-induced exacerbations of asthma indicate that the underlying disease is poorly controlled. Hence, inhaled corticosteroids are recommended for regular use in order to provide protection against exercise-induced asthma.[46] Indeed, HFA–beclometasone has been shown to reduce exercise-induced bronchoconstriction and exhaled nitric oxide (an expression of airway inflammation) in children with exercise-induced asthma.[47] Nonetheless, exercise may prove a particular problem in patients whose asthma is otherwise well-controlled by corticosteroids. In this case, supplementary use of other treatments such as long-acting β_2-agonists or leukotriene receptor antagonists is advised.[46]

Efficacy in clinical practice

The efficacy and safety of beclometasone in the clinical practice setting has been well established for some time. However, more experience is required on the potential implications of the impending phasing out of CFC-dependent inhaler devices. Structured evaluations of the efficacy and safety in clinical practice can be made using open-label studies, which may be of considerable duration as the ethical constraints of using a placebo group are lifted. Open-label trials generate more clinically relevant data than blinded trials, as patient awareness of treatment identity may contribute to compliance and perception of efficacy. Indeed, it is reported that the open-label transition from CFC–beclometasone to a non-CFC containing inhaled corticosteroid preparation causes an increase in practice-initiated healthcare utilisation by patients, and this is not due to any reduction in asthma control.[48]

One open-label study has compared the long-term efficacy and safety of switching patients who were stable on CFC–beclometasone (400–1600 µg/day) to half the dose of HFA–beclometasone (both delivered via a pressurised MDI), over a period of 12 months.[49] Symptomatic control was maintained, along with a comparable safety profile, in those who switched to HFA–beclometasone compared with those who were maintained on CFC-based therapy. The only indications of clinical superiority were slightly significant differences in favour of the HFA–beclometasone formulation in terms of the percentage of days without cough ($p=0.018$) and the proportion of nights without sleep disturbance (p=0.026) at certain time points within the study. Although CFC–beclometasone treatment was associated with greater mean morning plasma cortisol levels at month 2 (p=0.037), there was no significant difference by the end of the study. The number of patients instructed to start using a spacer due to severe dysphonia or oropharyngeal candidiasis was greater in the CFC–beclometasone group (7.6%) than in the HFA-beclometasone group (4.2%). It is noteworthy that 2% of patients who were switched to HFA–beclometasone reported adversely on the taste of the new inhaler. Pre-warning patients of the likelihood of this should smooth the transition between formulations.

A shorter open-label study also investigated the effects of switching to HFA–beclometasone, but patients in this case were being treated with any one of four inhaled corticosteroids prior to enrolment into this study (CFC–beclometasone, ≤2000 μg/day; budesonide ≤1600 μg/day; fluticasone ≤1000 μg/day; flunisolide ≤2000 μg/day).[50] All 716 adult participants were switched to HFA–beclometasone 800 μg/day, administered via an MDI or breath-actuated inhalation device for a total of 24 weeks. Pulmonary function was maintained at an equivalent level on switching from the higher doses of inhaled corticosteroids to HFA–beclometasone. The proportion of symptom-free days increased significantly relative to all previous treatments as did the proportion of symptom-free nights in all but those previously maintained on flunisolide. There was also a moderate reduction in the extent of rescue β-agonist use in all but those previously taking fluticasone. Prior to the study, quality of life was described as good or very good in 68.5% of study participants. This proportion increased to 81.3% following 24 weeks of treatment with HFA–beclometasone. Adverse events were generally low-to-moderate in severity, and caused 4.3% of participants to withdraw, with a similar distribution between all pre-treatment groups.

A further open-label study has focused specifically on the impact upon quality of life of switching from CFC–beclometasone to HFA–beclometasone treatment, arguing that this is a more clinically relevant parameter than tests of pulmonary function.[51] This 12-month study of 473 patients, who were maintained on CFC–beclometasone (400–1600 μg/day), was carried out across four countries. Patients were randomised to receive HFA–beclometasone, 200–800 μg/day, or to persist with their existing treatment. At every time point, both treatment groups demonstrated improved quality of life from baseline, as assessed by the AQLQ. At the 12-month study endpoint, the improvement over baseline was significantly greater for patients receiving HFA–beclometasone than CFC–beclometasone (p=0.019; Figure 4). The mean improvement during the entire course of the study was greater for HFA–beclometasone than CFC–beclometasone, though the difference did not reach statistical significance. Pulmonary function was also similar between the two groups. The investigators concluded that patients switched from a standard dose of CFC–beclometasone to approximately half the dose of HFA–beclometasone may experience significant improvements in quality of life even in the absence of significant changes to pulmonary function.

Patients switched from a standard dose of CFC-beclometasone to approximately half the dose of HFA-beclometasone may experience significant improvements to quality of life.

Figure 4. Mean change from baseline in overall Asthma Quality of Life Questionnaire (AQLQ) scores in patients treated with beclometasone formulated with either a hydrofluoroalkane (HFA) or chlorofluorocarbon (CFC) propellant.[51]

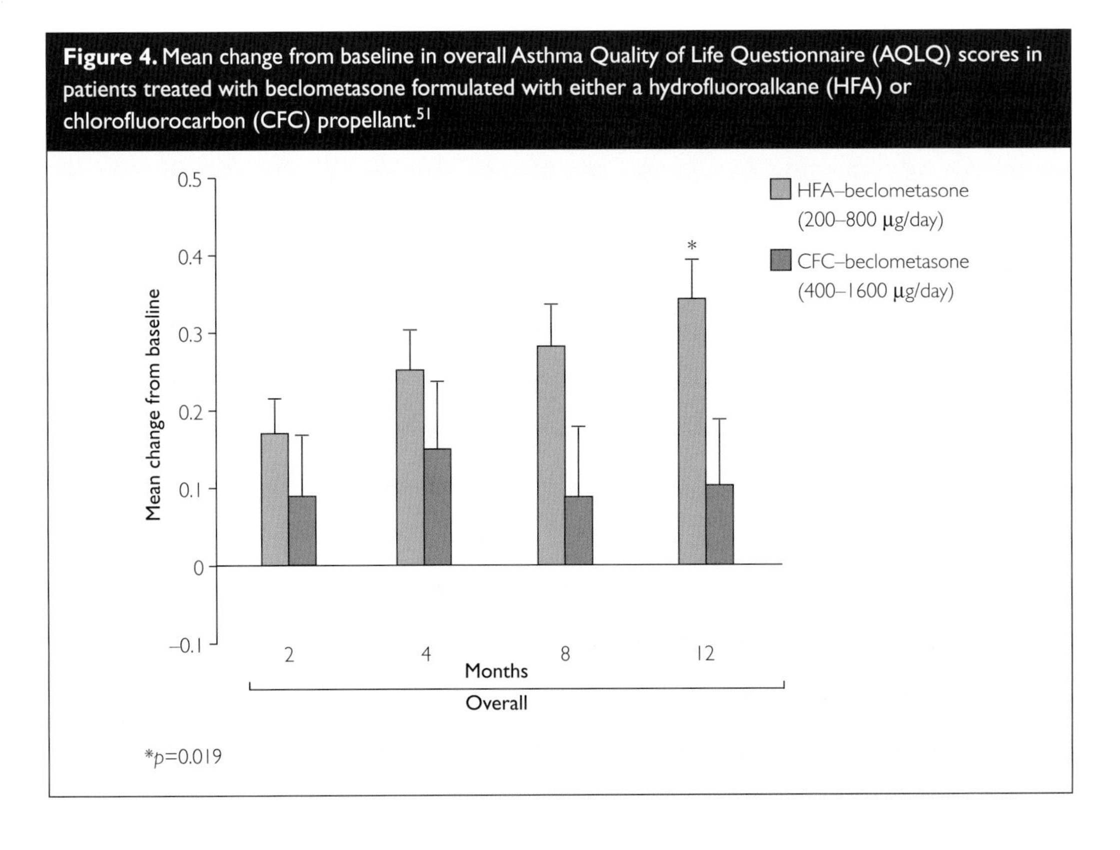

An open-label evaluation of the effects of switching from CFC–beclometasone to HFA–beclometasone therapy in children has been carried out over a period of 12 months.[52,53] This trial recruited 520 patients, aged between the ages of 5 and 11 years, whose asthma was well controlled with either CFC–beclometasone or budesonide at a dose of 200–800 μg/day. During the 4-week run-in period, all participants were treated with CFC–beclometasone (200–400 μg/day), administered via an MDI with a spacer, and then randomised to maintain this treatment or switch to half the dose of HFA–beclometasone, administered via a breath-actuated inhaler. In the first 6 months, the only significant difference between the two treatment groups was a greater morning PEF in the HFA–beclometasone group during weeks 7–8 (p=0.014). Other measures of pulmonary function, the incidence of asthma exacerbations and adverse events, and treatment compliance were comparable between the two groups. The clinical equivalence of the two treatment strategies was maintained throughout the 6-month study extension which followed.[53] Furthermore, there were no clinically meaningful differences between the groups in terms of growth or other systemic effects. Neither were there any significant differences between biochemical markers of bone formation and resorption. Although the study was not designed to detect dose–response relationships, the investigators commented that those patients on higher doses of both drugs experienced larger impairments in growth velocity. On comparison between the first and last 6 months of the trial, the investigators reported that growth velocity was significantly greater in the CFC group than the HFA group over the first 6 months, but that there was no significant difference in the second half of the trial. Furthermore, the mean change from baseline in height at the end of the study was not significantly different between the two groups at the study endpoint.

The use of HFA–beclometasone in clinical practice has also been assessed in an open-label study in comparison to the HFA–formulation of fluticasone.[54] This 8-week study evaluated the use of HFA–beclometasone, 800 µg/day, and HFA–fluticasone, 1000 µg/day, in 198 patients. Statistically equivalent improvements were observed in the two groups in terms of pulmonary function, β-agonist use, asthma symptom scores, sleep disturbance scores, percentage of days without asthma symptoms and percentage of days without sleep disturbance. HFA–beclometasone was superior in reducing mean eosinophil count and eosinophil cationic protein value, which is thought to reflect eosinophilic airway inflammation and asthma activity ($p<0.01$ for both at study endpoint). Adverse event profiles, as well as levels of treatment compliance and withdrawal, were similar in the two groups. The investigators concluded that HFA–beclometasone was at least as effective as a higher dose of HFA–fluticasone. This represents a shift in superiority from that reported with the CFC-based formulations of these two drugs.[32,33] Hence, beclometasone may prove to be a preferable choice of therapy amongst the new generation of non CFC-based inhaled corticosteroids.

HFA-beclometasone was at least as effective as a higher dose of HFA-fluticasone.

Safety and tolerability

In order to minimise the systemic side effect profile associated with corticosteroid therapy, it is important to achieve a wide margin between local activity on the lung surface and systemic activity.[33] It is superiority in this ratio which underlies the improved tolerability of inhaled over oral corticosteroid therapy.[8] Inhaled beclometasone has been consistently well tolerated in clinical trials, with the most commonly reported side-effects being headache, nausea and pharyngitis. Oral candidiasis is a recognised side-effect of beclometasone, the risk being directly associated with the extent of oral deposition. It might be expected that the HFA formulation of beclometasone, which demonstrates a much lower level of oral deposition than the CFC formulation due to the reduced particle size (see Figure 2), will be associated with a lower incidence of oral candidiasis.

There is no consistent evidence that inhaled beclometasone suppresses the hypothalamic–pituitary–adrenal axis, which is responsible for the generation of cortisol. Indeed, a double-strength MDI formulation of beclometasone had no significant impact on the response to cosyntropin.[55] This is a commonly used method to determine the capacity of the adrenal glands to respond to stimulation and to assess the functional reserve of the adrenal cortex.

Trials of the efficacy and safety of beclometasone in children have indicated that it may be responsible for retarding growth velocity.[44] A similar effect on growth has been observed with budesonide, and is suggested to be mediated by a reduction in insulin-like growth factors.[44,56] The effect of beclometasone on growth was further evaluated in the context of a comparative trial with fluticasone.[57] This 52-week trial of 343 children requiring regular inhaled corticosteroid therapy compared the effects of equal doses of beclometasone and fluticasone (200 μg, twice daily) on efficacy and safety, including growth velocity. The influence of the pubertal growth spurt in these patients was overcome by excluding all patients with a sexual maturity rating greater than Tanner stage 1 from the growth velocity analysis. Fluticasone was reported to be superior in terms of improving lung function, which was expected given the equal doses and recognised greater potency of fluticasone. Both drugs were well tolerated and had minimal effects on cortisol levels, but the adjusted mean growth velocity was significantly greater in fluticasone- than beclometasone-treated patients (Figure 5). Patients receiving beclometasone treatment were more likely to fall under a given growth percentile than those receiving fluticasone.

Longer-term data indicate that the impact of beclometasone on growth is most profound in the first year of treatment.[58] Further long-term studies of beclometasone and other inhaled corticosteroids are required to determine whether patients undergo a 'catch up' or whether their final absolute height is also impaired. The relationship between growth velocity and final height attainment in children is not well understood, and retardation of growth velocity by inhaled

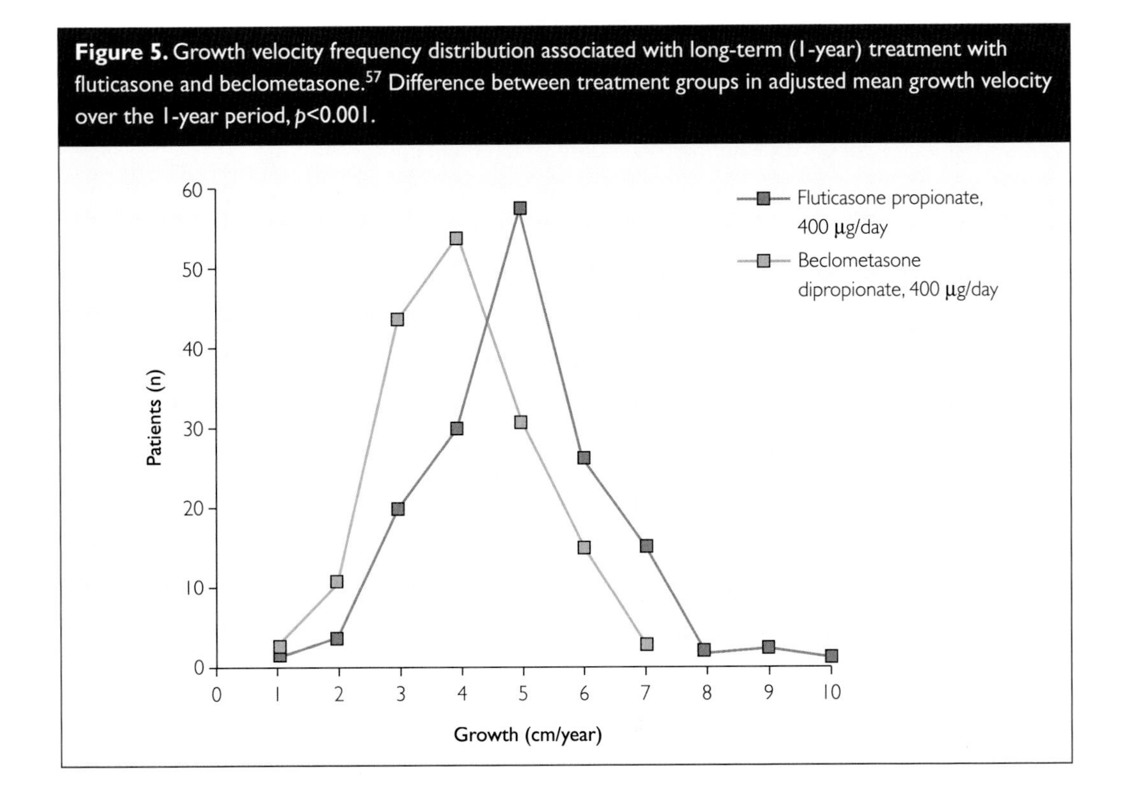

Figure 5. Growth velocity frequency distribution associated with long-term (1-year) treatment with fluticasone and beclometasone.[57] Difference between treatment groups in adjusted mean growth velocity over the 1-year period, $p<0.001$.

corticosteroids may prove to have no lasting impact on final height.[53] Studies of the effects of corticosteroid treatment on growth in asthmatic children are confounded by the fact that children with moderate-to-severe asthma generally show slower growth velocity and a later onset of puberty, regardless of treatment, whilst the use of placebo groups in long-term trials is subject to ethical constraints. Nevertheless, assessments of growth velocity will be a vital component in safety trials of new CFC-free inhaled corticosteroid formulations. Studies in adults have indicated that HFA–beclometasone is less systemically active than CFC–beclometasone, and as such the new formulation may have less impact on growth velocity.[59]

Another important patient population to consider is that of pregnant women. Asthma is probably the most common potentially serious medical complication occurring during pregnancy, with a prevalence in the US of approximately 6%.[60] Endocrinological and immunological changes that occur during pregnancy might be expected to alter a drug's efficacy and its pharmacokinetics. For example, it has been suggested that pregnancy may render tissues less responsive to corticosteroids. Hence, it is important to evaluate the use of beclometasone in this patient population. This has been done in the context of a comparative trial with oral theophylline, in female patients with a viable singleton pregnancy (less than 26 weeks gestational age with no major anomalies) and moderate asthma.[61] The data were found to be consistent with findings in non-pregnant patients, with beclometasone eliciting comparable symptomatic benefits, but fewer side-effects, than theophylline. There were no significant differences in maternal or perinatal outcomes between the two drugs. Given the benefits of beclometasone in terms of its superior adverse event profile, the investigators concluded that inhaled corticosteroids should be the maintenance therapy of choice for asthma during pregnancy.

Inhaled corticosteroids should be the maintenance therapy of choice for asthma during pregnancy.

Pharmacoeconomics

Asthma is recognised as one of the most costly conditions for the public health budget of many countries, and its incidence continues to rise.[33] Pharmacoeconomic assessments are complicated by the choice of drugs available, the choice of device and the variability in patient adherence, which is notoriously poor for inhaled corticosteroids.[39,40]

The impending phasing out of CFC-powered devices will also impact considerably upon the pharmacoeconomics of asthma therapy. Data from a 12-month open-label trial have been used in an attempt to estimate the cost implications of this change in the UK. A pragmatic trial such as this enables a reasonably accurate model of the true health economic impact of this shift in strategy.[49,62,63] Information was available from 473 patients over the age of 12 years, treated with CFC–beclometasone (400–1600 μg/day) or half the dose of HFA–beclometasone. The total healthcare costs per patient were shown to be very similar; the average cost of a symptom-free day was estimated to be £1.36 for HFA–beclometasone and £1.81 for CFC–beclometasone treatment. Approximately two-thirds of the total costs were accounted

The average cost of a symptom-free day was estimated to be £1.36 for HFA-beclometasone and £1.81 for CFC-beclometasone treatment.

for by drug acquisition costs. There was a clearer discrepancy between HFA–beclometasone and CFC–beclometasone when considering the cost of improving health-related quality of life over the study period (£13.24 and £29.38 per improved patient per week, respectively). In the majority of cases, HFA–beclometasone affords more effective asthma control at a similar cost to the CFC formulation.

Key points

- Beclometasone was the first inhaled corticosteroid to be licensed in the UK, and is now available in the UK in a CFC-free formulation, in line with international recommendations.
- Preclinical data indicate lower potency of beclometasone than other inhaled corticosteroids in terms of receptor binding. However, one of the primary metabolites has considerably greater receptor affinity and may contribute to the overall clinical efficacy of beclometasone.
- A wealth of data from placebo-controlled, comparative and open-label trials demonstrate that the HFA formulation of beclometasone is as effective as twice the dose of the CFC formulation, with a similar safety profile.
- The efficacy of the drug depends on the choice of administration device. Beclometasone is equally effective whether administered by an MDI or a DPI, but twice the dose is required for equivalent benefits when a nebuliser is used.
- When compared with other inhaled corticosteroids, beclometasone is comparable in efficacy to one-third the dose of mometasone furoate, one-half the dose of fluticasone propionate, and a slightly higher dose of budesonide.
- When compared with other anti-asthma treatments, beclometasone demonstrates comparable efficacy to theophylline at its optimum dose, though with fewer side-effects. It is at least as effective as one-quarter the dose of salmeterol, but data are inconclusive in terms of whether it is superior to montelukast (10 mg daily).
- Reformulation of other inhaled corticosteroids may alter the comparative data. In the reverse of the relationship between the CFC formulations, HFA–beclometasone is at least as effective as a slightly higher dose of HFA–fluticasone.
- HFA–beclometasone demonstrates good overall tolerability, and the adverse event profile is similar to that seen with double the dose of the CFC formulation.
- The major safety concern with beclometasone is relevant to its use in children. Beclometasone is reported to reduce growth velocity, particularly in boys. It is unclear, however, whether this treatment has any impact on final height attainment.
- It is likely that the phasing in of the HFA formulation will be associated with an overall reduction in treatment costs, as a lower dose is required to generate equivalent benefits to CFC–beclometasone.

References

A list of the published evidence which has been reviewed in compiling the preceding section of *BESTMEDICINE.*

1 D'Souza S. The Montreal Protocol and essential use exemptions. *J Aerosol Med* 1995; **8(Suppl 1)**: S13–17.

2 Price D, Valovirta E, Fischer J. The importance of preserving choice in inhalation therapy: the CFC transition and beyond. *Journal of Drug Assessment* 2004; 7: 45–61.

3 Bousquet J, Cantini L. Clinical studies in asthmatics with a new non-extra fine HFA formulation of beclometasone dipropionate (BDP Modulite). *Respir Med* 2002; **96(Suppl D)**: S17–27.

4 *British National Formulary (BNF) 48*. London: British Medical Association and Royal Pharmaceutical Society of Great Britain. September, 2004.

5 Boobis AR. Comparative physicochemical and pharmacokinetic profiles of inhaled beclomethasone dipropionate and budesonide. *Respir Med* 1998; **92(Suppl B)**: 2–6.

6 Taylor IK, Shaw RJ. The mechanism of action of corticosteroids in asthma. *Respir Med* 1993; **87**: 261–77.

7 Barnes PJ. Molecular mechanisms of corticosteroids in allergic diseases. *Allergy* 2001; **56**: 928–36.

8 Jackson LD, Polygenis D, McIvor RA, Worthington I. Comparative efficacy and safety of inhaled corticosteroids in asthma. *Can J Clin Pharmacol* 1999; **6**: 26–37.

9 Mondino C, Ciabattoni G, Koch P *et al.* Effects of inhaled corticosteroids on exhaled leukotrienes and prostanoids in asthmatic children. *J Allergy Clin Immunol* 2004; **114**: 761–7.

10 Colice GL. Comparing inhaled corticosteroids. *Respir Care* 2000; **45**: 846–53.

11 Seeto C, Namkung-Matthai H, Jayrams S *et al.* Differential potency of beclomethasone esters in-vitro on human T-lymphocyte cytokine production and osteoblast activity. *J Pharm Pharmacol* 2000; **52**: 417–23.

12 Shaw RJ. Inhaled corticosteroids for adult asthma: impact of formulation and delivery device on relative pharmacokinetics, efficacy and safety. *Respir Med* 1999; **93**: 149–60.

13 Rohatagi S, Appajosyula S, Derendorf H *et al.* Risk-benefit value of inhaled glucocorticoids: a pharmacokinetic/pharmacodynamic perspective. *J Clin Pharmacol* 2004; **44**: 37–47.

14 Electronic Medicines Compendium. *www.medicines.org.uk*

15 Devadason SG, Huang T, Walker S, Troedson R, Le Souef PN. Distribution of technetium-99m-labelled QVAR delivered using an Autohaler device in children. *Eur Respir J* 2003; **21**: 1007–11.

16 Leach CL. Improved delivery of inhaled steroids to the large and small airways. *Respir Med* 1998; **92(Suppl A)**: 3–8.

17 PDR Drug Information.

18 Brogden RN, Heel RC, Speight TM, Avery GS. Beclomethasone dipropionate. A reappraisal of its pharmacodynamic properties and therapeutic efficacy after a decade of use in asthma and rhinitis. *Drugs* 1984; **28**: 99–126.

19 Nathan RA, Nolop KB, Cuss FM, Lorber RR. A comparison of double-strength beclomethasone dipropionate (84 microg) MDI with beclomethasone dipropionate (42 microg) MDI in the treatment of asthma. *Chest* 1997; **112**: 34–9.

20 Nayak A, Lanier R, Weinstein S, Stampone P, Welch M. Efficacy and safety of beclomethasone dipropionate extrafine aerosol in childhood asthma: a 12-week, randomized, double-blind, placebo-controlled study. *Chest* 2002; **122**: 1956–65.

21 Hampel F, Lisberg E, Guerin JC. Effectiveness of low doses (50 and 100 microg b.i.d) of beclomethasone dipropionate delivered as a CFC-free extrafine aerosol in adults with mild to moderate asthma. Study Group. *J Asthma* 2000; **37**: 389–98.

22 Stradling JR, Pearson MG, Morice AH, Peake MD, Barnes NC. Efficacy and safety of a novel beclomethasone dipropionate dry powder inhaler (Clickhaler) for the treatment of adult asthma. Amsterdam Clinical Study Group. *J Asthma* 2000; **37**: 183–90.

23 Grzelewska-Rzymowska I, Kroczynska-Bednarek J, Zarkovic J. Comparison of the efficacy and safety of high doses of beclometasone dipropionate suspension for nebulization and beclometasone dipropionate via a metered-dose inhaler in steroid-dependent adults with moderate to severe asthma. *Respir Med* 2003; **97(Suppl B)**: S21–6.

24 Bisca N, Cernatescu I, Dragomir D *et al.* Comparison of the efficacy and safety of beclometasone dipropionate suspension for nebulization and beclometasone dipropionate via a metered-dose inhaler in paediatric patients with moderate to severe exacerbation of asthma. *Respir Med* 2003; **97(Suppl B)**: S15–20.

25 Price D, Thomas M, Mitchell G, Niziol C, Featherstone R. Improvement of asthma control with a breath-actuated pressurised metred dose inhaler (BAI): a prescribing claims study of 5556 patients using a traditional pressurised metred dose inhaler (MDI) or a breath-actuated device. *Respir Med* 2003; **97**: 12–19.

26 Hawkins G, McMahon AD, Twaddle S *et al.* Stepping down inhaled corticosteroids in asthma: randomised controlled trial. *BMJ* 2003; **326**: 1115.

27 Busse WW, Brazinsky S, Jacobson K *et al.* Efficacy response of inhaled beclomethasone dipropionate in asthma is proportional to dose and is improved by formulation with a new propellant. *J Allergy Clin Immunol* 1999; **104**: 1215–22.

28 Boulet LP, Cartier A, Ernst P, Larivee P, Laviolette M. Safety and efficacy of HFA-134a beclomethasone dipropionate extra-fine aerosol over six months. *Can Respir J* 2004; **11**: 123–30.

29 Juniper EF, Buist AS. Health-related quality of life in moderate asthma: 400 microg hydrofluoroalkane beclomethasone dipropionate *vs* 800 microg chlorofluorocarbon beclomethasone dipropionate. The Study Group. *Chest* 1999; **116**: 1297–303.

30 Nathan RA, Nayak AS, Graft DF *et al.* Mometasone furoate: efficacy and safety in moderate asthma compared with beclomethasone dipropionate. *Ann Allergy Asthma Immunol* 2001; **86**: 203–10.

31 Chervinsky P, Nelson HS, Bernstein DI, Berkowitz RA, Siegel SC. Comparison of mometasone furoate administered by metered dose inhaler with beclomethasone dipropionate. *Int J Clin Pract* 2002; **56**: 419–25.

32 Terzano C, Ricci A, Burinschi V, Nekam K, Lahovsky J. Comparison of the efficacy of beclometasone dipropionate and fluticasone propionate suspensions for nebulization in adult patients with persistent asthma. *Respir Med* 2003; **97(Suppl B)**: S35–40.

33 Gustafsson P, Tsanakas J, Gold M *et al.* Comparison of the efficacy and safety of inhaled fluticasone propionate 200 micrograms/day with inhaled beclomethasone dipropionate 400 micrograms/day in mild and moderate asthma. *Arch Dis Child* 1993; **69**: 206–11.

34 Terzano C, Allegra L, Barkai L, Cremonesi G. Beclomethasone dipropionate versus budesonide inhalation suspension in children with mild to moderate persistent asthma. *Eur Rev Med Pharmacol Sci* 2001; **5**: 17–24.

35 Baumgartner RA, Martinez G, Edelman JM *et al.* Distribution of therapeutic response in asthma control between oral montelukast and inhaled beclomethasone. *Eur Respir J* 2003; **21**: 123–8.

36 Israel E, Chervinsky PS, Friedman B *et al.* Effects of montelukast and beclomethasone on airway function and asthma control. *J Allergy Clin Immunol* 2002; **110**: 847–54.

37 Malmstrom K, Rodriguez-Gomez G, Guerra J *et al.* Oral montelukast, inhaled beclomethasone, and placebo for chronic asthma. A randomized, controlled trial. Montelukast/ Beclomethasone Study Group. *Ann Intern Med* 1999; **130**: 487–95.

38 Laviolette M, Malmstrom K, Lu S *et al.* Montelukast added to inhaled beclomethasone in treatment of asthma. Montelukast/Beclomethasone Additivity Group. *Am J Respir Crit Care Med* 1999; **160**: 1862–8.

39 Carter ER, Ananthakrishnan M. Adherence to montelukast versus inhaled corticosteroids in children with asthma. *Pediatr Pulmonol* 2003; **36**: 301–4.

40 Maspero JF, Duenas-Meza E, Volovitz B *et al.* Oral montelukast versus inhaled beclomethasone in 6- to 11-year-old children with asthma: results of an open-label extension study evaluating long-term safety, satisfaction, and adherence with therapy. *Curr Med Res Opin* 2001; **17**: 96–104.

41 Williams B, Noonan G, Reiss TF *et al.* Long-term asthma control with oral montelukast and inhaled beclomethasone for adults and children 6 years and older. *Clin Exp Allergy* 2001; **31**: 845–54.

42 The NHS Health Technology Assessment Programme.

43 Reed CE, Offord KP, Nelson HS, Li JT, Tinkelman DG. Aerosol beclomethasone dipropionate spray compared with theophylline as primary treatment for chronic mild-to-moderate asthma. The American Academy of Allergy, Asthma and Immunology Beclomethasone Dipropionate-Theophylline Study Group. *J Allergy Clin Immunol* 1998; **101**: 14–23.

44 Tinkelman DG, Reed CE, Nelson HS, Offord KP. Aerosol beclomethasone dipropionate compared with theophylline as primary treatment of chronic, mild to moderately severe asthma in children. *Pediatrics* 1993; **92**: 64–77.

45 Simons FE. A comparison of beclomethasone, salmeterol, and placebo in children with asthma. Canadian Beclomethasone Dipropionate-Salmeterol Xinafoate Study Group. *N Engl J Med* 1997; **337**: 1659–65.

46 British Thoracic Society and Scottish Intercollegiate Guidelines Network. British Guideline on the Management of Asthma. 2004. *www.sign.ac.uk*

47 Petersen R, Agertoft L, Pedersen S. Treatment of exercise-induced asthma with beclomethasone dipropionate in children with asthma. *Eur Respir J* 2004; **24**: 932–7.

48 Haughney J, Roberts J, Stearn R, Lee A, Price D. Transition from CFC-BDP to non-CFC steroid increases scheduled but not unscheduled healthcare. British Thoracic Society Winter Meeting 2004. Queen Elizabeth Conference Centre, London, 2004.

49 Fireman P, Prenner BM, Vincken W *et al.* Long-term safety and efficacy of a chlorofluorocarbon-free beclomethasone dipropionate extrafine aerosol. *Ann Allergy Asthma Immunol* 2001; **86**: 557–65.

50 Ederle K. Improved control of asthma symptoms with a reduced dose of HFA-BDP extrafine aerosol: an open-label, randomised study. *Eur Rev Med Pharmacol Sci* 2003; **7**: 45–55.

51 Juniper EF, Price DB, Stampone PA *et al.* Clinically important improvements in asthma-specific quality of life, but no difference in conventional clinical indexes in patients changed from conventional beclomethasone dipropionate to approximately half the dose of extrafine beclomethasone dipropionate. *Chest* 2002; **121**: 1824–32.

52 Szefler SJ, Warner J, Staab D *et al.* Switching from conventional to extrafine aerosol beclomethasone dipropionate therapy in children: a 6-month, open-label, randomized trial. *J Allergy Clin Immunol* 2002; **110**: 45–50.

53 Pedersen S, Warner J, Wahn U *et al.* Growth, systemic safety, and efficacy during 1 year of asthma treatment with different beclomethasone dipropionate formulations: an open-label, randomized comparison of extrafine and conventional aerosols in children. *Pediatrics* 2002; **109**: e92.

54 Aubier M, Wettenger R, Gans SJ. Efficacy of HFA-beclomethasone dipropionate extra-fine aerosol (800 microg day$^{(-1)}$) versus HFA-fluticasone propionate (1000 microg day$^{(-1)}$)) in patients with asthma. *Respir Med* 2001; **95**: 212–20.

55 Brannan MD, Herron JM, Reidenberg P, Affrime MB. A systemic bioactivity comparison of double-strength and regular-strength beclomethasone dipropionate MDI formulations. *Ann Allergy Asthma Immunol* 1998; **80**: 39–44.

56 Wolthers OD, Pedersen S. Growth of asthmatic children during treatment with budesonide: a double blind trial. *BMJ* 1991; **303**: 163–5.

57 de Benedictis FM, Teper A, Green RJ *et al.* Effects of 2 inhaled corticosteroids on growth: results of a randomized controlled trial. *Arch Pediatr Adolesc Med* 2001; **155**: 1248–54.

58 Saha MT, Laippala P, Lenko HL. Growth of asthmatic children is slower during than before treatment with inhaled glucocorticoids. *Acta Paediatr* 1997; **86**: 138–42.

59 Randell TL, Donaghue KC, Ambler GR *et al.* Safety of the newer inhaled corticosteroids in childhood asthma. *Paediatr Drugs* 2003; **5**: 481–504.

60 Kwon HL, Belanger K, Bracken MB. Asthma prevalence among pregnant and childbearing-aged women in the United States: estimates from national health surveys. *Ann Epidemiol* 2003; **13**: 317–24.

61 Dombrowski MP, Schatz M, Wise R *et al.* Randomized trial of inhaled beclomethasone dipropionate versus theophylline for moderate asthma during pregnancy. *Am J Obstet Gynecol* 2004; **190**: 737–44.

62 Price D, Haughney J, Duerden M, Nicholls C, Moseley C. The cost effectiveness of chlorofluorocarbon-free beclomethasone dipropionate in the treatment of chronic asthma: a cost model based on a 1-year pragmatic, randomised clinical study. *Pharmacoeconomics* 2002; **20**: 653–64.

63 Cleland J, Thomas M, Price D. Pharmacoeconomics of asthma treatment. *Expert Opin Pharmacother* 2003; **4**: 311–18.

Acknowledgements

Figure 2 is adapted from Leach, 1998.[16]
Figure 3 is adapted from Laviolette *et al.*, 1999.[38]
Figure 4 is adapted from Juniper *et al.*, 2002.[51]
Figure 5 is adapted from de Benedictis *et al.*, 2001.[57]

3. Drug review – Budesonide (Pulmicort®)

Dr Eleanor Bull
CSF Medical Communications Ltd

Summary

Budesonide is an inhaled corticosteroid with high local anti-inflammatory activity. Compared with other reference corticosteroids (e.g. beclometasone dipropionate), budesonide demonstrates a high ratio of topical-to-systemic activity. Owing to a unique esterification process, budesonide is retained in airways tissue longer than any other inhaled corticosteroid, thus prolonging the duration of its anti-inflammatory effects. When administered via the Turbohaler® dry powder inhaler, approximately 34% of a metered dose of budesonide is deposited in the lungs. Extensive clinical trials of budesonide have demonstrated that it effectively controls mild-to-severe persistent asthma in children and adults, eliciting significant improvements in lung function (forced expiratory volume in 1 second [FEV_1] and peak expiratory flow [PEF]) and asthma symptoms, and also reduces the frequency of nocturnal awakenings and the use of β_2-adrenoceptor (β_2-agonist) rescue medication. These improvements are generally dose-dependent and budesonide is clinically effective at low doses (e.g. 200–400 μg). Budesonide reduces the need for oral corticosteroids in patients with more severe asthma. Moreover, budesonide is associated with a comparatively low incidence of clinically relevant systemic adverse events (e.g. adrenal suppression, growth retardation, metabolic disturbances). Instead, sore throat, hoarseness and an irritant cough are the most common side-effects associated with long-term treatment. As with all inhaled corticosteroids, the budesonide treatment regimen should be tailored to the individual patient, and the dose of budesonide should be maintained at the minimum effective dose necessary to maintain good asthma control.

Introduction

Inhaled corticosteroids are used as prophylactic therapy in all but the mildest cases of asthma with persistent symptoms.

Inhaled corticosteroids have played a central role in asthma therapy for the last 30 years and relieve the symptoms of asthma by reducing inflammation of the airways.[1] Their development represented a major breakthrough in asthma therapy, limiting the need for long-term systemic corticosteroids and their associated systemic side-effects, and paving the way towards routine maintenance (or preventer) therapy of asthma, rather than as-needed rescue therapy. Today, inhaled corticosteroids are used as prophylactic therapy in all but the mildest cases of asthma with persistent symptoms.

Beclometasone dipropionate was first introduced in the UK in 1972 and quickly became the standard therapy for patients with asthma inadequately controlled with bronchodilators alone. Fluticasone propionate and budesonide followed, with mometasone furoate the most recent inhaled corticosteroid to be introduced in the UK. In general, the inhaled corticosteroids have similar clinical effectiveness with regard to asthma and, therefore, their relative safety profiles are critical in differentiating between them on the basis of therapeutic margin.[2] Guidelines jointly issued by the Scottish Intercollegiate Guidelines Network (SIGN) and the British Thoracic Society (BTS) in 2004, recommend the regular use of inhaled corticosteroids (usual maintenance dose of 400 μg/day for adults and 200 μg/day for children aged 5–12 years of beclometasone dipropionate or equivalent) when an inhaled short-acting β_2-agonist alone fails to control asthma adequately.[3] According to these guidelines, the starting dosage of any inhaled corticosteroid should always be tailored to the severity of the asthma and be kept to the minimum dosage necessary for good asthma control.

Concerns regarding the safety of the regular inhalation of corticosteroids, particularly in children, have been well-documented. Adrenal suppression, bone loss, skin thinning, decreased linear growth, metabolic changes and behavioural abnormalities, have all been reported following long-term administration of corticosteroids, and pertain largely to the systemic effects of these drugs.[4] Although much controversy remains, there is no clear evidence that conventional doses of inhaled corticosteroids significantly retard bone growth in children.[4]

Ideally, an inhaled corticosteroid would exhibit high local therapeutic activity in the airways, whilst showing minimal systemic effects.

Ideally, an inhaled corticosteroid would exhibit high local therapeutic activity in the airways, whilst possessing minimal systemic effects. Prolonged lung retention, high affinity and potency for glucocorticoid receptors, low oral bioavailability, rapid clearance and systemic elimination are also desirable characteristics.[5,6]

Budesonide is a second-generation corticosteroid indicated for the prophylaxis of asthma and exercise-induced asthma.[7,8] A glucocorticosteroid with high local anti-inflammatory action, budesonide is a well-established and widely used anti-asthma drug and demonstrates many of the features of an ideal inhaled corticosteroid.[1] Budesonide can be administered once or twice daily, and its full therapeutic effect is apparent within a few days of treatment initiation. The current review discusses the pharmacological properties of budesonide and its efficacy in controlled clinical trials in adults and children with asthma. In line with other reviews of anti-asthma drugs previously published in the journal *Drugs in Context*, clinical trials of budesonide in patients with Chronic Obstructive Pulmonary Disease (COPD) are beyond the scope of the review and are not discussed herein.

Budesonide can be administered via a pressurised metered dose inhaler (pMDI) and a dry powder inhaler (DPI; Pulmicort® Turbohaler®; Novoliser®; Budesonide Cyclocaps®).[7,9] It is also available as a nebuliser suspension (Pulmicort Respules®) for use in patients for whom a pMDI or DPI is inappropriate (e.g. young children).[10] In this section, we have focused primarily on data specific to the Pulmicort Turbohaler – the most widely used budesonide delivery device available worldwide. References to the budesonide nebuliser suspension have been included where appropriate. Symbicort®, the combination of budesonide with the long-acting β_2-agonist, formoterol, is discussed in detail later in this edition of *BESTMEDICINE.*

Pharmacology

Chemistry

The chemical structure of budesonide is illustrated in Figure 1. The formulation of budesonide available for clinical use is a racemic mixture of two epimers, 22R and 22S, that do not interconvert.[11] Of these, the 22R epimer has a two-fold greater affinity for the glucocorticoid receptor than the 22S epimer and is also less water soluble, thus prolonging its retention in the lung.[11] Budesonide is non-halogenated, in contrast to many of the other inhaled corticosteroids currently available (e.g. beclometasone dipropionate), which may promote its inactivation by biotransformation and thus contribute to its high topical-to-systemic activity ratio.[5]

The chemistry of budesonide is of essentially academic interest and most healthcare professionals will, like you, skip this section.

Mechanism of action

The inhaled corticosteroids exert their effects through cytoplasmic glucocorticoid receptors. When bound together, the corticosteroid–receptor complex translocates to the cell nucleus where it

Figure 1. The chemical structure of budesonide.

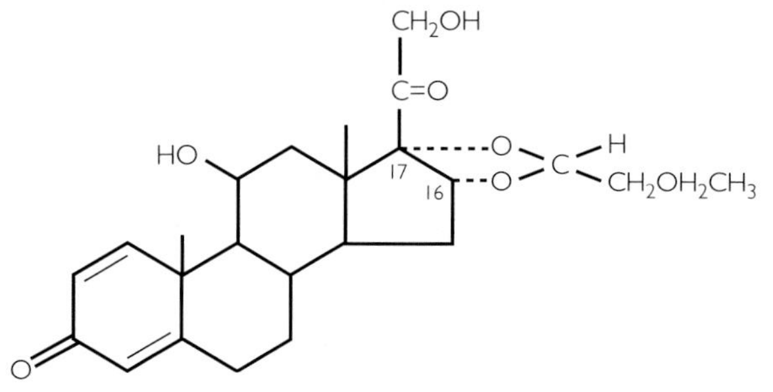

modifies the transcription of a wide range of inflammatory mediators (e.g. cytokines, histamine, eicosanoids, leukotrienes) and thereby inhibits the inflammatory component of chronic asthma.[5,6] Corticosteroids also inhibit the activation of inflammatory cells including lymphocytes, eosinophils, mast cells, neutrophils and macrophages.[5] Budesonide has also been shown to improve airway hyper-responsiveness, manifested as a reduction in airway reactivity to histamine and methacholine in susceptible patients.[7]

Budesonide undergoes esterification, primarily in the lungs and bronchial cells, a process that ultimately sustains its local anti-inflammatory activity and improves its airway selectivity.

Esterification

The prolonged exposure of a corticosteroid to the glucocorticoid receptors in the airways will increase its anti-inflammatory effects. Although budesonide demonstrates a slightly lower affinity for glucocorticoid receptors than fluticasone propionate or mometasone furoate, it is retained in airways tissue to a greater extent.[1,5] This is due to the fact that budesonide undergoes esterification, primarily in the lungs and bronchial cells, a process that ultimately sustains its local anti-inflammatory activity and improves its airway selectivity.[12] Following administration and passage into the lungs, excess budesonide is esterified to budesonide oleate in a rapid, reversible process to form an essentially inactive intracellular ester pool (Figure 2).[13] As the intracellular concentration of budesonide decreases, the esterified budesonide is hydrolysed and active budesonide is released from the depot in a continuous manner, thus prolonging its duration of effect (Figure 2).[13]

Figure 2. The reversible process of budesonide esterification in the airways.[13]

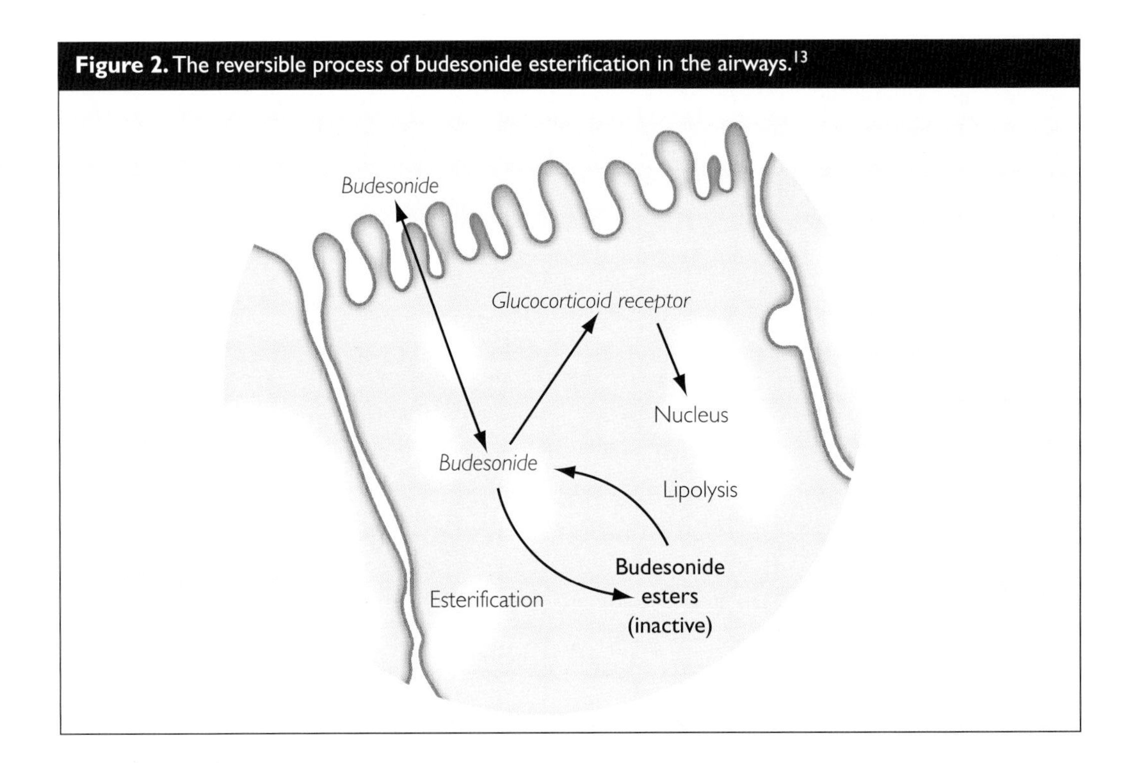

Testament to the rapidity of this process, experiments performed in rats showed that 80% of radiolabelled budesonide located within the trachea and main bronchi was associated with budesonide esters within 20 minutes of inhalation.[14]

Pharmacokinetics

The pharmacokinetic properties of budesonide are shown in Table 1.[5,7,11,15] Following inhalation, budesonide is rapidly and extensively absorbed through the lung, though there is considerable inter-individual variability in the degree of lung absorption.[11] Budesonide reaches the systemic circulation either through the lungs or via gastrointestinal absorption of the small amount of drug that is inadvertently swallowed. Ninety per cent of budesonide undergoes biotransformation in the liver.[7] The major metabolites of budesonide – 6β-hydroxybudesonide and 16α-hydroxyprednisolone – are relatively inactive, demonstrating less than 1% of the anti-inflammatory activity of budesonide. The metabolism of budesonide is primarily mediated by cytochrome P450 (CYP) 3A4.[7]

The pharmacokinetics of a drug are of interest to healthcare professionals because it is important for them to understand the action of a drug on the body over a period of time.

Budesonide has a relatively short systemic half-life and a low volume of distribution, which suggests that it may be associated with fewer systemic adverse events than other inhaled corticosteroids (e.g. fluticasone propionate and mometasone furoate).[1] Budesonide's high rate of clearance and linear pharmacokinetics further enhance its tolerability profile.[1]

Table 1. The pharmacokinetic properties of budesonide.[5,7,11,15]

Pharmacokinetic parameter	
Inhalation bioavailability (%)	28
Oral bioavailability (%)	11
Systemic bioavailability (%)	73
C_{max} (nmol/L)	3.5 (following dose of 1000 μg)
t_{max} (minutes)	15–45
Volume of distribution at steady-state (L)	183
Plasma protein binding (%)	90
First-pass inactivation of delivered dose (%)	89
Total clearance (L/hour)	84
$t_{1/2}$ (hours)	3
Excretion (%)	41 (mouth or inhaler) 32 (urine) 15 (faeces)

t_{max}, time to reach maximum drug plasma concentration (C_{max}); $t_{1/2}$, elimination half-life.

Delivery device

The mean pulmonary bioavailability for inhaled budesonide is 28% of the nominal dose (compared with 39% for fluticasone propionate), although bioavailability is greatly influenced by the efficiency of the inhaler device used.[11] Budesonide can be inhaled via a number of delivery devices, including the Turbohaler, a breath-actuated metered dose DPI, available as doses of 100, 200 and 400 μg per actuation.[7] The Turbohaler is inspiratory flow driven and follows inspired air into the airways. The deposition of budesonide is more efficient when using the Turbohaler, with 25–30% of the metered dose reaching the lungs, compared with only 15% when using a pMDI.[7,11] The dose of budesonide delivered by a nebuliser is highly dependent on the nebulising equipment used. An air flow rate of 6–8 L/minute and a fill volume of 2–4 mL are recommended.[10]

Dosage

The dose of inhaled budesonide should always be tailored to the individual patient and should be maintained at the minimum necessary dose to maintain good asthma control.

The dose of inhaled budesonide should always be tailored to the individual patient and should be maintained at the minimum necessary dose to maintain good asthma control.[7] If asthma control deteriorates, patients should be advised to contact their physician immediately.[7] When transferring from oral corticosteroids, treatment should be initiated with high-dose budesonide, given in combination with the previous dose of oral corticosteroid, for approximately 10 days, followed by the gradual reduction of the oral corticosteroid dose. In many cases, it is possible to completely substitute budesonide for the oral corticosteroid. Rarely during the transfer procedure, the lower systemic steroidal action may result in the emergence of allergic or arthritic symptoms (e.g. rhinitis, eczema, muscle and joint pain).[7]

When administering budesonide via the Turbohaler, treatment should be initiated at a starting dose of 200–1600 μg daily, given in two divided doses, with the dose selected according to the severity of asthma symptoms.[8] The daily dose recommended by SIGN and BTS, is 200–800 μg/day.[3] In less severe cases of asthma, a single daily dose of 200–400 μg, administered in the evening, should be sufficient to maintain asthma control. For children under the age of 12 years, budesonide can be administered as two divided daily doses of between 200–800 μg, or a single daily dose of 200–400 μg.[8] Again, the recommended dose, in accordance with current guidelines, is 200–400 μg/day.[3] In light of the systemic side-effects that have been associated with inhaled corticosteroids in the past (e.g. growth suppression and adrenal insufficiency), it is particularly important in children that the dose of inhaled steroid used is the lowest compatible with maintaining disease control.[3]

When budesonide is administered via nebuliser suspension, the licensed starting dose is 1000–2000 μg twice daily, or 500–1000 μg twice daily for children aged between 3 months and 12 years. The recommended maintenance dose of budesonide is 500–1000 μg twice daily in adults and for children aged over 12 years, and 250–500 μg twice daily in children younger than 12 years.[8]

Clinical efficacy

Placebo-controlled studies

The placebo-controlled studies which have evaluated the efficacy of budesonide in adults with asthma are summarised in Table 2.[16–21] In general, compared with placebo, budesonide significantly improved measures of PEF and FEV_1 in a dose-dependent manner (Figure 3), and also significantly reduced asthma symptom scores. Furthermore, the rate of premature study discontinuation generally decreased with increasing dosage of budesonide.

Compared with placebo, budesonide significantly improved measures of PEF and FEV_1 in a dose-dependent manner.

The START study was the first large-scale, long-term clinical trial to investigate the effect of early intervention with inhaled corticosteroids in patients with newly diagnosed mild persistent asthma.[22] It is also the largest placebo-controlled trial of budesonide to report to date. The patient population comprised a mixture of 7241 adults and children from 32 countries who had been diagnosed with mild persistent asthma for less than 2 years and had not previously been treated regularly with corticosteroids. Participants were randomised to receive either budesonide, 400 μg once daily administered via Turbohaler (or 200 μg for children younger than 11 years), or placebo, for 3 years, in addition to their normal asthma medication. At baseline, mean pre-bronchodilator FEV_1 values were 86.3 and 86.6% of the predicted normal for budesonide and placebo treatment groups, respectively. Over the course of this 3-year study, the rates of premature treatment discontinuation were 27.5 and 28.5% for budesonide and placebo treatment groups, respectively (*p*-value not reported). Clinical efficacy, evaluated primarily as the time to the first severe asthma-related event, was significantly prolonged by budesonide treatment ($p<0.0001$; Figure 4). The risk of a first severe asthma-related event was reduced by 44% following budesonide treatment (hazard ratio 0.56; $p<0.0001$). In addition, patients treated with budesonide experienced significantly more symptom-free days than those receiving placebo ($p<0.0001$; Figure 5). The percentage of patients requiring a course of oral corticosteroids was significantly higher for the placebo group (23 *vs* 15% for placebo and budesonide, respectively; $p<0.0001$). Compared with placebo, budesonide-treated patients exhibited significantly greater increases in post-bronchodilator FEV_1 from baseline after both 1 and 3 years of treatment (1.48 and 0.88%; $p<0.0001$ and $p=0.0005$, respectively). The corresponding increases in pre-bronchodilator FEV_1 were 2.24 and 1.71% for 1 and 3 years, respectively ($p<0.0001$ for both time-points). Although budesonide was generally well tolerated, the rate of linear growth was significantly reduced amongst children under 11 years receiving budesonide (mean difference –0.43 cm per year; $p<0.0001$). Interestingly, this study failed to highlight any benefits in terms of the effect of budesonide on airway remodelling, as evidenced by the lack of difference between post-bronchodilator FEV_1 values. The authors proposed that this lack of response may have been due to a masking of any improvement in FEV_1 by the natural resolution of asthma in children during adolescence.

The time to the first severe asthma-related event was significantly prolonged by budesonide treatment.

Table 2. Summary of placebo-controlled trials of budesonide in adult patients with mild-to-moderate asthma.[16–21]

Study and dosage regimen	Asthma severity at baseline	Main outcomes
Busse *et al.*, 1998[16] Double-blind n=473 12 weeks Budesonide, 200, 400, 800 or 1600 μg daily, or placebo	Mean FEV_1 63–66% of predicted normal Mean morning PEF 360 L/minute	• Premature treatment discontinuation due to exacerbation and worsening of asthma: 61, 20, 11, 8 and 7% for placebo, 200, 400, 800 and 1600 μg budesonide, respectively ($p<0.001$ *vs* placebo for all comparisons). • Mean change from baseline in morning PEF showed significant improvement in all budesonide treatment groups ($p<0.001$ *vs* placebo, Figure 3). • The onset of action of budesonide was noted within 1 week of initiation. • There were no differences between any treatment groups in the change in mean basal morning plasma cortisol levels over the course of the study.
McFadden *et al.*, 1999[17] Double-blind n=309 18 weeks Budesonide, 200 or 400 μg daily, for first 6 weeks, 200 μg thereafter, or placebo	Mean FEV_1 81.9% of predicted normal Mean reversibility 23%	• Total premature treatment discontinuations: 26, 15 and 10% for placebo, and budesonide, 200 and 400/200 μg groups, respectively ($p=0.005$ for 400/200 μg group *vs* placebo; $p>0.05$ for 200 μg group *vs* placebo). • Mean increases in FEV_1 were 0.10 and 0.11 L in the budesonide, 200 and 400/200 μg groups, respectively, compared with a decrease of 0.09 L in the placebo group ($p<0.001$ *vs* placebo). • Mean changes in morning PEF were 0.7, 21.0 and 22.0 L/minute for placebo, and budesonide, 200 and 200/400 μg groups, respectively ($p\leq0.01$ *vs* placebo). • Daytime asthma symptom scores improved by 21 and 34% in the budesonide, 200 and 200/400 μg groups, respectively ($p\leq0.05$ and $p\leq0.001$ *vs* placebo).
Casale *et al.*, 2003[18] (Quality of life analysis of McFadden *et al.*, 1999[17])	Mean AQLQ score 4.7	• Mean overall AQLQ scores improved significantly from baseline in both budesonide treatment groups to week 18 (0.14, 0.51 and 0.78 points for placebo, and budesonide, 200 and 400/200 μg groups, respectively; $p\leq0.001$ *vs* placebo). • The percentage of patients showing clinically important improvements (≥0.5 unit) in overall AQLQ at week 18 was 43 and 55% for budesonide, 200 and 400/200 μg, treatment groups, respectively. • There was significant correlation between the AQLQ score and measures of clinical efficacy (e.g. morning PEF, β_2-agonist use, asthma symptoms; $p\leq0.001$).

AQLQ, Asthma Quality of Life Questionnaire; FEV_1, forced expiratory volume in 1 second; PEF, peak expiratory flow.

Table 2. Continued

Study and dosage regimen	Asthma severity at baseline	Main outcomes
Kemp *et al.*, 1999[19] Double-blind n=273 12 weeks Budesonide, 200 or 400 μg twice daily or placebo	Mean FEV_1 67% of predicted normal Mean reversibility 33.9%	• Total premature drug withdrawals 20.2, 9.7 and 5.5% for placebo, and budesonide, 200 and 400 μg groups, respectively (p=0.003 for budesonide, 400 μg, *vs* placebo; p>0.05 for 200 μg group *vs* placebo). • Mean differences from placebo in morning PEF were 43.6 and 40.1 L/minute for the 200 and 400 μg budesonide groups, respectively (p<0.001 *vs* placebo). • Mean differences from placebo in FEV_1 were 0.44 and 0.50 L for the 200 and 400 μg budesonide groups, respectively (p<0.001 *vs* placebo). • Mean differences from placebo in day- and night-time asthma symptom scores were –0.33 and –0.38 (day) and –0.43 and –0.54 (night) for the 200 and 400 μg budesonide groups, respectively (p<0.001 *vs* placebo). • The onset of action (determined by morning PEF) of budesonide occurred within 2 days of treatment initiation.
Metzger *et al.*, 2002[20] Double-blind n=184 12 weeks Budesonide, 400 μg once daily, or placebo	Mean FEV_1 77.9% of predicted normal Mean reversibility 23.3%	• Mean improvement in FEV_1 from baseline was significantly greater than placebo following treatment with budesonide (p<0.001). • Mean improvements in morning and evening PEF from baseline were significantly greater following budesonide treatment than with placebo up to 4 weeks, and these persisted throughout the 12 weeks of treatment (p<0.001). • Mean day- and night-time asthma symptom scores improved from baseline by a greater extent following treatment with budesonide compared with placebo (p=0.035 and p=0.029 for day- and night-time, respectively *vs* placebo).
Hampel *et al.*, 2004[21] (Quality of life analysis of Metzger et al., 2002[20])	Mean AQLQ score 4.8	• The improvement in overall AQLQ score associated with budesonide treatment was significant at weeks 4 (0.29 *vs* –0.29) and 12 (0.38 *vs* –0.38) (p≤0.001 *vs* placebo). • Differences in AQLQ score were clinically important (≥0.5 unit) amongst budesonide-treated patients (43 *vs* 16%, for budesonide and placebo-treated patients, respectively; p-value not reported). • There was significant correlation between AQLQ score and measures of clinical efficacy (e.g. morning PEF, β_2-agonist use, asthma symptoms; p≤0.016).

AQLQ, Asthma Quality of Life Questionnaire; FEV_1, forced expiratory volume in 1 second; PEF, peak expiratory flow.

Figure 3. Mean change from baseline in morning Peak Expiratory Flow (PEF) over 12 weeks (top) and at week 12 (bottom) of treatment with budesonide (100–800 μg twice daily) or placebo.[16]

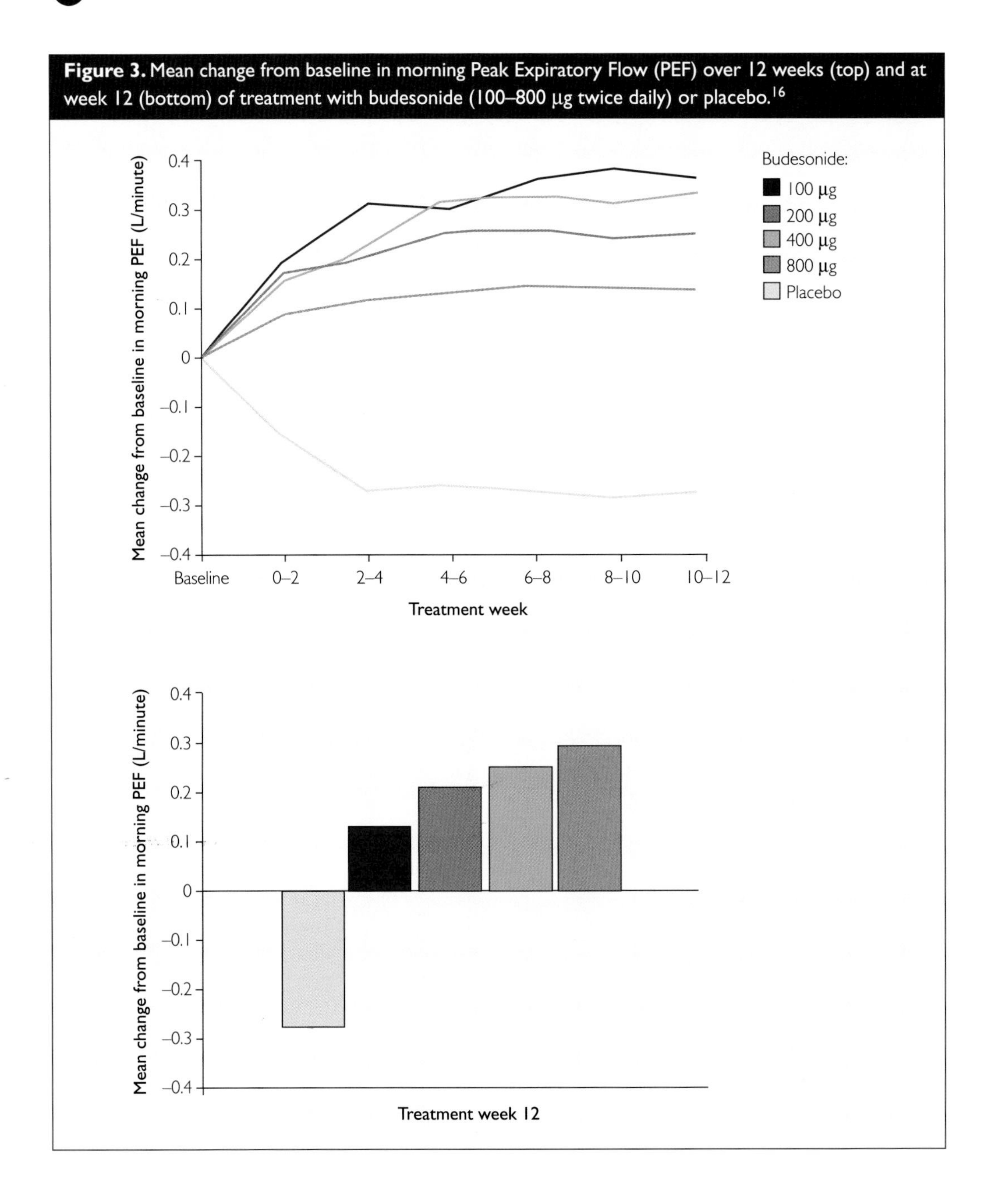

Dosage regimen

A double-blind study conducted in 682 adult patients with asthma, compared the level of asthma control achieved following a static dose of budesonide (400 μg once daily for 18 weeks) with that achieved using an initial loading dose (400 μg twice daily for 6 weeks followed by 400 μg once daily for 12 weeks).[23] At baseline, the mean PEF was 413 L/minute with greater than 15% reversibility. Following 18 weeks' treatment, mean morning PEF had improved significantly by

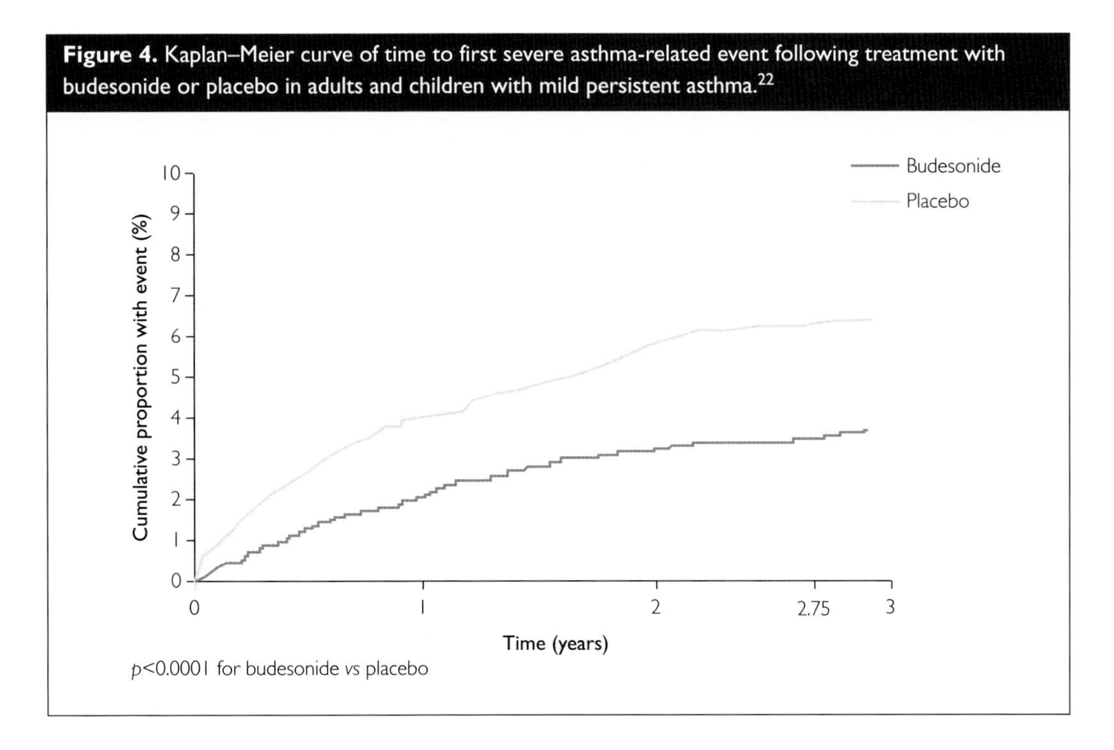

Figure 4. Kaplan–Meier curve of time to first severe asthma-related event following treatment with budesonide or placebo in adults and children with mild persistent asthma.[22]

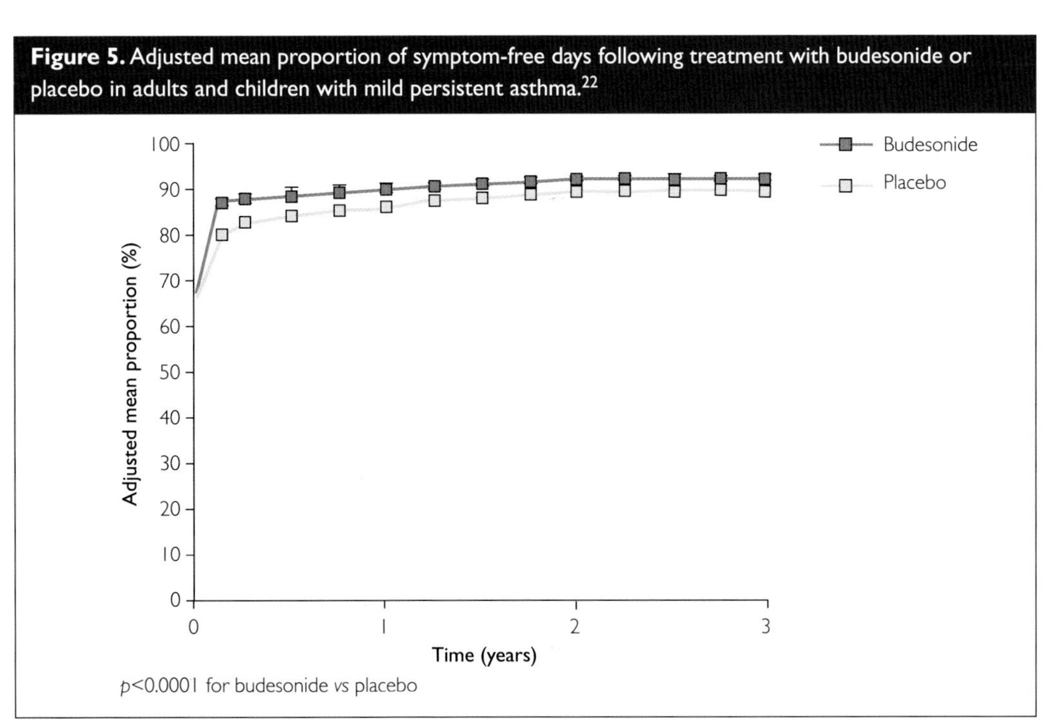

Figure 5. Adjusted mean proportion of symptom-free days following treatment with budesonide or placebo in adults and children with mild persistent asthma.[22]

45 L/minute from baseline in both budesonide treatment groups (p=0.0001 for both comparisons). The treatment-related reductions from baseline values in the mean clinic symptom scores for cough,

Improvements in both morning PEF and β_2-agonist use appeared to be more pronounced in the budesonide loading dose group after 6 weeks of treatment.

wheeze, breathlessness and chest tightness were also highly significant and comparable between the two treatment groups (cough: –0.54 *vs* –0.49; wheeze: –0.70 *vs* –0.57; breathlessness: –0.68 *vs* –0.71; chest tightness: –0.65 *vs* –0.56; all data are budesonide loading *vs* static doses, respectively; p=0.0001 *vs* baseline for all comparisons). Day- and night-time symptom scores were also reduced significantly from baseline following 18 weeks' treatment with both budesonide treatment regimens (–0.57 *vs* –0.49 for day- and –0.42 *vs* –0.45 for night-time symptoms, for loading and static doses, respectively; p=0.0001 *vs* baseline for all comparisons). Sleep disturbance was improved and the use of β_2-agonist rescue medication reduced from baseline following both budesonide treatment regimens (–1.21 *vs* –1.06 nights/week sleep disturbance; –1.36 *vs* –1.06 puffs/day of β_2-agonist for loading and static doses, respectively; p=0.0001 *vs* baseline for all comparisons). Although the overall level of asthma control did not differ according to the type of treatment regimen employed, the improvements in both morning PEF and β_2-agonist use appeared to be more pronounced in the budesonide loading dose group after 6 weeks of treatment (36.1 *vs* 26 L/minute for morning PEF and –1.10 *vs* –0.94 puffs per day of β_2-agonist for loading and static doses, respectively; $p<0.05$ *vs* static dose). Thus, this study highlights some early clinical advantages gained from employing an initial higher loading dose of budesonide.

A longer-term, double-blind study investigated the effects of two different budesonide treatment regimens over 6 months, in 213 patients with moderate asthma, who were previously treated with beclometasone dipropionate.[24] Initially, all patients received high-dose budesonide, 800 µg twice daily, for a 1-month period. Thereafter, study participants were randomised to receive one of the following treatments for 6 months: low-dose budesonide (100 µg twice daily) plus placebo in case of an exacerbation; standard-dose budesonide (400 µg twice daily) plus placebo in case of an exacerbation; low-dose budesonide (100 µg twice daily) plus 200 µg budesonide in case of an exacerbation. At study baseline, the mean FEV_1 across all treatment groups was 74.2% of the predicted normal value. The initial 1-month treatment period with high-dose budesonide markedly reduced all symptoms of asthma. Thus, the overall percentages of patients still reporting continuous wheeze, cough and shortness of breath after 1 month of treatment were 8, 10 and 7%, respectively, compared with 55, 56 and 55% at the end of the run-in period. The percentages of patients exhibiting these symptoms during the randomised treatment phase were similar in the different treatment groups ($p>0.05$). For example, the percentages of patients reporting wheeze on more than 30% of days were 1.5, 2.9 and 1.3% for standard-dose budesonide plus placebo, low-dose budesonide plus budesonide and low-dose budesonide plus placebo, respectively ($p>0.05$). Lung function, measured by the forced vital capacity (FVC), FEV_1 and PEF, improved slightly and remained stable during randomised treatment, across all treatment groups. The majority of patients in each group reported no asthma exacerbations (84, 82 and 68% for standard-dose budesonide plus placebo, low-dose budesonide plus budesonide and low-dose budesonide plus placebo, respectively; $p \leq 0.04$ *vs* low-dose budesonide plus placebo). To summarise, these data show that when patients have been stabilised following treatment initiation with high-dose budesonide, a low-dose of budesonide, with additional budesonide made available for cases of asthma exacerbations, is as effective as a standard-dose at controlling symptoms and lung function over several months.

Meta-analysis

A meta-analysis of six placebo-controlled studies of budesonide in 1435 adolescents or adults with mild-to-moderately severe asthma[16,19,25–28] investigated the relationship between budesonide dose, administered via a pMDI or Turbohaler, and the clinical response observed.[29] The dose of budesonide used in these studies ranged from 200–1600 μg/day, and at baseline, the mean FEV_1 of enrolled patients was 69% of the predicted normal value. Most of the clinical benefit associated with budesonide treatment was achieved at a dose of 200–500 μg/day, with little further improvement shown with higher doses. Using a negative exponential model, it was shown that 80% of the benefit of 1600 μg/day budesonide would have been achieved at doses of approximately 200–400 μg/day, and 90% at doses of 300–600 μg/day. The authors concluded that the majority of therapeutic benefit of budesonide when delivered either by a DPI or a pMDI, was achieved at a dose of 400 μg/day, and that a maximum effect was obtained using a dose of approximately 1000 μg/day. These data contrast with the COMPACT (Clinical Outcomes with Montelukast as a Partner Agent to Corticosteroid Therapy) study, which reported that patients who were symptomatic on doses of 800 μg/day showed further improvement, in terms of asthma control and lung function, when their dose was increased to 1600 μg/day.[30] These discrepancies may be attributable to the existence of patient subgroups that display different dose–response relationships to the 'normal' patient population. A further study in patients with moderate-to-severe asthma highlighted the benefits of an aggressive tailored anti-inflammatory treatment approach in terms of reducing the number of severe asthma exacerbations in a sub-population of severely affected patients.[31]

The majority of therapeutic benefit of budesonide was achieved at a dose of 400 μg/day and a maximum effect was obtained using a dose of approximately 1000 μg/day.

Open-label study

A large study of open-label design recruited 1133 adults and children with mild-to-severe persistent asthma from four placebo-controlled studies of budesonide, and extended the budesonide treatment period to 52 weeks.[16,19,32–34] The double-blind treatment period of each study ranged from 2 weeks to 5 months, and the dosage of budesonide, administered via Turbohaler, ranged between 100–800 μg twice daily, with 200 μg the dose most commonly administered. At baseline, the mean FEV_1 was 68.2% of the predicted normal value and by the end of the double-blind treatment phase, this had increased to 74.4%. By week 52, the mean FEV_1 had improved further to 81.3%. The rate of premature treatment discontinuation was 14.1%, with asthma exacerbations and adverse events the most common causes of withdrawal. Of the 144 oral corticosteroid-dependent patients included in the study, 64 entered the open-label treatment period having discontinued their oral steroidal treatment in accordance with recommended guidelines. Ninety-one per cent of these patients remained free from oral corticosteroids at the end of the open-label phase. There was no evidence of suppression of basal or adrenocorticotropic hormone (ACTH)-stimulated cortisol levels over the course of the study (mean increase from baseline of 4 and 3 nmol/L for basal and ACTH-stimulated cortisol levels, respectively). Thus, this study has demonstrated that improvements in pulmonary function observed during controlled studies of budesonide were maintained over 1 year of continued treatment.

Improvements in pulmonary function observed during controlled studies of budesonide were maintained over 1 year of continued treatment.

Comparative studies

Budesonide *vs* montelukast

The COMPACT study examined the therapeutic consequences of adding the leukotriene receptor antagonist, montelukast, to the treatment regimen of adult patients inadequately controlled on inhaled budesonide, compared with a doubling of budesonide dose.[30] Patients (n=889) received either a daily dose of montelukast, 10 mg, plus budesonide, 800 μg, or budesonide, 1600 μg, for a total period of 16 weeks. The rates of premature treatment discontinuation were 4.5 and 5.9%, for montelukast/budesonide and double-dose budesonide treatment groups, respectively (*p*-value not reported). At baseline, mean FEV_1 was 68.7% of the predicted normal value and mean morning PEF was 384 L/minute. During the last 10 weeks of treatment, mean morning PEF improved significantly from baseline by a comparable degree in the montelukast/budesonide and double-dose budesonide groups (33.5 and 30.1 L/minute, respectively; *p*-value not reported). The change in morning PEF during the first 3 days of treatment was more rapid and more pronounced in the montelukast/budesonide combination group compared with those receiving double-dose budesonide (20.1 *vs* 9.61 L/minute, respectively, $p<0.001$). Changes from baseline in the use of β_2-agonist rescue medication and daytime asthma symptom scores were similar in the different treatment groups (β_2-agonist use: –0.78 *vs* –0.75 puffs/day; $p=0.51$; symptom scores: –0.34 *vs* –0.35; $p=0.91$; all comparisons for montelukast/budesonide *vs* double-dose budesonide, respectively). The improvement in the number of nocturnal awakenings, median days with asthma exacerbations, asthma-free days, quality of life scores and the proportion of patients requiring oral steroids or hospital admission did not differ significantly between the two treatment groups ($p>0.05$). Both treatments were well tolerated and there were no differences between groups in terms of the number of patients experiencing adverse events (37.1 *vs* 41.3% for montelukast/budesonide and double-dose budesonide, respectively; *p*-value not reported). Overall, with the notable exception of morning

PEF, the improvements in lung function and asthma symptom management associated with adding montelukast to an existing budesonide treatment regimen were similar to those achieved by doubling the dose of budesonide.

Improvements in lung function and asthma symptom management associated with adding montelukast to existing budesonide treatment were similar to those achieved by doubling the dose of budesonide.

Budesonide *vs* mometasone furoate

The most recently introduced inhaled corticosteroid, mometasone furoate (hereafter referred to as mometasone), has been compared with budesonide in a number of studies, two of which are reported here. In the first study, in 730 patients with moderate persistent asthma, mometasone, 100, 200 or 400 μg twice daily, was compared with budesonide, 400 μg twice daily, over a period of 12 weeks.[35] Although both drugs elicited significant improvements from baseline in FEV_1, the changes associated with mometasone, 200 and 400 μg twice daily, were significantly greater than those associated with budesonide 400 μg twice daily (increases of 0.16, 0.16 and 0.06 L, respectively; $p<0.05$ for both doses of mometasone *vs* budesonide). There were no significant differences between treatment groups in terms of FVC, the incidence of cough or nocturnal awakenings ($p>0.05$), though the use of β_2-agonist rescue medication was significantly less frequent in the 200 μg twice-daily mometasone group than in the budesonide group (–90.66 *vs* –33.9 μg/day salbutamol; $p<0.05$).

This study has attracted criticism, primarily because only one dose of budesonide was compared with three doses of mometasone.[36] Moreover, since the budesonide dose was as high as the highest dose of mometasone, it was not possible to ascertain what impact a lower dose of budesonide could have made in this patient population.

The second study comparing mometasone with budesonide was placebo-controlled and included 262 patients with moderate persistent asthma previously using twice-daily inhaled corticosteroids.[37] Patients were randomised to receive either budesonide, 400 μg metered dose once daily, or mometasone, 440 μg metered dose once daily, for a period of 8 weeks. At baseline, mean FEV_1 ranged from 71.6–75.1% of the predicted normal value. More patients in the placebo group than in either the budesonide or mometasone treatment groups discontinued treatment early because of treatment failure (35, 10 and 6%, respectively; *p*-value not reported). After 8 weeks, the percentage improvement in FEV_1 from baseline associated with mometasone treatment significantly exceeded that associated with either budesonide or placebo treatment (8.9, 2.1 and –3.9% for mometasone, budesonide and placebo, respectively; $p<0.01$ and $p<0.001$). Although both active treatments improved aspects of morning and evening asthma symptoms, and reduced the use of β_2-agonist rescue medication, in general, the improvements associated with mometasone were superior to those associated with budesonide (change in salbutamol use: –0.91 *vs* –0.21 inhalations/day for mometasone and budesonide, respectively; $p<0.01$ *vs* placebo for both comparisons and $p<0.05$ *vs* budesonide).

Although both active treatments improved aspects of asthma control, in general, the improvements associated with mometasone were superior to those associated with budesonide.

Efficacy in paediatric asthma

Placebo-controlled studies

A double-blind, placebo-controlled study in 404 children aged 6–18 years, with moderate-to-severe persistent asthma who had previously been treated with inhaled corticosteroids, examined the efficacy of budesonide when administered twice daily at doses of 100, 200 or 400 µg over a period of 12 weeks.[32] At baseline, mean FEV_1 was 74.6% of the predicted normal value. A significantly larger proportion of budesonide- than placebo-treated participants completed the study (15–18 *vs* 49%; $p<0.001$), with worsening asthma accounting for the majority of patient withdrawals. After 12 weeks of treatment, morning PEF values had increased significantly from baseline amongst those patients receiving budesonide compared with placebo (mean changes of 4.4, 5.6, 6.7 and –3.9%, for budesonide, 100, 200, 400 µg, twice daily, and placebo, respectively; $p<0.001$ *vs* placebo). Budesonide-treated patients responded within 2 weeks of treatment and a maximum effect was achieved by 2–4 weeks and was sustained over 12 weeks. The mean change from baseline in FEV_1 was also significantly greater amongst budesonide-treated patients and again was more pronounced with the higher doses (mean changes of 3.1, 7.7, 7.3 and –4.6% of the predicted value for budesonide, 100, 200, 400 µg, twice daily, and placebo, respectively; $p<0.001$ *vs* placebo). Budesonide treatment significantly reduced the frequency of day- and night-time asthma symptoms ($p<0.001$) and limited the use of β_2-agonist rescue medication (mean change in the number of inhalations per day of –24, –30, –40 and +26% for budesonide, 100, 200, 400 µg twice daily, and placebo, respectively; $p<0.001$ *vs* placebo). Importantly, none of the budesonide treatment regimens were associated with significant changes in basal or mean cosynotropin-stimulated plasma cortisol concentrations over the 12-week period.

Budesonide-treated patients responded within 2 weeks of treatment and a maximum effect was achieved by 2–4 weeks and was sustained over 12 weeks.

A similar study conducted in 274 children aged between 6 and 17 years, investigated the efficacy of once-daily budesonide treatment in patients who had previously been maintained on a twice-daily inhaled corticosteroid treatment schedule.[38] Participants, who had a history of persistent asthma, received either budesonide, 200 or 400 µg once daily, or placebo for a period of 12 weeks. Mean baseline FEV_1 readings were 77.5, 77.0 and 76.6% of the predicted normal value, for budesonide, 200 and 400 µg, and placebo treatment groups, respectively (*p*-value not reported). The rate of premature treatment discontinuation due to disease deterioration or lack of improvement was significantly lower amongst patients receiving budesonide (11, 10 and 24% for budesonide, 200 and 400 µg once daily, and placebo, respectively; $p\leq0.024$ *vs* placebo). The change in FEV_1 over the course of the study was significantly greater for both doses of budesonide than with placebo (mean changes of 2.65, 3.29 and –1.49% of the predicted value for budesonide, 200 and 400 µg once daily, and placebo, respectively; $p=0.015$ and $p=0.005$ *vs* placebo). Both morning and evening PEF improved significantly from baseline following budesonide treatment ($p\leq0.041$; Figure 6). The incidence of day- and night-time asthma symptoms was also reduced significantly following budesonide treatment (–0.03 and –0.12 *vs* 0.19 for daytime symptoms, and –0.12 and –0.11 *vs* 0.14 for night-time symptoms, for budesonide, 200 and 400 μg once daily, *vs* placebo, respectively; $p \leq 0.001$ *vs* placebo).

The question of treatment adherence was addressed in a double-blind study in 122 children with mild asthma (mean FEV_1 103.7% of predicted).[39] Participants were randomised to receive either budesonide,

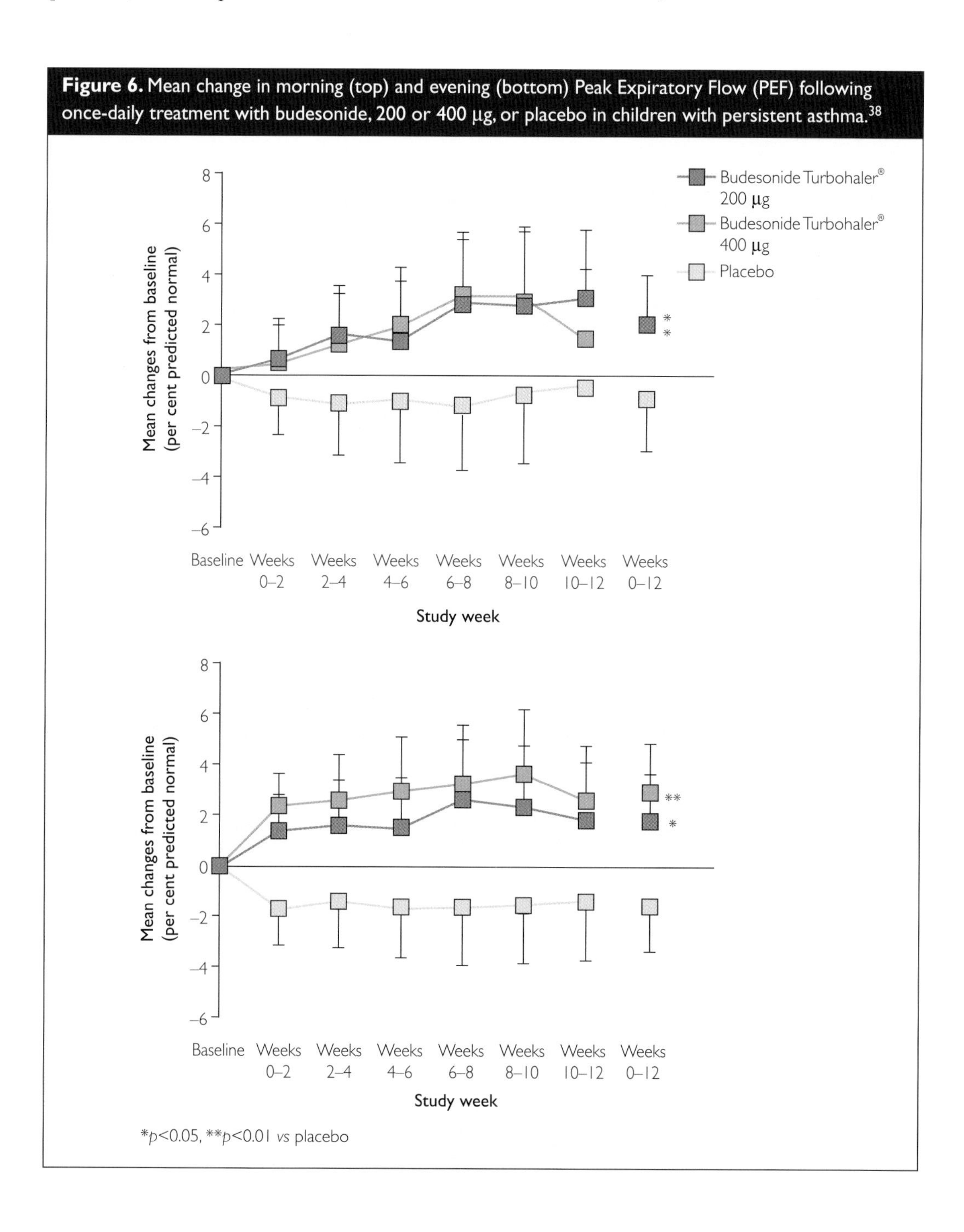

Figure 6. Mean change in morning (top) and evening (bottom) Peak Expiratory Flow (PEF) following once-daily treatment with budesonide, 200 or 400 μg, or placebo in children with persistent asthma.[38]

100 or 200 μg daily, or placebo for 27 months and drug adherence was assessed by counting the number of remaining doses in the inhaler when study medication was returned at 6-month intervals. Overall, drug adherence declined progressively over the course of the study, a trend that was evident from 3–9 months onwards (mean values of 40.6 and 46.9% for morning and evening medication, respectively). Drug adherence declined more rapidly in the placebo group than in the budesonide treatment groups, a difference that became significant during the last 6 months of the study (32.2 *vs* 48.8% compliance for placebo and budesonide, respectively; $p=0.039$). Treatment adherence was always higher for evening compared with morning medication at all study intervals, reaching significance after 9 months (51.7 *vs* 58.8% for morning and evening, respectively; $p<0.001$).

Drug adherence declined more rapidly in the placebo group than in the budesonide treatment groups.

Budesonide *vs* nedocromil sodium

Nedocromil sodium and the related drug, sodium cromoglycate, are non-steroidal drugs most frequently used in children for asthma prophylaxis.

The relative efficacies of budesonide and nedocromil for the long-term control of asthma were compared in the Childhood Asthma Management Programme (CAMP), a large placebo-controlled study of 1041 children, 5–12 years of age, with mild-to-moderate asthma.[40] Patients received either budesonide, 200 μg, nedocromil, 8 mg, or placebo, twice daily for a period of 4–6 years. The mean duration of follow-up was 4.3 years. The mean changes in spirometric measures, asthma severity and physical development over the duration of the study are presented in Table 3. Whilst budesonide was associated with significant improvements in a number of measurements of asthma control, there was no appreciable difference between either of the active treatments and placebo with regard to the degree of change in FEV_1, the primary outcome measure. Budesonide was associated with a significant reduction in linear growth over the course of the study; the mean increase in height was 1.1 cm less following budesonide than placebo treatment (22.7 *vs* 23.8 cm; $p=0.005$). Nedocromil was not associated with such a reduction in linear growth.

Budesonide nebuliser suspension

The clinical trials examining the efficacy of budesonide inhalation suspension in infants and small children with asthma are summarised in Table 4.[41–44] In general terms, budesonide, when administered as a nebuliser suspension, elicited significant and sustained improvements in asthma symptoms and measures of clinical efficacy (PEF and FEV_1), whilst reducing the use of β_2-agonist rescue medication and increasing the time to the first asthma exacerbation. Importantly for a paediatric patient population, budesonide was consistently well tolerated, exhibiting an adverse event profile comparable with that of placebo treatment.

Budesonide, when administered as a nebuliser suspension, elicited significant and sustained improvements in asthma symptoms and measures of clinical efficacy.

Table 3. The mean changes in spirometric measures, asthma severity and physical development following 4–6 years of treatment with budesonide, 200 μg, nedocromil, 8 mg or placebo.[40]

Outcome measure	Mean value			*p*-value	
	Budesonide (n=311)	Nedocromil (n=312)	Placebo (n=418)	Budesonide *vs* placebo	Nedocromil *vs* placebo
Post-bronchodilator FEV_1					
(% of predicted)	0.6	–0.5	–0.1	0.36	0.56
FVC (L)	1.27	1.29	1.33	0.05	0.25
Pre-bronchodilator FEV_1					
(% of predicted)	2.9	0.4	0.9	0.02	0.57
FVC (L)	1.29	1.28	1.35	0.07	0.06
Asthma symptom score	–0.44	–0.38	–0.37	0.005	0.80
Episode-free days (per month)	11.3	9.3	9.3	0.01	0.97
Use of salbutamol for symptoms					
(puffs per week)	–7.4	–5.7	–5.3	<0.001	0.42
Nocturnal awakenings	–0.7	–0.6	–0.6	0.14	0.48
Hospitalisations due to asthma					
(per 100 person-year)	2.5	4.3	4.4	0.04	0.99
Change in height (cm)	22.7	23.7	23.8	0.005	0.65
Change in bone density (g/cm^2)	0.17	0.17	0.18	0.53	0.15

FEV_1, forced expiratory volume in 1 second; FVC, forced vital capacity.

Safety and tolerability

Although inhaled corticosteroids have considerably fewer systemic effects than oral corticosteroids, adverse events have been reported following regular use.[8] High doses in particular have been associated with an increased risk of adrenal suppression, reduced bone mineral density, glaucoma, cataracts, hoarseness and candidiasis of the mouth or throat.[8] The use of a DPI or a spacer may minimise oropharyngeal deposition, whilst candidiasis responds well to antifungal lozenges without the need to discontinue corticosteroid therapy.[8] Gargling with water or brushing teeth after administration may also limit such effects. In general, the linear growth retardation associated with oral corticosteroid therapy does not appear to be a significant problem when using recommended doses of inhaled corticosteroids.[8] As with all inhaled medications, the potential for paradoxical bronchospasm should also be considered when prescribing corticosteroids. Mild bronchospasm may be prevented by inhalation of a short-acting β_2-agonist, or by transfer from an aerosol inhalation to a dry powder inhalation.[8]

Budesonide itself is generally well tolerated when administered at therapeutic doses. Hoarseness, sore throat and local irritation causing cough are amongst the most common side-effects reported.[7,8,15] Furthermore, at therapeutic doses, budesonide, delivered either via a pMDI or DPI, produced little or no reduction in plasma cortisol levels

Table 4. Summary of clinical trials examining the efficacy of budesonide inhalation suspension in infants and young children with asthma.[41–44]

Study and dosage regimen	Asthma severity at baseline	Main outcomes
Kemp *et al.*, 1999[41] Placebo-controlled Double-blind n=359 12 weeks Children 6 months to 8 years Budesonide, 250, 500 or 1000 µg daily	Mild persistent asthma Mean FEV_1 83.1% of predicted normal Mean reversibility 27.7%	• All doses of budesonide significantly improved day- and night-time symptoms of asthma ($p \leq 0.049$ *vs* placebo). • All doses of budesonide significantly reduced the use of rescue medication (6.26, 6.31, 5.98 day reductions *vs* 4.19 puffs/day for placebo; $p \leq 0.038$ *vs* placebo). • FEV_1 improved significantly following budesonide, 500 and 1000 µg (both 0.03 L *vs* –0.07 L for placebo; $p \leq 0.044$). • Adverse events and cortisol levels were similar in all treatment groups. • Discontinuations were significantly greater in placebo group *vs* 1000 µg budesonide group (28 *vs* 14%, respectively; $p=0.02$).
Baker *et al.*, 1999[42] Placebo-controlled Double-blind n=481 12 weeks Children 6 months to 8 years Budesonide, 250 µg once daily, 250 µg twice daily, 500 µg twice daily, or 1000 µg once daily	Moderate persistent asthma Mean FEV_1 80% of predicted normal. Mean reversibility 29% Mean asthma symptom score 1.3 (maximum 3)	• Budesonide (250 µg twice daily, 500 µg twice daily and 1000 µg) significantly improved day-time symptoms (–0.4, –0.46 and –0.37; $p \leq 0.05$ *vs* placebo [–0.19]). • Budesonide (250 µg twice daily, 500 µg twice daily and 1000 µg) significantly improved night-time symptoms (–0.49, –0.42 and –0.4; $p \leq 0.01$ *vs* placebo [–0.13]). • Budesonide (250 µg twice daily, 500 µg twice daily and 1000 µg) significantly improved morning PEF 23.0, 24.8 and 17.1 L/minute; $p \leq 0.05$ *vs* placebo [–0.2]). • Only budesonide 500 µg twice daily significantly improved FEV_1 (0.17 *vs* 0.04 L/minute; $p \leq 0.05$ *vs* placebo). • Adverse events and cortisol levels were similar between all treatment groups.

FEV_1, forced expiratory volume in 1 second; PACQLQ, Paediatric Asthma Caregiver's Quality of Life Questionnaire; PEF, peak expiratory flow.

either in healthy individuals or in patients with persistent asthma, compared with other inhaled corticosteroids.[2] The lower incidence of systemic effects associated with budesonide may be due, in part, to its short systemic half-life and limited volume of distribution.[1]

Table 4. Continued

Study and dosage regimen	Asthma severity at baseline	Main outcomes
Leflein *et al.*, 2002[43] Open-label n=335 52 weeks Children aged 2–6 years Budesonide, 500 μg daily, or cromolyn sodium nebuliser solution, 20 mg, four-times daily	Mean asthma symptom severity score 1.4 (daytime) and 1.3 (night-time), based on a scale of 1 to 3	• The mean yearly asthma exacerbation rate was significantly lower following budesonide treatment (1.23 *vs* 2.41 exacerbations for budesonide and cromolyn sodium, respectively; $p<0.001$). • The mean time to first asthma exacerbation was significantly longer in the budesonide group (216.6 *vs* 147.8 days, respectively; $p<0.001$). • The mean time to the first use of additional long-term asthma medication was significantly longer in the budesonide group (320.5 *vs* 235.1 days, respectively; $p<0.001$) • Day- and night-time asthma symptoms were significantly improved following treatment with budesonide ($p<0.001$ *vs* cromolyn sodium). • Rate of study completion was significantly higher in the budesonide treatment group (92 *vs* 80%, respectively; $p=0.01$).
Murphy *et al.*, 2003[44] Quality of life analysis of Leflein *et al.*, 2002[43]	Mean PACQLQ score 4.8	• The improvement in total PACQLQ score was significantly greater in the budesonide treatment group (1.15 *vs* 0.77; $p=0.001$). • Caregivers expressing the greatest burden at baseline experienced the greatest improvements in PACQLQ score following treatment. • 90.7% of caregivers in the budesonide group were 'completely or very satisfied' compared with 53.4% in the cromolyn sodium group.

FEV_1, forced expiratory volume in 1 second; PACQLQ, Paediatric Asthma Caregiver's Quality of Life Questionnaire; PEF, peak expiratory flow.

Safety in paediatric populations

Budesonide is the most extensively studied inhaled corticosteroid in children with asthma, with a wealth of safety data.[1] Analyses of clinical safety data derived from the worldwide budesonide inhalation suspension development programme included over 1600 children from double-blind studies of 12 weeks and their open-label extensions up to 52 weeks.[43,45,46] No incidence of posterior subcapsular cataracts were reported in any study and the frequencies of oropharyngeal events or infection were comparable with those reported following treatment with other conventional corticosteroids. The degree of adrenal suppression did not reach significance, with no major differences in basal or ACTH-stimulated cortisol levels reported. The most common adverse events following long-term treatment with budesonide, which occurred in at least 10% of children, were respiratory infections (58 *vs* 49% for budesonide and conventional corticosteroid therapy, respectively), sinusitis (33 *vs* 27%), fever (28% *vs* 20%), otitis media (22 *vs* 19%), pharyngitis (19 *vs* 17%), rhinitis (17 *vs* 11%), headache (11 *vs* 10%) and bronchitis (11 *vs* 8%).

Effect on adult height

Some of the controlled clinical trials included in the safety analyses outlined previously, have reported small but significant differences in short-term growth velocity between children receiving inhaled budesonide and those receiving conventional asthma therapies. For example, the previously mentioned CAMP study reported a significant reduction in linear growth following long-term budesonide treatment.[40] Over the course of this 4–6-year investigation, the mean increase in height was 1.1 cm less following budesonide than placebo treatment (22.7 *vs* 23.8 cm; p=0.005).

A prospective analysis of 211 children who had attained adult height, 142 of whom had undergone long-term budesonide treatment for asthma, further investigated the effects of budesonide treatment on adult height.[47] Children treated with budesonide attained adult height after a mean of 9.2 years of treatment at a mean daily dose of 412 μg budesonide. The mean differences between measured and target adult heights were +0.3 cm for budesonide, –0.2 cm for control children with asthma who had never received inhaled corticosteroid treatment, and –0.9 cm for the healthy siblings of patients in the budesonide treatment group. There was no significant correlation between the duration of treatment (p=0.16) or the cumulative dose of budesonide (p=0.14) and the difference between measured and target adult heights. The adult height attained depended significantly on the child's height before initiating budesonide treatment (p<0.001). Overall, the changes in growth rate observed during the first years of budesonide treatment were not associated with final adult height (p=0.44) and children treated with budesonide attained normal adult height.

Although budesonide treatment has been associated with a slowing of initial growth velocity, there appears to be no effect on achieving normal adult height.

Thus, although budesonide treatment has been associated with a slowing of initial growth velocity, there appears to be no effect on achieving normal adult height. Regular monitoring of height is, however, advocated in children receiving prolonged treatment with inhaled corticosteroids.

Precautions for use

Budesonide is contra-indicated in patients with active pulmonary tuberculosis or hypersensitivity to budesonide.[7] Caution should also be observed when administering budesonide to patients with quiescent lung tuberculosis or fungal or viral infections of the airways.[7] Those patients transferring from oral corticosteroid therapy to inhaled budesonide may experience unmasking of allergic or arthritic symptoms such as rhinitis, eczema and muscle and joint pain. As mentioned previously, the routine monitoring of height in children receiving long-term budesonide treatment is recommended.[7] Asthma is one of the most common medical conditions that can complicate pregnancy and adequate control of asthma is vital to prevent maternal and foetal hypoxia. However, the benefits of budesonide use during pregnancy should be weighed against the potential risk to the foetus, and doses should be kept to the absolute minimum.[7]

Drug interactions

No specific drug interaction data are available regarding budesonide, although in view of its metabolic pathway, drugs that markedly inhibit CYP3A4 (e.g. ketoconazole) have the potential to increase systemic exposure to budesonide.[7,8] Thus, the concurrent use of these compounds with budesonide should be avoided where possible. The action of corticosteroids in general may be adversely affected by co-administration with amphotericin, barbiturates, carbamazepine, coumarins, methotrexate, phenytoin, primidone and rifamycins.[8] High doses of corticosteroids may also impair the immune response to live vaccines and concomitant use should therefore be avoided.

Pharmacoeconomics

The major financial costs associated with asthma management are principally related to the medical cost of hospitalisation, emergency care and drug therapy.[48] Indirectly, asthma also accounts for costs attributed to the loss of school or work days.[48] In theory, an effective anti-asthma drug would lower the number of hospitalisations and emergency pharmacological treatments, thereby reducing the economic burden associated with the condition. Patients with well-managed asthma can expect to live a near-normal lifestyle with minimal or no adverse events. It is worth considering, however, that inhaled corticosteroids, in common with other anti-asthma agents, are not curative and so any costs incurred in treatment will persist for the lifetime of the individual patient.

Pharmacoeconomic analyses of budesonide have demonstrated a marked reduction in oral prednisolone requirements, hospital admissions and days spent in the clinic associated with regular treatment.[49] In addition, adverse events associated with budesonide treatment are usually mild-to-moderate in intensity and do not necessitate further treatment.[49] Patients with mild-to-moderate asthma have shown improvement in sleep and lifestyle indices following treatment with budesonide and are more able to perform hard physical work. Data derived from the quality of life studies described previously have shown significant and consistent improvements in patients' overall satisfaction with their lifestyle.[18,21,44]

Analyses of budesonide have demonstrated a marked reduction in oral prednisolone requirements, hospital admissions and days spent in the clinic associated with regular treatment.

The cost-effectiveness of early intervention with budesonide was assessed in an economic analysis of the START study, described

The addition of budesonide to an asthma treatment regimen decreased the number of days spent in hospital by 68% and the number of emergency department visits by 67% compared with the placebo treatment.

previously.[22,50] Patients continued with their usual asthma medication and in addition, received either budesonide, 200 or 400 μg daily, or placebo for a period of 3 years. Compared with those patients receiving their usual therapy plus placebo, patients treated with budesonide gained an average of 14.1 extra symptom-free days per year (p<0.001 *vs* placebo). The addition of budesonide to the asthma treatment regimen also decreased the number of days spent in hospital by 68% (p<0.001) and the number of emergency department visits by 67% (p<0.05) compared with the placebo treatment group.

Key points

- Budesonide is an inhaled corticosteroid indicated for the long-term prevention of asthma exacerbations in both adults and children.
- The unique mechanism by which budesonide undergoes reversible esterification, prolongs its airways retention and thereby increases its duration of effect.
- Budesonide may be administered once or twice daily via a DPI, a pMDI or nebuliser. The deposition characteristics of the DPI appear to offer a good balance between therapeutic effects and unwanted systemic events.
- In placebo-controlled studies, budesonide elicited dose-dependent improvements in PEF and FEV_1, reduced asthma symptom scores, reduced β_2-agonist use and prolonged the time to the first severe asthma-related event.
- The early initiation of budesonide treatment in patients with recently diagnosed asthma provided pronounced benefits. Further trials have demonstrated that an initial loading dose of budesonide increases the short-term response to treatment.
- The efficacy of budesonide was sustained for up to 3 years in placebo-controlled studies.
- Controlled paediatric studies have shown that budesonide is effective and well tolerated, whether administered via a DPI or as a nebuliser suspension.
- Budesonide is generally well tolerated with cough, local irritation and hoarseness amongst the most commonly reported side-effects. Budesonide demonstrates limited systemic effects, in contrast with oral corticosteroids.
- Although the short-term growth rate of children may be impaired by long-term budesonide treatment, the overall adult height attained is unaffected.

References

A list of the published evidence which has been reviewed in compiling the preceding section of *BESTMEDICINE.*

1 Pearlman D. Preclinical properties of budesonide: translation to the clinical setting. *Clin Ther* 2003; **25**: C75–91.

2 Skoner D. Therapeutic margin of budesonide in patients with mild to severe asthma. *Clin Ther* 2003; **25**: C61–74.

3 Scottish Intercollegiate Guidelines Network and British Thoracic Society. British Guidelines on the Management of Asthma. SIGN, Edinburgh, 2004.

4 Hanania N, Chapman K, Kesten S. Adverse effects of inhaled corticosteroids. *Am J Med* 1995; **98**: 196–208.

5 O'Connell E. Review of the unique properties of budesonide. *Clin Ther* 2003; **25**: C61–74.

6 Boobis A. Comparative physicochemical and pharmacokinetic profiles of inhaled beclomethasone dipropionate and budesonide. *Respir Med* 1998; **92**: B2–6.

7 AstraZeneca UK Limited. Pulmicort® Turbohaler® 100. *Summary of product characteristics.* Luton, Bedfordshire, 2004.

8 *British National Formulary (BNF) 48.* London: British Medical Association and Royal Pharmaceutical Society of Great Britain. September, 2004.

9 Viatris Pharmaceuticals Ltd. Novolizer Budesonide 200 micrograms Inhalation Powder. Cambridge, UK, 2004.

10 AstraZeneca UK Limited. Pulmicort® Respules® 0.5 mg and 1 mg. *Summary of product characteristics.* Luton, Bedfordshire, 2004.

11 Donnelly R, Seale J. Clinical pharmacokinetics of inhaled budesonide. *Clin Pharmacokinet* 2001; **40**: 427–40.

12 Banov C. The role of budesonide in adults and children with mild-to-moderate persistent asthma. *J Asthma* 2004; **41**: 5–17.

13 Edsbacker S, Brattsand R. Budesonide fatty-acid esterification: a novel mechanism prolonging binding to airway tissue. Review of available data. *Ann Allergy Asthma Immunol* 2002; **88**: 609–16.

14 Miller-Larsson A, Mattsson H, Hjertberg E *et al.* Reversible fatty acid conjugation of budesonide. Novel mechanism for prolonged retention of topically applied steroid in airway tissue. *Drug Metab Dispos* 1998; **26**: 623–30.

15 Brogden R, McTavish D. Budesonide. An updated review of its pharmacological properties, and therapeutic efficacy in asthma and rhinitis. *Drugs* 1992; **44**: 375–407.

16 Busse W, Chervinsky P, Condemi J *et al.* Budesonide delivered by Turbuhaler is effective in a dose-dependent fashion when used in the treatment of adult patients with chronic asthma. *J Allergy Clin Immunol* 1998; **101**: 457–63.

17 McFadden E, Casale T, Edwards T *et al.* Administration of budesonide once daily by means of turbuhaler to subjects with stable asthma. *J Allergy Clin Immunol* 1999; **104**: 46–52.

18 Casale T, Nelson H, Kemp J *et al.* Budesonide Turbuhaler delivered once daily improves health-related quality of life and maintains improvements with a stepped-down dose in adults with mild to moderate asthma. *Ann Allergy Asthma Immunol* 2003; **90**: 323–30.

19 Kemp J, Wanderer A, Ramsdell J *et al.* Rapid onset of control with budesonide Turbuhaler in patients with mild-to-moderate asthma. *Ann Allergy Asthma Immunol* 1999; **82**: 463–71.

20 Metzger W, Hampel F, Sugar M. Once-daily budesonide inhalation powder (Pulmicort Turbuhaler) is effective and safe in adults previously treated with inhaled corticosteroids. *J Asthma* 2002; **39**: 65–75.

21 Hampel F, Sugar M, Parasuraman B, Uryniak T, Liljas B. Once-daily budesonide inhalation powder (Pulmicort Turbuhaler) improves health-related quality of life in adults previously receiving inhaled corticosteroids. *Adv Ther* 2004; **21**: 27–38.

22 Pauwels R, Pedersen S, Busse W *et al.* Early intervention with budesonide in mild persistent asthma: a randomised, double-blind trial. *Lancet* 2003; **361**: 1071–6.

23 Campbell L, Gooding T, Aitchison W, Smith N, Powell J. Initial loading (400 micrograms twice daily) versus static (400 micrograms nocte) dose budesonide for asthma management. PLAN Research Group. *Int J Clin Pract* 1998; **52**: 361–8.

24 Foresi A, Morelli M, Catena E. Low-dose budesonide with the addition of an increased dose during exacerbations is effective in long-term asthma control. On behalf of the Italian Study Group. *Chest* 2000; **117**: 440–6.

25 Miyamoto T, Takahashi T, Nakajima S *et al.* A double-blind, placebo-controlled dose-response study with budesonide Turbuhaler in Japanese asthma patients. Japanese Pulmicort Turbuhaler study group. *Respirology* 2000; **5**: 247–56.

26 Lorentzson S, Boe J, Eriksson G, Persson G. Use of inhaled corticosteroids in patients with mild asthma. *Thorax* 1990; **45**: 733–5.

27 O'Byrne P, Cuddy L, Taylor D *et al.* Efficacy and cost benefit of inhaled corticosteroids in patients considered to have mild asthma in primary care practice. *Can Respir J* 1996; **3**: 169–75.

28 Pirozynski M, Kulaga Z, Karlstrom R. Pulmicort Turbuhaler in mild to moderate asthma: comparison of initial high dose, constant low dose and placebo. *Am J Respir Crit Care Med* 1996; **153**: A343.

29 Masoli M, Holt S, Weatherall M, Beasley R. Dose-response relationship of inhaled budesonide in adult asthma: a meta-analysis. *Eur Respir J* 2004; **23**: 552–8.

30 Price D, Hernandez D, Magyar P *et al.* Randomised controlled trial of montelukast plus inhaled budesonide versus double dose inhaled budesonide in adult patients with asthma. *Thorax* 2003; **58**: 211–6.

31 Green R, Brightling C, McKenna S *et al.* Asthma exacerbations and sputum eosinophil counts: a randomised controlled trial. *Lancet* 2002; **360**: 1715–21.
32 Shapiro G, Bronsky E, LaForce C *et al.* Dose-related efficacy of budesonide administered via a dry powder inhaler in the treatment of children with moderate to severe persistent asthma. *J Pediatr* 1998; **132**: 976–82.
33 Nelson H, Bernstein I, Fink J *et al.* Oral glucocorticosteroid-sparing effect of budesonide administered by Turbuhaler: a double-blind, placebo-controlled study in adults with moderate-to-severe chronic asthma. Pulmicort Turbuhaler Study Group. *Chest* 1998; **113**: 1264–71.
34 Tinkelman D, Bronsky E, Gross G, Schoenwetter W, Spector S. Efficacy and safety of budesonide inhalation powder (Pulmicort Turbuhaler) during 52 weeks of treatment in adults and children with persistent asthma. *J Asthma* 2003; **40**: 225–36.
35 Bousquet J, D'Urzo A, Hebert J *et al.* Comparison of the efficacy and safety of mometasone furoate dry powder inhaler to budesonide Turbuhaler. *Eur Respir J* 2000; **16**: 808–16.
36 Carlsson L, Edsbacker S. Comparative efficacy and safety of mometasone furoate dry powder inhaler and budesonide Turbuhaler. *Eur Respir J* 2001; **17**: 1332–3.
37 Corren J, Berkowitz R, Murray J, Prenner B. Comparison of once-daily mometasone furoate versus once-daily budesonide in patients with moderate persistent asthma. *Int J Clin Pract* 2003; **57**: 567–72.
38 Shapiro G, Mendelson L, Pearlman D. Once-daily budesonide inhalation powder (Pulmicort Turbuhaler) maintains pulmonary function and symptoms of asthmatic children previously receiving inhaled corticosteroids. *Ann Allergy Asthma Immunol.* 2001; **86**: 633–40.
39 Jonasson G, Carlsen K, Mowinckel P. Asthma drug adherence in a long term clinical trial. *Arch Dis Child* 2000; **83**: 330–3.
40 Long-term effects of budesonide or nedocromil in children with asthma. The Childhood Asthma Management Program Research Group. *New Eng J Med* 2000; **343**: 866–72.
41 Kemp J, Skoner D, Szefler S *et al.* Once-daily budesonide inhalation suspension for the treatment of persistent asthma in infants and young children. *Ann Allergy Asthma Immunol* 1999; **83**: 231–9.
42 Baker J, Mellon M, Wald J *et al.* A multiple-dosing, placebo-controlled study of budesonide inhalation suspension given once or twice daily for treatment of persistent asthma in young children and infants. *Pediatrics* 1999; **103**: 414–21.
43 Leflein J, Szefler S, Murphy K *et al.* Nebulized budesonide inhalation suspension compared with cromolyn sodium nebulizer solution for asthma in young children: results of a randomized outcomes trial. *Pediatrics* 2002; **109**: 866–72.
44 Murphy K, Fitzpatrick S, Cruz-Rivera M, Miller C, Parasuraman B. Effects of budesonide inhalation suspension compared with cromolyn sodium nebulizer solution on health status and caregiver quality of life in childhood asthma. *Pediatrics* 2003; **112**: 212–19.
45 Scott M, Skoner D. Short-term and long-term safety of budesonide inhalation suspension in infants and young children with persistent asthma. *J Allergy Clin Immunol* 1999; **104**: 200–9.
46 Szefler S, Lyzell E, Fitzpatrick S, Cruz-Rivera M. Safety profile of budesonide inhalation suspension in the pediatric population: worldwide experience. *Ann Allergy Asthma Immunol.* 2004; **93**: 83–90.
47 Agertoft L, Pedersen S. Effect of long-term treatment with inhaled budesonide on adult height in children with asthma. *N Engl J Med* 2000; **343**: 1064–9.
48 Cleland J, Thomas M, Price D. Pharmacoeconomics of asthma treatment. *Expert Opin Pharmacother* 2003; **4**: 311–18.
49 Davis R, McTavish D. Budesonide. An appraisal of the basis of its pharmacoeconomic and quality-of-life benefits in asthma. *Pharmacoeconomics* 1995; **7**: 457–70.
50 Sullivan S, Buxton M, Andersson L *et al.* Cost-effectiveness analysis of early intervention with budesonide in mild persistent asthma. *J Allergy Clin Immunol* 2003; **112**: 1229–36.

Acknowledgements

Figure 2 is adapted from Edsbacker *et al.*, 2002.[13]
Figure 3 is adapted from Busse *et al.*, 1998.[16]
Figures 4 and 5 are adapted from Pauwels *et al.*, 2003.[22]
Figure 6 is adapted from Shapiro *et al.*, 2001.[38]

4. Drug review – Ciclesonide (Alvesco®)

Dr Eleanor Bull
CSF Medical Communications Ltd

You are strongly urged to consult your doctor before taking, stopping or changing any of the products reviewed or referred to in *BESTMEDICINE* or any other medication that has been prescribed or recommended by your doctor.

Summary

Ciclesonide is an inhaled corticosteroid indicated for the treatment of persistent asthma in adults aged 18 years and over. As a soft steroid, ciclesonide is converted in the lung to its active metabolite – desmethylpropionyl ciclesonide (des-CIC) – to provide potent local anti-inflammatory effects, and thereafter undergoes predictable metabolism to its inactive metabolites. Des-CIC displays high affinity for pulmonary glucocorticoid receptors, low oral bioavailability, high plasma protein binding and is rapidly eliminated from the body. The rational design of ciclesonide, with its predictable metabolism, is intended to reduce systemic exposure to the steroid, thereby limiting its propensity for eliciting the clinically significant systemic adverse events implicated with corticosteroid use (e.g. adrenal suppression, bone loss, skin thinning, decreased growth, metabolic changes). Ciclesonide is administered via a metered dose inhaler (MDI) as a solution-aerosol with a high lung deposition (~52%). In controlled clinical studies of patients with persistent asthma, ciclesonide (administered one or twice daily) elicited similar improvements in lung function, asthma symptoms and use of β_2-adrenoceptor agonist (β_2-agonist) rescue medication, to those associated with the more widely used inhaled corticosteroid, fluticasone propionate. Ciclesonide is generally well tolerated and is associated with a low incidence of oropharyngeal adverse events.

Introduction

Inhaled corticosteroids relieve the symptoms of asthma by reducing inflammation of the airways. Their development represented a major breakthrough in asthma therapy, limiting the need for long-term treatment with oral corticosteroids and the associated systemic side-effects (e.g. adrenal suppression, bone loss, skin thinning, decreased linear growth, metabolic changes and behavioural abnormalities). Today, inhaled corticosteroids are used as prophylactic therapy in all but the mildest cases of asthma with persistent symptoms. Guidelines jointly issued by the Scottish Intercollegiate Guidelines Network (SIGN) and the British Thoracic Society (BTS) in 2004, recommend the regular use of inhaled corticosteroids – at daily doses of 200–800 μg for adults and 200–400 μg for children aged 5–12 years – when an inhaled short-acting β_2-agonist alone fails to adequately control asthma.[1]

In general, the inhaled corticosteroids (e.g. budesonide, beclometasone dipropionate, fluticasone propionate, and mometasone furoate [hereafter, referred to as beclometasone, fluticasone and mometasone) have similar clinical effectiveness with regard to asthma control and, therefore, their relative safety profiles are critical in differentiating between them on the basis of therapeutic margin. Concerns regarding the safety of regular inhalation of corticosteroids, particularly in children, have been well-documented and pertain largely to systemic effects of these drugs.[2] Over the years, attempts have been made to develop corticosteroids, which retain potent local anti-inflammatory activity but with improved safety profiles. Ideally, an inhaled corticosteroid would exhibit high local therapeutic activity in the airways, whilst possessing minimal systemic effects. Prolonged lung retention, high affinity and potency for glucocorticoid receptors, low oral and high pulmonary bioavailability, high pulmonary deposition, rapid systemic clearance and elimination are also highly desirable characteristics.[3]

Ideally, an inhaled corticosteroid would exhibit high local therapeutic activity in the airways, whilst possessing minimal systemic effects.

The development of 'soft steroids' (e.g. loteprednol etabonate, fluocortin-21 butyl ester and butixocort propionate[a]) has the potential to revolutionise the clinical safety profile of the inhaled corticosteroids as a drug class.[4,5] Soft steroids are specifically designed so that they are delivered near to their site of action where they exert their pharmacological effects and then undergo predictable metabolism to inactive metabolites.[4,6] This approach therefore limits the systemic availability of the corticosteroid and drastically reduces the likelihood of unwanted side-effects.[6]

Ciclesonide is a soft steroid that is delivered as a prodrug, and is indicated in the prophylactic management of persistent asthma.[7] The parent compound itself demonstrates negligible anti-inflammatory activity and requires cleavage by endogenous esterases in the lung to create its pharmacologically active metabolite, des-CIC.[7] Preclinical data published to date have shown that ciclesonide exhibits many of the ideal characteristics of an inhaled corticosteroid described previously.[8] This review discusses the pharmacological properties of ciclesonide and its reported efficacy in controlled clinical trials in both adults and children with asthma, although ciclesonide is not licensed for use in paediatric populations.

---

[a]These drugs are currently under development and consequently are not licensed in the UK.

Pharmacology

Chemistry

The chemical structures of ciclesonide and its active metabolite, des-CIC, are illustrated in Figure 1.[3] Des-CIC is derived from ciclesonide by esterase cleavage at the C21 position, a process that occurs once the drug has reached the airways.[3] This reversible fatty acid conjugation process is thought to prolong ciclesonide's pulmonary residence time, by providing a local depot for the slow release of the active compound.[3,7]

The chemistry of ciclesonide is of essentially academic interest and most healthcare professionals will, like you, skip this section.

Mechanism of action

As an inhaled corticosteroid, ciclesonide exerts its physiological effects through cytoplasmic glucocorticoid receptors. When bound together, the corticosteroid–receptor complex translocates to the cell nucleus where it modifies the transcription of a wide range of inflammatory mediators (e.g. cytokines, histamine, eicosanoids, leukotrienes), and thereby inhibits the inflammatory component of chronic asthma.[6] Corticosteroids also inhibit the activation of inflammatory cells including lymphocytes, eosinophils, mast cells, neutrophils and macrophages.[6]

What distinguishes ciclesonide mechanistically from the other inhaled corticosteroids is that it is only converted to its active form once it has reached the airways. Ciclesonide itself exhibits a low binding affinity for the glucocorticoid receptor, yet in the airways it is enzymatically converted to its active metabolite, des-CIC, which displays high affinity for pulmonary glucocorticoid receptors and thus pronounced anti-inflammatory activity.[7] *In vitro* studies of rat lung preparations have shown that the relative glucocorticoid receptor binding affinities of ciclesonide and des-CIC are 12 and 1212, respectively, compared with the receptor binding affinity of

Ciclesonide is only converted to its active form once it has reached the airways.

Figure 1. The chemical structure of ciclesonide (left) and its active metabolite, desmethylpropionyl-ciclesonide (des-CIC; right).

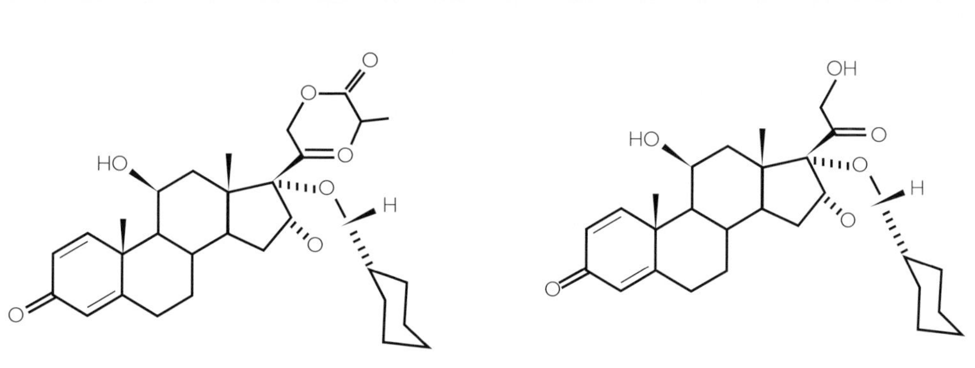

dexamethasone (defined as 100).[9] The receptor binding affinity of the des-CIC metabolite is comparable with that of the inhaled corticosteroid, budesonide (1212 *vs* 905, respectively).[9]

Animal models of asthma/inflammation

A series of experiments have been performed in order to determine the *in vitro* and *in vivo* anti-inflammatory activity profile of ciclesonide, as detailed below.

- Ciclesonide potently inhibited the activation of murine and human lymphocytes in a series of *in vitro* experiments.[9] Des-CIC was more potent than the parent compound and compared favourably with budesonide.
- Ciclesonide, des-CIC and budesonide (by intratracheal administration) all inhibited antigen-induced accumulation of eosinophils, total protein and tumour necrosis factor (TNF)-α in bronchoalveolar lavage fluid of ovalbumin-sensitised and challenged Brown-Norway rats (ED_{50}[b] ranged from 0.4–1.3 mg/kg for all drugs).[9]
- Ciclesonide and budesonide both inhibited bradykinin-induced protein leakage into rat trachea (ED_{25}[c] of 14.7 and 39.6 μM for ciclesonide and budesonide, respectively).[9]
- Ciclesonide inhibited granuloma formation (ED_{50} of 2 μg/pellet) in the rat cotton pellet model (the final weight of the cotton pellet after subcutaneous implantation for 7 days is used as a measure of granuloma formation and thus the anti-inflammatory response) whilst budesonide and des-CIC were 15- and 20-fold less active, respectively.[9] Thymus involution was also induced with ED_{50} values of 303, 279 and 154 μg/pellet for ciclesonide, des-CIC and budesonide, respectively.[9]
- Following 28 days of oral administration, ciclesonide exhibited a low potency in reducing the weights of the thymus and adrenal glands of rats, suggesting a low oral availability.[9]

Anti-inflammatory effects in humans

The effect of repeated inhalation of ciclesonide on the early- and late-phase immune responses after allergen challenge, was investigated in a double-blind, placebo-controlled, cross-over study of 13 patients with mild allergic asthma (mean forced expiratory volume in 1 second [FEV_1] of 91% of the predicted normal value).[10] Participants received either ciclesonide, 800 μg twice daily, or placebo for 1 week, with 3–5 weeks between treatment sequences. Participants underwent allergen challenge at the end of each treatment sequence. The expected reductions in FEV_1, recorded 0–2 or 2–12 hours following allergen challenge, were significantly limited by ciclesonide treatment (reductions of 0.193 and

---

[b]ED_{50}, concentration causing a 50% increase relative to the maximal response.

[c]ED_{25}, concentration causing a 25% increase relative to the maximal response.

0.23 L for early and late phase reactions, respectively; $p<0.05$ *vs* placebo). Furthermore, ciclesonide was well tolerated and had no effect on cortisol excretion in 24-hour urine samples. Thus, compared with placebo, ciclesonide significantly lowered the severity of both the early and late phase reactions to allergen challenge, confirming its anti-inflammatory profile in patients with asthma. The lack of hypothalamic–pituitary–adrenal (HPA) axis suppression also highlighted its low propensity for systemic effects.

Ciclesonide significantly lowered the severity of both the early and late phase reactions to allergen challenge.

Effect on airway responsiveness

The effect of ciclesonide on airway responsiveness to bronchoprovocation with adenosine-5-monophosphate (AMP) was examined in a double-blind, placebo-controlled, cross-over study in 29 patients with mild-to-moderate asthma.[11] Three doses of ciclesonide were tested: 50, 200 and 800 μg administered twice daily via dry powder inhaler (DPI)[d] for 2 weeks, with 3–8 weeks' wash-out between consecutive treatment periods. Patients were challenged with AMP before and after each treatment phase, and sputum samples were collected for analysis. Compared with placebo treatment, ciclesonide (total doses: 400 and 1600 μg/day) significantly reduced airway responsiveness to AMP (expressed as the doubling dose [dd] shift from respective baselines), by 2.0 and 3.4 dd, respectively ($p<0.05$ for both comparisons). This reduction in airway responsiveness demonstrated significant dose dependency ($p=0.039$). The percentage of sputum eosinophils was reduced significantly following the 400 and 1600 μg total daily doses of ciclesonide compared with placebo (median reductions of 6 and 2.7%, respectively; $p<0.05$ and $p<0.01$ *vs* baseline, respectively).

The percentage of sputum eosinophils was reduced significantly following the 400 and 1600 μg total daily doses of ciclesonide compared with placebo.

The comparative effects of ciclesonide and fluticasone on airway hyper-responsiveness were examined in a double-blind, cross-over study of 19 patients with mild-to-moderate asthma.[12] Both drugs were administered via a hydrofluoroalkane (HFA)-pressurised MDI. Having discontinued their usual inhaled corticosteroid and following 2 weeks' treatment with salmeterol, 50 μg twice daily, and montelukast, 10 mg once daily, patients were randomised to receive either ciclesonide, 200 μg (two inhalations, once daily) or fluticasone propionate, 125 μg (two inhalations, twice daily) for 4 weeks. Participants were also instructed to take placebo formulations at appropriate points throughout the day, so that the overall number of inhalations remained constant between the two treatment groups. No differences were detected between ciclesonide and fluticasone, in terms of methacholine PC_{20}[e] values, expressed as the doubling dose (dd) shift from respective baselines (difference of 0.4 dd; $p>0.05$). In addition, the sequence in which the patients received ciclesonide and fluticasone had no bearing on PC_{20} outcome. No differences between ciclesonide and fluticasone were

[d]The administration of ciclesonide via a dry powder inhaler is currently not licensed.
[e]The provocative dose causing a 20% reduction from baseline FEV_1.

observed for secondary parameters of pulmonary function, including FEV_1 (improvements of 2 and 4% respectively; $p>0.05$). Thus, 4 weeks of once-daily treatment with ciclesonide elicited comparable improvements to twice-daily fluticasone in terms of methacholine-induced hyper-responsiveness in patients with mild-to-moderate persistent asthma.

Effect on serum cortisol

A pooled analysis of data derived from nine phase 1 studies in both healthy and asthmatic populations (n=151), demonstrated that both ciclesonide and des-CIC caused negligible cortisol suppression at doses ranging from 340 to 3600 µg.[13]

The effect of ciclesonide on the circadian rhythm of serum cortisol levels was assessed in 12 healthy male volunteers in a placebo-controlled, cross-over study, with each treatment phase conducted over a 7-day period.[14] Participants were randomised to one of three ciclesonide treatment regimens (800 µg in the morning, 800 µg in the evening or 400 µg twice daily), with at least 7 days between each treatment arm. Twenty-four-hour serum cortisol profiles were measured on the seventh treatment day. Overall, all serum cortisol profiles showed typical circadian rhythms (i.e. peaks at 08:00 hours and troughs observed between 21:00 and 02:00 hours of the following day). The geometric mean of the 24-hour mesor (area under concentration–time curve [$AUC_{0-24\ hours}$]) measured 7.22, 6.75, 7.08 and 6.75 µg/dL for placebo, morning, evening and twice-daily doses, respectively (*p*-values not reported). Cortisol amplitude and acrophase (time of maximum) did not differ significantly between treatment groups (Figure 2). Thus, ciclesonide treatment was judged to have no significant effect on serum cortisol levels, and thus the HPA axis when administered over a 24-hour period.

Ciclesonide treatment was judged to have no significant effect on serum cortisol levels, and thus the HPA axis when administered over a 24-hour period.

Pharmacokinetics

The pharmacokinetic properties of ciclesonide are presented in Table 1.[7,15] The negligible oral bioavailability of ciclesonide, relative to some of the other inhaled corticosteroids, minimises its systemic absorption and consequently enhances its tolerability profile (Figure 3).[3,7] Similarly, the high serum clearance of ciclesonide and its high plasma protein binding, again limits the propensity for associated systemic effects and further improves ciclesonide's safety profile.[7]

The negligible oral bioavailability of ciclesonide minimises its systemic absorption and consequently enhances its tolerability profile.

Ciclesonide is metabolised to its active metabolite, des-CIC, by lung esterases. Further metabolism to hydroxylated inactive metabolites is catalysed by cytochrome P450 (CYP) 3A4. Ciclesonide undergoes almost complete first-pass metabolism in the liver and is therefore undetectable in serum after oral administration.[16]

Ciclesonide can be administered to elderly patients and patients with hepatic or renal impairment without dosage adjustment.[7] A lack of data in children and adolescents under the age of 17 years, currently precludes the use of ciclesonide in younger patient populations.[7]

Figure 2. Mean 24-hour profiles of serum cortisol following 7 days of treatment with ciclesonide (morning, evening or twice-daily administration), or placebo.[14]

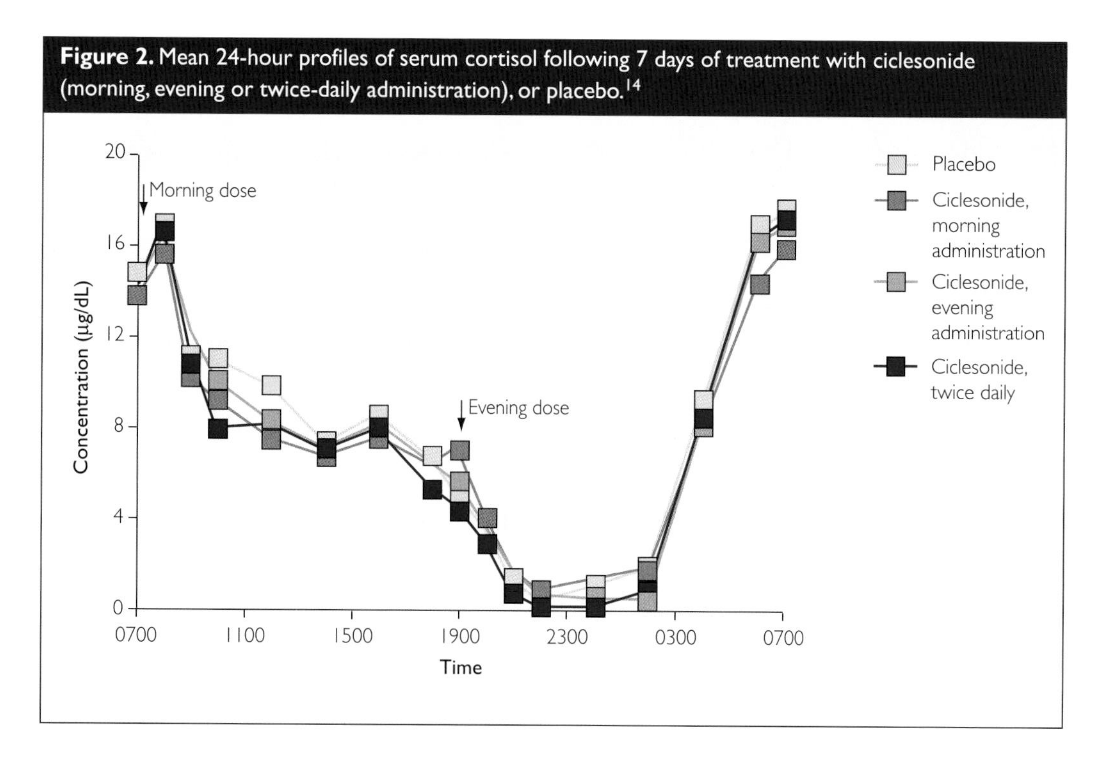

Table 1. The pharmacokinetic properties of ciclesonide.[7,15]

Pharmacokinetic parameter	
Oral bioavailability (%)	<0.5
Systemic bioavailability (%)	
Ciclesonide	18%
des-CIC	50%
Lung deposition (%)	52
Plasma protein binding (%)	99
Volume of distribution (L/kg)	2.9
Total serum clearance (L/hour/kg)	2.0
$t_{1/2}$ (hours)	ciclesonide 0.71
	des-CIC 3.5
Excretion (%)	faeces – 77.9%

des-CIC, C21-desmethylpropionyl-ciclesonide; $t_{1/2}$, elimination half-life.

Drug delivery and deposition

Ciclesonide is delivered in solution form via an HFA-MDI, which demonstrates a linear relationship between different doses, puff strengths and systemic exposure.[7] The use of a spacer device does not appear to alter the pharmacokinetics of ciclesonide or its active metabolite.[17] Approximately 50% of ciclesonide inhaled via an MDI is deposited in the lungs in both healthy and asthmatic individuals.[3,18]

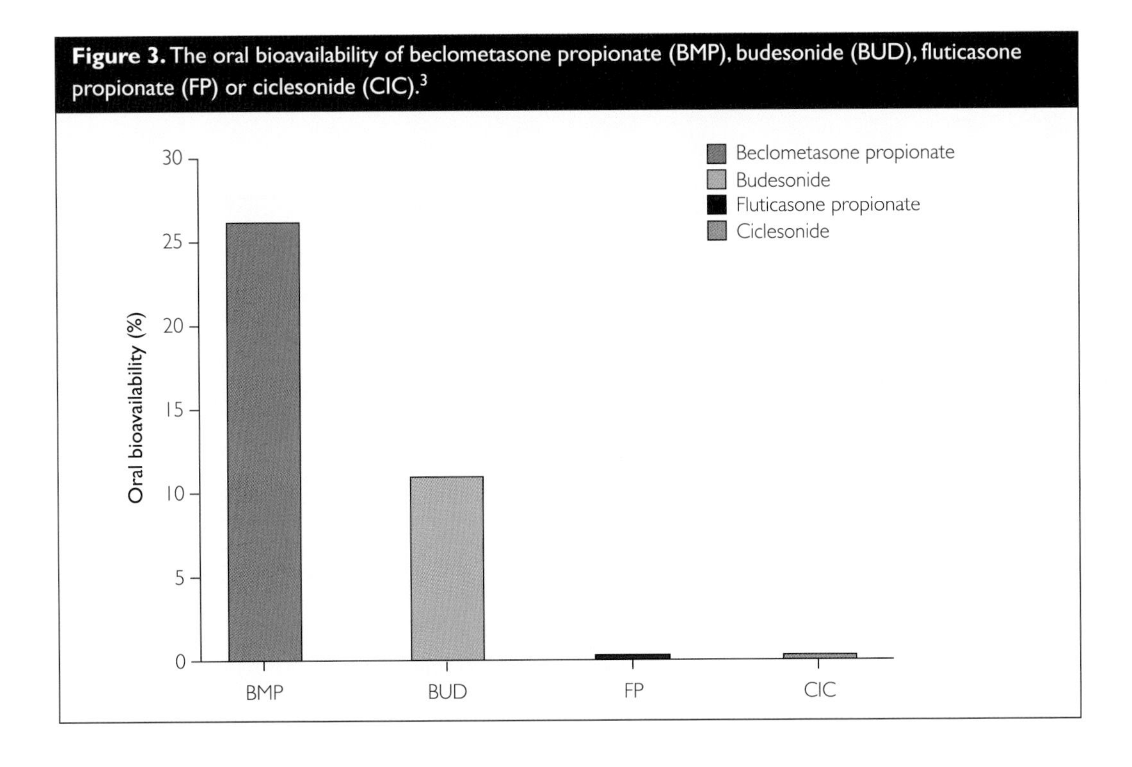

Figure 3. The oral bioavailability of beclometasone propionate (BMP), budesonide (BUD), fluticasone propionate (FP) or ciclesonide (CIC).[3]

52% of the administered dose of ciclesonide reached the lung, 38% of the dose was deposited in the mouth or pharynx, whilst the remainder was exhaled.

An imaging study of eight healthy individuals, used 99m technetium (^{99m}Tc)-labelled ciclesonide (50 µg via MDI) to investigate the pulmonary deposition of ciclesonide.[18] Deposition was assessed using two-dimensional gamma scintigraphy. Overall, 52% of the administered dose of ciclesonide reached the lung, 38% of the dose was deposited in the mouth or pharynx, whilst the remainder was exhaled. Ciclesonide was distributed evenly throughout the lung, with mean depositions of 34, 36 and 30% for the peripheral, middle and central lung regions, respectively.

Dosage

The recommended starting dosage of ciclesonide is 160 µg once daily (the maximum recommended dose).[7] Once asthma control is achieved, the dose of ciclesonide should be individualised and titrated to the minimum dose necessary for adequate asthma control. A daily dose of 80 µg has proved to be an effective maintenance dose in a wide number of patients.[7] Although evening administration of ciclesonide is preferred, this is usually left to the discretion of the physician and the preferences of the individual patient.[7]

Close monitoring is advocated for those patients transferring to ciclesonide after using regular treatment with oral corticosteroids. Oral steroids should be withdrawn gradually; a 1 mg reduction in the daily dose of prednisolone (or its equivalent) is recommended at weekly intervals. During the transfer procedure, the lower systemic steroidal action may result in the emergence of allergic or arthritic symptoms (e.g. rhinitis, eczema, muscle and joint pain) and patients should be made aware of the likelihood of this.

Clinical efficacy

Dosage regimen

The relative efficacies of morning and evening ciclesonide administration were examined in an 8-week double-blind study in 209 adult patients with asthma, characterised by an FEV_1 between 50 and 90% of the predicted normal value.[19] Following a 1–4-week baseline period, patients were randomly allocated to treatment with either a single morning or evening dose of ciclesonide, 200 μg. At baseline, mean FEV_1 was 77% of the predicted normal value and mean reversibility was 23%. The overall difference from baseline in morning peak expiratory flow (PEF) between morning and evening ciclesonide administration groups after 8 weeks, was 27 L/minute ($p<0.05$ between morning and evening groups). The corresponding changes in evening PEF were 7 and 16 L/minute for morning and evening administration, respectively, amounting to a mean difference between treatments of 9 L/minute ($p>0.05$). FEV_1 and forced vital capacity (FVC) improved significantly from baseline in both treatment groups after 8 weeks' treatment (FEV_1 increased by 0.31 L in both groups and FVC increased by 0.19 and 0.22 L for morning and evening administration, respectively; $p\leq0.05$ *vs* baseline). Improvements in asthma symptom scores were also comparable between groups, measuring –0.38 and –0.50 for morning and evening ciclesonide administration, respectively ($p<0.001$ *vs* baseline for both comparisons). The daily use of short-acting β_2-agonist rescue medication declined by the same extent in both treatment groups after 8 weeks (–0.36 inhalations/day; $p\leq0.05$ *vs* baseline). Both dosage regimens were well tolerated and no differences in tolerability were reported between groups. Neither regimen significantly affected mean 24-hour urinary cortisol excretion (differences from baseline of 1.98 and 5.78 nmol/mmol creatinine for morning and evening administration respectively; $p>0.05$ *vs* baseline and between groups).

Thus, ciclesonide significantly improved asthma control – in terms of evening PEF, FEV_1, FVC, asthma symptoms and rescue medication use – regardless of whether it was administered in the morning or in the evening. The improvements in morning PEF were more pronounced following administration of ciclesonide in the evening. Since either regimen is effective, administration time should be selected according to the individual needs and preferences of the patient.

Ciclesonide significantly improved asthma control regardless of whether it was administered in the morning or in the evening.

Comparative studies

The effectiveness of a once-daily ciclesonide treatment regimen was compared with that of twice-daily fluticasone in a double-blind study of 451 adult patients with asthma.[20] All patients had previously been managed on beclometasone, 500 μg/day, or equivalent. All previous treatments were discontinued and participants were randomised to

Once-daily ciclesonide was as effective as twice-daily fluticasone in terms of lung function parameters, asthma symptoms and the use of rescue medication.

receive either ciclesonide, 160 µg once daily, or fluticasone propionate, 88 µg twice daily, for a period of 12 weeks. At baseline, mean FEV_1 measured 2.42 L and mean reversibility was 75%. Both treatment regimens elicited comparable improvements in FEV_1 over the course of the study (Figure 4; $p<0.0001$ *vs* baseline for both comparisons). The improvements in FVC and morning PEF followed similar trends (increases in FVC of 531 and 523 mL; increases in morning PEF of 29 and 36 L/minute; both for ciclesonide and fluticasone, respectively; $p<0.0001$ *vs* baseline for all comparisons). Asthma symptom scores improved by a comparable extent between treatment groups (–0.55 *vs* –0.75 for ciclesonide and fluticasone, respectively; $p<0.0001$ *vs* baseline for both comparisons). Similarly, the overall use of rescue medication (in line with standard clinical practice) decreased significantly following both treatments (–0.9 *vs* –1.25 puffs/day for ciclesonide and fluticasone, respectively; $p<0.0001$ *vs* baseline for both comparisons). Both asthma symptoms and rescue medication use improved within 24 hours of treatment. In summary, once-daily ciclesonide was as effective as twice-daily fluticasone in terms of lung function parameters, asthma symptoms and the use of rescue medication. The improved convenience of the ciclesonide regimen may further enhance patient adherence to therapy.

Figure 4. The time course of the forced expiratory volume in 1 second (FEV_1) over 12 weeks of treatment with either ciclesonide (160 µg once daily) or fluticasone propionate (88 µg twice daily).[20]

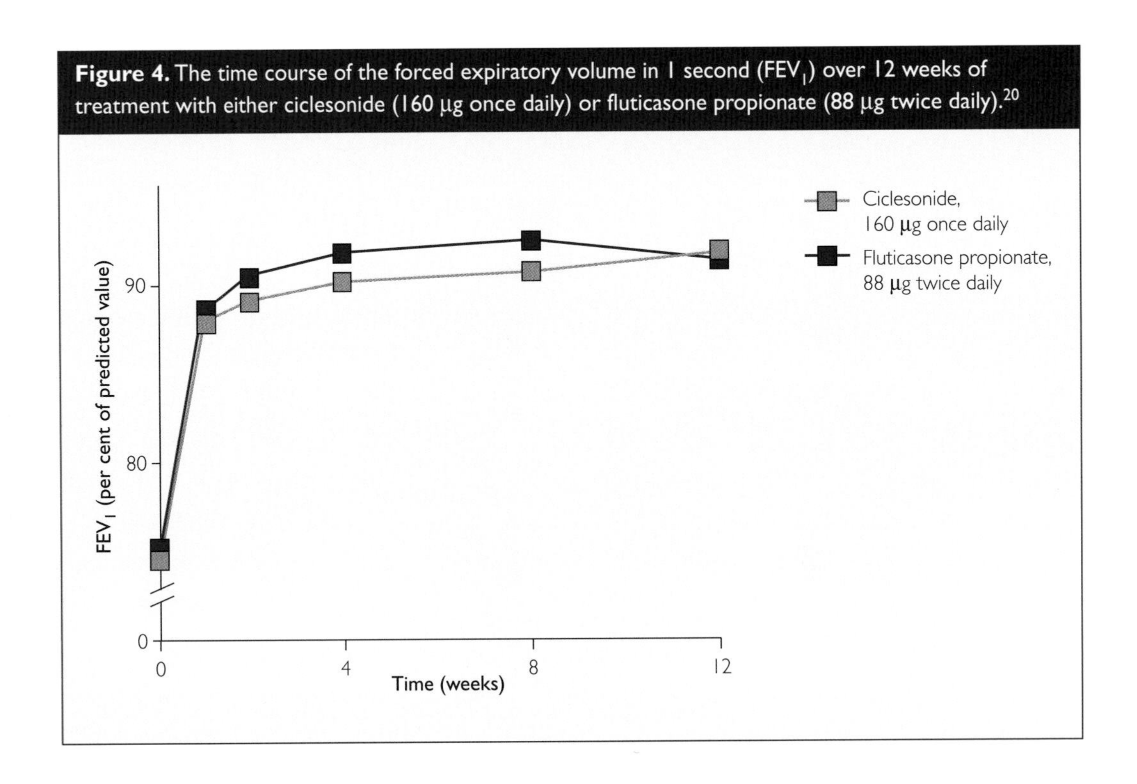

Efficacy in children

The efficacy of ciclesonide was compared with that of fluticasone in a large double-blind study in children and adolescents (n=556) aged between 6 and 15 years (mean age 10 years) with persistent asthma.[21] Following a 2–4-week run-in phase, during which time patients received inhaled salbutamol only, participants were randomised to receive either ciclesonide, 80 µg twice daily, or fluticasone propionate, 88 µg twice daily, for 12 weeks. At baseline, mean FEV_1 was 1.68 L and the majority of participants were considered to have moderate-to-severe asthma. Overall, FEV_1 improved significantly in both treatment groups, such that mean increases of 298 and 297 mL were reported following ciclesonide and fluticasone, respectively ($p<0.0001$ *vs* baseline for both comparisons). The percentage value of the predicted FEV_1 improved from baseline by a similar extent in ciclesonide and fluticasone treatment groups (16 *vs* 12% and 14 *vs* 14% in patients under and over 12 years of age, respectively; *p*-values not reported). Treatment-associated improvements in asthma symptoms and the use of rescue medication (in line with standard clinical practice) are presented in Figure 5 ($p<0.0001$ *vs* baseline for both comparisons). In summary, ciclesonide and fluticasone proved equally effective in the treatment of children with moderate-to-severe persistent asthma.[f]

Figure 5. Changes in asthma symptoms and rescue medication use (puffs per day) following 12 weeks of treatment with either ciclesonide (80 µg twice daily) or fluticasone propionate (88 µg twice daily) in children with persistent asthma.[21]

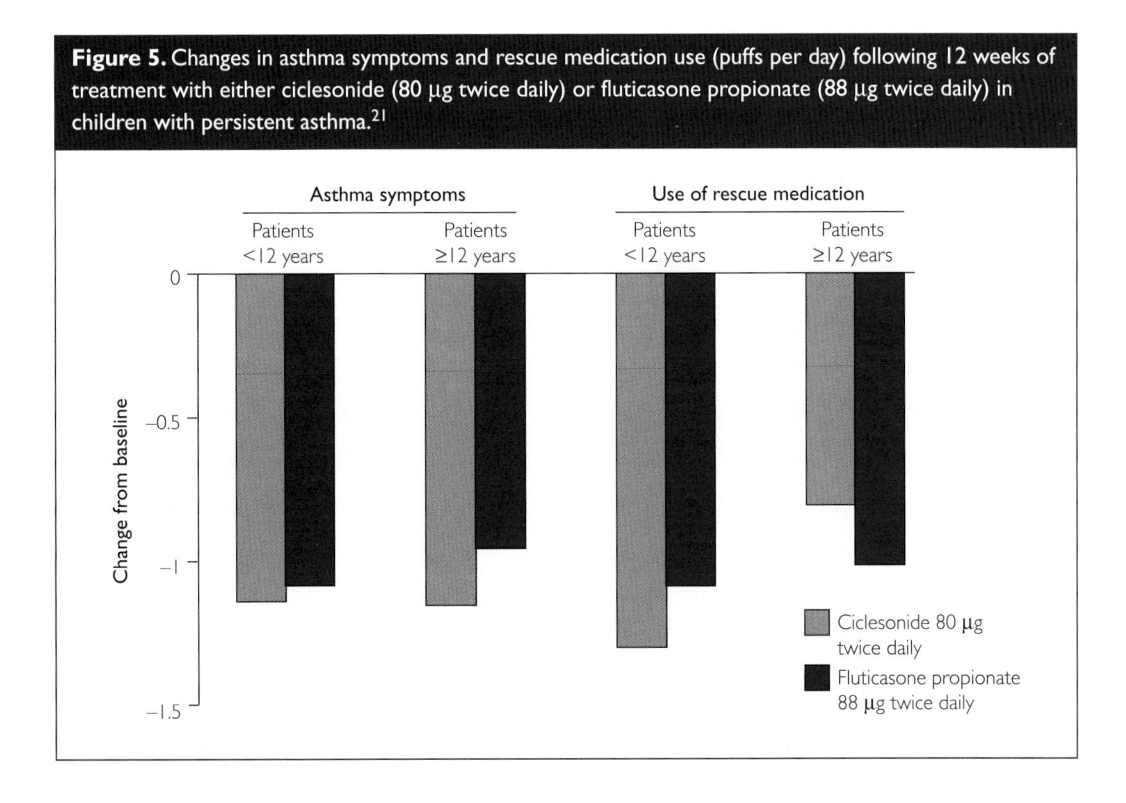

[f]Ciclesonide is currently not licensed for use in children.

You are strongly urged to consult your doctor before taking, stopping or changing any of the products reviewed or referred to in *BESTMEDICINE* or any other medication that has been prescribed or recommended by your doctor.

Safety and tolerability

Although inhaled corticosteroids have considerably fewer systemic effects than their orally delivered equivalents, adverse events have been reported following their regular use.[22] High doses in particular have been associated with an increased risk of adrenal suppression, reduced bone mineral density, glaucoma, cataracts, hoarseness and candidiasis of the mouth or throat.[22] The use of a DPI or a spacer may minimise oropharyngeal deposition, whilst candidiasis responds well to antifungal lozenges without the need to discontinue corticosteroid therapy.[22] Gargling with water or brushing teeth after administration of an inhaled corticosteroid may also limit such effects. As with all inhaled medications, the potential for paradoxical bronchospasm should also be considered when prescribing corticosteroids. Mild bronchospasm may be prevented by inhalation of a short-acting β_2-agonist, or by transfer from an aerosol inhalation to a dry powder inhalation.[7,22]

Data derived from clinical studies of ciclesonide conducted to date, have shown that only 4% of patients, receiving ciclesonide in the dose range 80–1280 μg/day, experienced adverse events and in the majority of cases, these were mild in severity (Table 2).[7]

Effect on cortisol levels

The safety of long-term administration of ciclesonide, up to daily doses of 1280 μg, was determined in an open-label, 40-week extension of a 12-week double-blind trial, in patients with persistent asthma (FEV_1 60–90% of predicted normal value).[23] Prior to enrolment in the double-blind phase, patients had previously been managed with a constant dose of an inhaled corticosteroid, ranging from 400 to 800 μg/day of beclometasone dipropionate, or equivalent. At randomisation, patients (n=329) were allocated to either ciclesonide, 160 μg once daily, ciclesonide, 640 μg twice daily, or placebo for 12 weeks. Those patients

Table 2. The nature and frequency of adverse events reported in clinical trials with ciclesonide (dose range 80–1280 μg/day).[7]

Adverse event	Percentage of patients affected
Common (1–10%)	
Paradoxical bronchospasm	1.0
Uncommon (0.1–1%)	
Hoarseness	0.9
Application site reactions (burning, inflammation, irritation)	0.6
Bad taste	0.4
Application site dryness	0.3
Rash and eczema	0.3
Cough after inhalation	0.3

who completed the double-blind treatment phase or discontinued due to lack of efficacy, entered the open-label phase (n=283) and received ciclesonide, 640 μg once or twice daily, for 4 weeks followed by an individualised dose of ciclesonide for a further 36 weeks. At study endpoint, the mean daily dose of ciclesonide was 776 μg, with 94.7% patients receiving daily doses of between 320 and 1280 μg. The overall incidence of oropharyngeal adverse events was low and included pharyngitis (4%), voice alteration (2%) and oral candidiasis (1%). Urine cortisol increased significantly by 28% over the open-label phase of the study ($p<0.05$ *vs* start of extension). However, the change in serum cortisol over this period was not significant (–4%; $p>0.05$). Neither urine nor serum cortisol altered significantly over the double-blind period of ciclesonide treatment. The authors concluded that long-term treatment with ciclesonide, over a total period of 1 year, was not associated with clinically relevant cortisol suppression, as supported by a lack of systemic side-effects.

Long-term treatment with ciclesonide, over a total period of 1 year, was not associated with clinically relevant cortisol suppression, as supported by a lack of systemic side-effects.

Safety in children

The safety profile of ciclesonide was compared with that of fluticasone propionate in the paediatric study described earlier.[21,24] Patients treated with ciclesonide showed elevated levels of free cortisol in 24-hour urine samples adjusted for creatinine (increase of 1.05 nmol/mmol creatinine *vs* baseline; *p*-value not reported). In contrast, fluticasone-treated patients displayed an average decrease of –1.07 nmol/mmol creatinine ($p=0.0732$ between treatment groups). Those patients with 24-hour creatinine values within the normal range, showed significant treatment-related differences in urine cortisol excretion (+1.5 *vs* –1.75 nmol/mmol creatinine for ciclesonide and fluticasone, respectively; $p=0.0062$ between groups). The overall incidence of adverse events was comparable for both treatment groups. In summary, ciclesonide-treated patients showed no reduction in cortisol levels, in contrast to patients treated with fluticasone.

Ciclesonide-treated patients showed no reduction in cortisol levels, in contrast to patients treated with fluticasone.

Precautions for use

Caution should be observed when administering ciclesonide to patients with active or quiescent pulmonary tuberculosis, fungal or viral infections.[7] Ciclesonide is not indicated for the treatment of *status asthmaticus* or other acute episodes of asthma, or for the relief of acute asthma symptoms.[7] Physicians should advise patients of the risk of adrenal suppression, growth retardation in children, reduced bone mineral density, cataract and glaucoma; all of which are associated with the inhaled corticosteroids. For this reason, treatment should always be maintained at the lowest dose necessary for optimal asthma control.[7] Patients transferring from long-term treatment with oral corticosteroids may remain at risk of adverse events relating to impaired adrenal reserves, for some time following transfer.[7] Oral steroid withdrawal may also unmask allergies that were previously controlled (e.g. allergic rhinitis, eczema), and patients should be made aware of this possibility.[7]

Drug interactions

The propensity for clinically relevant drug–drug interactions associated with ciclesonide treatment is minimal, since serum levels of ciclesonide and its active metabolite remain characteristically low. However, in view of its metabolic pathway, the co-administration of ciclesonide with potent inhibitors of CYP3A4 isoenzyme (e.g. ketoconazole and ritonavir) should be undertaken with caution.

Key points

- Ciclesonide is an inhaled corticosteroid that is indicated for the prophylactic treatment of asthma in adults aged 18 years and over.
- The recommended starting dosage of ciclesonide is 160 μg once daily, which is also the maximum recommended daily dose. Patients can be titrated down to a lower maintenance dose of 80 μg once asthma control is achieved.
- As a soft-steroid, ciclesonide is converted by esterases in the lung into its active metabolite, des-CIC.
- Des-CIC shows high affinity for glucocorticoid receptors, low oral and high pulmonary bioavailability, and rapid systemic clearance.
- In animal models of inflammation, ciclesonide reduced lymphocyte activation, eosinophil accumulation, granuloma formation and thymus involution.
- In humans with asthma, ciclesonide decreased the severity of the early and late phase immune responses to allergen challenge, and lowered airway hyper-responsiveness to AMP and methacholine.
- Following inhalation via an MDI, ciclesonide is distributed evenly throughout the lung.
- In controlled clinical trials of up to 12 weeks' duration, ciclesonide elicited similar improvements in lung function, asthma symptoms and use of β_2-agonist rescue medication to fluticasone propionate, both in adults and children with persistent asthma.
- Ciclesonide treatment has not been associated with any clinically relevant alterations in serum cortisol production.

References

A list of the published evidence which has been reviewed in compiling the preceding section of *BESTMEDICINE.*

1. Scottish Intercollegiate Guidelines Network and the British Thoracic Society. British Guidelines on the Management of Asthma. SIGN, Edinburgh, 2004.
2. Hanania N, Chapman K, Kesten S. Adverse effects of inhaled corticosteroids. *Am J Med* 1995; **98**: 196–208.
3. Derendorf H. Relevant pharmacokinetic parameters for determining efficacy and safety in inhaled corticosteroids. *Eur Respir Rev* 2004; **13**: 62–5.
4. Bodor N, Buchwald P. Soft drug design: general principles and recent applications. *Med Res Rev* 2000; **20**: 58–101.
5. Szelenyi I, Hochhaus G, Heer S *et al.* Loteprednol etabonate: a soft steroid for the treatment of allergic diseases of the airways. *Drugs Today* 2004; **36**: 313–20.
6. Belvisi M, Hele D. Soft steroids: a new approach to the treatment of inflammatory airways diseases. *Pulm Pharmacol Ther* 2003; **16**: 321–5.
7. Altana Pharma AG. Alvesco® 80 (ciclesonide). *Summary of product characteristics.* Konstanz, Germany, 2004.
8. Belvisi M. Preclinical pharmacology of ciclesonide. *Eur Respir Rev* 2004; **13**: 66–8.
9. Stoeck M, Riedel R, Hochhaus G *et al. In vitro* and *in vivo* anti-inflammatory activity of the new glucocorticoid ciclesonide. *J Pharmacol Exp Ther* 2004; **309**: 249–58.
10. Larsen B, Nielsen L, Engelstatter R, Steinijans V, Dahl R. Effect of ciclesonide on allergen challenge in subjects with bronchial asthma. *Allergy* 2003; **58**: 207–12.
11. Taylor D, Jensen M, Kanabar V *et al.* A dose-dependent effect of the novel inhaled corticosteroid ciclesonide on airway responsiveness to adenosine-5'-monophosphate in asthmatic patients. *Am J Respir Crit Care Med* 1999; **160**: 237–43.
12. Lee D, Haggart K, Currie G, Bates C, Lipworth B. Effects of hydrofluoroalkane formulations of ciclesonide 400 microg once daily vs fluticasone 250 microg twice daily on methacholine hyper-responsiveness in mild-to-moderate persistent asthma. *Br J Clin Pharmacol* 2004; **58**: 26–33.
13. Rohatagi S, Arya V, Zech K *et al.* Population pharmacokinetics and pharmacodynamics of ciclesonide. *J Clin Pharmacol* 2003; **43**: 365–78.
14. Weinbrenner A, Huneke D, Zschiesche M *et al.* Circadian rhythm of serum cortisol after repeated inhalation of the new topical steroid ciclesonide. *J Clin Endocrinol Metab* 2002; **87**: 2160–3.
15. Reynolds N, Scott L. Ciclesonide. *Drugs* 2004; **64**: 511–19.
16. Nave R, Bethke T, van Marle S, Zech K. Pharmacokinetics of [14C]ciclesonide after oral and intravenous administration to healthy subjects. *Clin Pharmacokinet.* 2004; **43**: 479–86.
17. Nave R, Baumgartner E, Bethke T, Steinijans V, Drollmann A. Equivalent pharmacokinetics of the active metabolite of ciclesonide when using the ciclesonide-MDI with and without a spacer. *14th Annual Congress of the European Respiratory Society. Glasgow, Scotland,* 2004.
18. Bethke T, Boudreau R, Hasselquist B *et al.* High lung deposition of ciclesonide in 2D and 3D imaging. *12th Annual Congress of the European Respiratory Society. Stockholm, Sweden,* 2002.
19. Postma D, Sevette C, Martinat Y *et al.* Treatment of asthma by the inhaled corticosteroid ciclesonide given either in the morning or evening. *Eur Respir J* 2001; **17**: 1083–8.
20. Buhl R, Vinkler I, Magyar P *et al.* Once daily ciclesonide and twice daily fluticasone propionate are equally effective in the treatment of patients with asthma. *14th Annual Congress of the European Respiratory Society.* Glasgow, United Kingdom, 2004.
21. Pedersen S, Garcia Garcia M, Manjra A *et al.* Ciclesonide and fluticasone propionate show comparable efficacy in children and adolescents with asthma. 14th Annual Congress of the European Respiratory Society. Glasgow, United Kingdom, 2004.
22. *British National Formulary (BNF) 48.* London: British Medical Association and Royal Pharmaceutical Society of Great Britain. September, 2004.
23. Chapman K, Boulet L, D'Urzo A, Oedekoven C, Engelstatter R. Long-term administration of ciclesonide is safe and well tolerated in patients with persistent asthma. *4th Triennial World Asthma Meeting. Bangkok, Thailand,* 2004.
24. Pedersen S, Gyurkovits K, von Delft K, Boss H, Engelstatter R. Safety profile of ciclesonide as compared with fluticasone propionate in the treatment of children and adolescents with asthma. *14th Annual Congress of the European Respiratory Society.* Glasgow, Scotland, 2004.

Acknowledgements

Figure 2 is adapted from Weinbrenner *et al.,* 2002.[14]

Figure 3 is adapted from Derendorf, 2004.[3]

Figure 4 is adapted from Buhl *et al.,* 2004.[20]

Figure 5 is adapted from Pedersen *et al.,* 2004.[21]

5. Drug review – Fluticasone (Flixotide®)

Dr Anna Palmer
CSF Medical Communications Ltd

You are strongly urged to consult your doctor before taking, stopping or changing any of the products reviewed or referred to in *BESTMEDICINE* or any other medication that has been prescribed or recommended by your doctor.

Summary

Fluticasone propionate (hereafter referred to as fluticasone) is a potent inhaled corticosteroid indicated for the maintenance treatment of asthma. Fluticasone appears to be effective at much lower doses than other commonly used inhaled corticosteroids and has the advantage of a low oral bioavailability. Fluticasone, administered at doses as low as 100 µg twice daily, has been shown to improve peak expiratory flow (PEF), forced expiratory volume in 1 second (FEV_1) and also reduces symptom scores, use of rescue bronchodilator therapy and the incidence of disturbed nights, in both children (aged 4–11 years) and adults. Fluticasone appears to be more effective when it is administered in a twice-daily, rather than a once-daily regimen. Improvements in lung function, after twice-daily fluticasone, are observed rapidly and as early as the first day after initiation of treatment although maximal benefits are not observed until at least two weeks of treatment. The maximum recommended dose of fluticasone (1000 µg/day, twice daily) is also effective in improving lung function in patients with more severe asthma. Fluticasone is available for administration via a dry powder inhaler (DPI) or when formulated with aerosols for delivery by a metered dose inhaler (MDI). Both formulations are equally effective and well tolerated. Comparative studies have demonstrated that fluticasone has enhanced efficacy in improving lung function than older inhaled corticosteroids such as beclometasone dipropionate (hereafter referred to as beclometasone) and budesonide. Fluticasone is also more effective than the oral agents, theophylline, montelukast and zafirlukast in the treatment of mild-to-moderate asthma. Treatment with fluticasone is generally well tolerated and at low doses (<200 µg/day in children or <800 µg/day in adults) is rarely associated with clinically significant effects upon adrenal function, bone mineral density or linear growth rates in children.

Introduction

Corticosteroids are widely regarded as the most effective anti-inflammatory agents for the treatment of the underlying symptoms of asthma. This is reflected in treatment guidelines that recommend inhaled corticosteroids as the preferred preventer therapy for the maintenance treatment of asthma.[1] UK guidelines on the management of asthma recommend that daily corticosteroid preventer therapy should be initiated in all patients requiring β_2-agonist bronchodilator therapy more frequently than once per day.[1] Fluticasone is a highly potent, inhaled glucocorticoid with negligible oral bioavailability and a high therapeutic index.[2] In addition to its use as an inhaled asthma therapy, fluticasone is also available in topical formulations for the treatment of skin disorders and as nasal droplets for the relief of allergic rhinitis. Fluticasone is indicated for the preventative treatment of asthma of all severities and is available both as dry powder formulation and as an aerosol for delivery by an MDI. Fluticasone is recommended for administration in a twice-daily regimen, with an initial recommended dose in adults (aged over 16 years) of 200–500 μg/day up to a maximum total daily dose of 2000 μg/day, given according to the severity of asthma symptoms. The recommended starting dose in children aged 4–16 years, is 100–200 μg/day, with a maximum daily dose of 400 μg.[3]

Pharmacology

Chemistry

☛ *The chemistry of fluticasone is of essentially academic interest and most healthcare professionals will, like you, skip this section.*

The structure of all corticosteroids is based upon the structure of cortisol, with appropriate chemical modifications made on the basis of structure–function relationships (Figure 1).[4] Fluticasone was developed specifically in an attempt to identify a corticosteroid that exhibited improved potency and airway selectivity, with minimal systemic effects. Fluticasone's structure ensures a combination of high lipophilicity (to aid rapid cell entry and binding to glucocorticoid receptors) with rapid clearance (to minimise systemic side-effects).

Mechanism of action

Corticosteroids exert their effects through their interaction with glucocorticoid receptors located within the cell cytoplasm of many different cell types (Figure 2).[2] The glucocorticoid receptor exists in an inactive state bound to chaperone proteins called heat shock proteins that dissociate once the agonist (i.e. fluticasone) binds. The activated receptor–agonist complex then dimerises and the homodimer complex translocates to the nucleus where it binds to DNA sequences known as glucocorticoid response elements. Binding of the complex to positive glucocorticoid response elements activates gene transcription and initiates a variety of other events including the up-regulation of β_2-adrenoceptors. Conversely, when the complex binds to negative glucocorticoid response elements or interacts directly with nuclear transcription factors (e.g. nuclear factor κB, nuclear factor of activated

Figure 1. Chemical structures of cortisol, dexamethasone, triamcinolone, beclometasone and fluticasone.

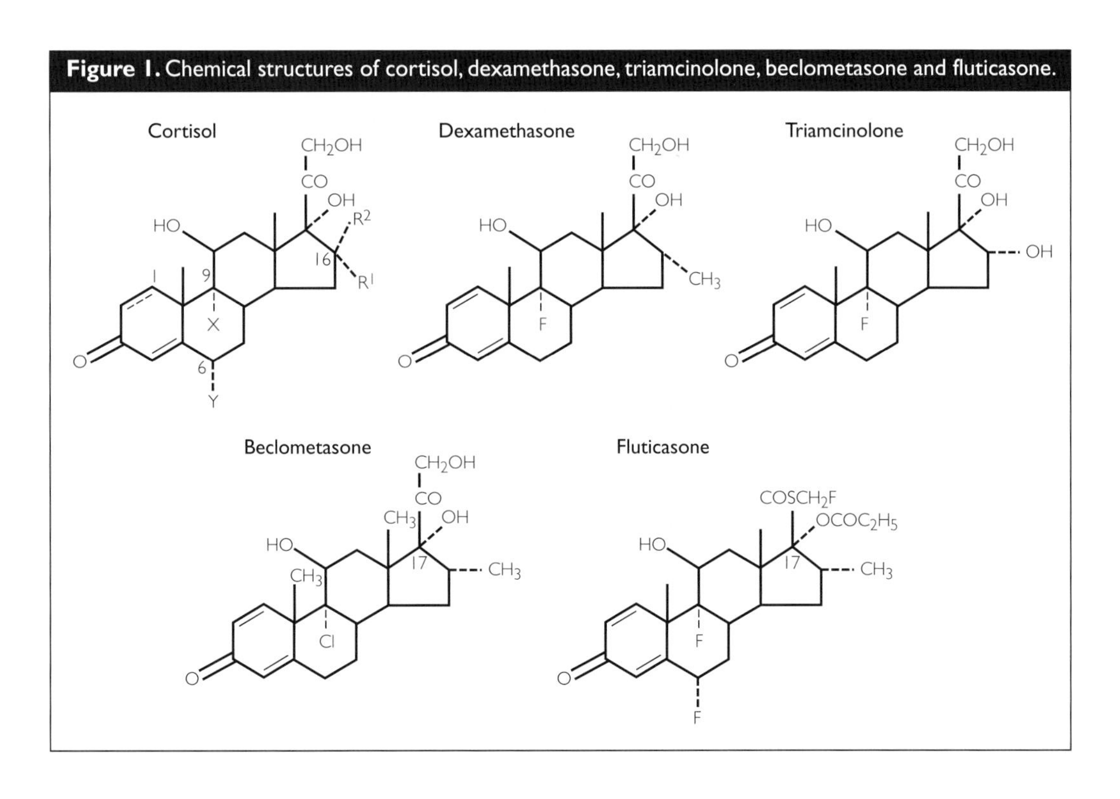

Figure 2. Interaction of glucocorticoids (GC) such as fluticasone, with glucocorticoid receptor (GR). HSP, heat shock protein; GRE, glucocorticoid response element; NFκB, nuclear factor κB; NF-AT, nuclear factor of activated T-cells; AP-1, activator protein-1.[2]

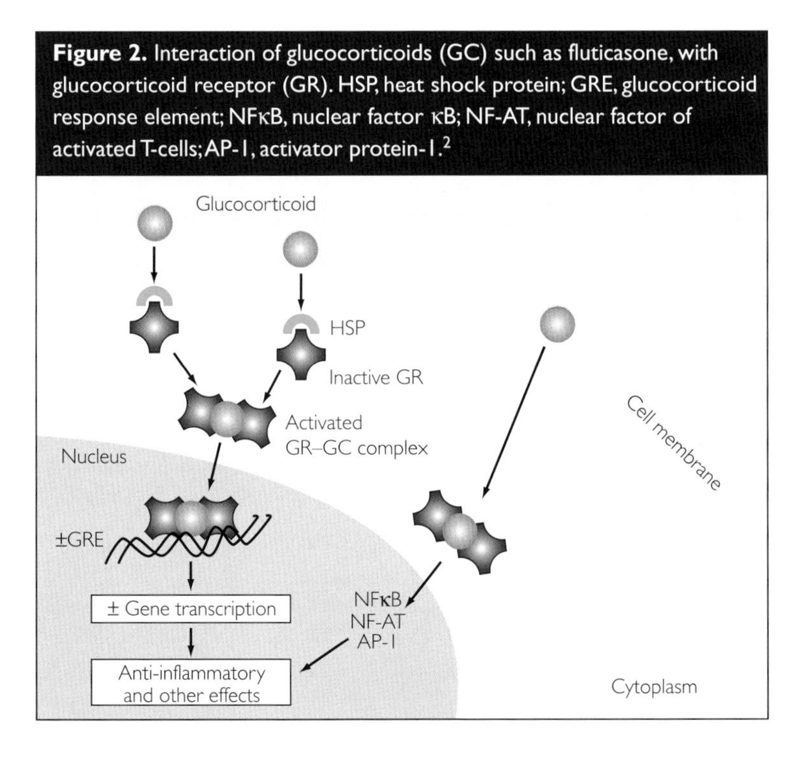

T cells or activator protein-1) gene transcription is suppressed. The sum effect of these interactions is an anti-inflammatory response. These mechanisms also account for the associated adverse effects of corticosteroids upon metabolism (e.g. glucose intolerance) and arterial hypertension.[2] In addition to these genomic effects, there is some evidence for more rapid and direct effects of the glucocorticoids, which involve either binding to plasma membrane receptors or a direct steroid–membrane interaction without glucocorticoid receptor involvement.[2]

Potency and selectivity

Fluticasone has also been shown to have the greatest degree of binding to lung tissue in comparison with beclometasone, budesonide, flunisolide and hydrocortisone.

Fluticasone has a significantly higher therapeutic index than that of beclometasone or flucinolone acetonide (91 *vs* 0.4 and 1.0 respectively). Thus, in comparison with these older-generation corticosteroids, this would predict a greater potency and a lower potential for side-effects with fluticasone. In addition, fluticasone is also highly lipophilic (e.g. >1000 times higher lipophilicity than triamcinolone acetonide [hereafter referred to as triamcinolone]), which promotes its entry into cells and allows rapid binding to glucocorticoid receptors.[5] This property also helps to increase deposition in the lung and aids retention in lung tissue, since it is only slowly released from the lung compartment.[4] Fluticasone has also been shown to have the greatest degree of binding to lung tissue in comparison with beclometasone, budesonide, flunisolide and hydrocortisone.[6]

Fluticasone has a high affinity for human lung glucocorticoid receptors (0.5 nmol/L), which is ten-fold higher than that for triamcinolone and three-fold higher than that for budesonide.[4] In addition to its high affinity, fluticasone also exhibits high selectivity for the receptor together with fast association and slow dissociation rates. These factors are likely to mediate a high degree of binding to, and retention within, lung tissue, and also accounts for its relatively long terminal elimination half-life.[6]

Pharmacokinetics

Absorption and distribution

Steady state concentrations are achieved within 1 week of twice-daily treatment with either 100 or 500 μg doses of inhaled fluticasone. The maximum plasma concentration (C_{max}) of fluticasone at the higher dose was 0.096 μg/L, but was undetectable with the 100 μg dose.[7] Inhaled fluticasone is highly protein bound (90%), with only the unbound portion of the drug available for interaction with the glucocorticoid receptor. Fluticasone also has a high volume of distribution (4.2 L/kg).[2] Systemic exposure to fluticasone occurs either as a result of its absorption after inhalation in the lungs or from oral absorption after a portion of the administered dose is inadvertently swallowed. The high rate of metabolism of fluticasone ensures a low oral systemic bioavailability of less than 1% and absolute bioavailability ranging from 15% with the dry powder formulation to 29% when delivered from an MDI.[5,8] Studies have shown that it is the inhaled portion of fluticasone rather than the swallowed fraction that leads to the greatest systemic exposure.[8]

Metabolism and elimination

Fluticasone has an extended elimination half-life ($t_{1/2}$) in plasma. The $t_{1/2}$ of the fluticasone–glucocorticoid receptor complex exceeds 10 hours, compared with 3.5, 4.0, 5.0, and 7.5 hours for the receptor interactions with flunisolide, triamcinolone, budesonide and beclometasone, respectively.[4] After inhalation of a single 1000 μg dose of fluticasone, the $t_{1/2}$ was reported as 14.4 hours. This dropped to 11.1 hours after twice-daily dosing of 1000 μg for 7 days.[8] Fluticasone undergoes complete (>99%) first-pass metabolism in the liver to the 17β-carboxylic acid. This metabolite has negligible pharmacologic activity and a low receptor binding affinity.[4] Fluticasone undergoes oxidative metabolism via cytochrome P450 (CYP) 3A4 in the gut and liver, whilst renal clearance accounts for less than 0.02% of total fluticasone elimination.[8]

In summary, fluticasone has a favourable pharmacological profile, including:

- a high degree of lipophilicity
- a high receptor affinity for the glucocorticoid receptor
- fast association/slow dissociation from the glucocorticoid receptor
- a high degree of deposition and retention in lung tissue
- a long elimination half-life
- minimal systemic bioavailablity
- a high therapeutic index.

Anti-inflammatory effects of fluticasone

The anti-inflammatory actions of corticosteroids in asthma relate to direct inhibition of cells involved in the inflammatory process (i.e. mast cells, eosinophils, basophils and lymphocytes), and to the inhibition of inflammatory mediators produced by these cells (i.e. histamine, leukotrienes and cytokines).[5] *In vitro* studies have shown that fluticasone is the most potent of a range of corticosteroids in combating inflammation in various human inflammatory cell system (Table 1).[4]

Fluticasone is the most potent of a range of corticosteroids in combating inflammation in various human inflammatory cell systems.

Further *in vivo* evidence has shown that 2-month treatment with inhaled fluticasone (1000 μg, twice daily) reduced the numbers of mast cells (by 80.2%), eosinophils (by 93.6%) and T cells (by an average of 86.5%) in bronchial biopsy specimens.[4] Fluticasone also effectively inhibited the release of interleukin (IL)-5 from stimulated CD4+ lymphocytes isolated from the peripheral blood of healthy volunteers (Table 1).[4,5] In addition, fluticasone (500 μg twice daily for 8 weeks) decreased bronchoalveolar lavage levels of metalloproteinase and increased levels of tissue inhibitors of the matrix metalloproteinases. Both factors have been implicated in matrix protein deposition and basement membrane thickening.[4] This implies a potential role of fluticasone in attenuating both inflammation and airway remodelling.

Table 1. Corticosteroid-induced inhibition of human inflammatory cells.[4]

Corticosteroid	IC_{50} (nmol/L)			
	IL-5 release from T cells	T-cell proliferation	Histamine release from basophils	Eosinophil apoptosis
Beclometasone dipropionate	7.7	10.0	1.0	138.7
Triamcinolone acetonide	9.8	1.0	20.0	23.8
Budesonide	1.7	0.2	0.6	8.5
Mometasone furoate	0.3	N/D	0.3	N/D
Fluticasone propionate	0.2	0.05	0.03	1.7

IL, interleukin; N/D, not determined.

Overall, fluticasone effectively inhibits T-cell proliferation, cytokine release (including IL-1β, IL-4, IL-6, IL-8, tumour necrosis factor [TNF]-α), adhesion molecule expression (such as E-selectin and vascular cell adhesion molecule), and promotes apoptosis of eosinophils and endogenous anti-inflammatory mechanisms (e.g. production of secretory leucocyte protease inhibitor).[6]

Clinical efficacy

Placebo-controlled studies

Dose-ranging studies

Dose-ranging studies are particularly important to ensure that the optimum dose of a drug can be determined in order that benefit can be realised with the least risk of side-effects.

The high therapeutic index of fluticasone and its resulting high potency in comparison with other inhaled glucocorticoids ensures that it is clinically effective at low doses.[5,6] Many *in vivo* and *in vitro* studies examining the anti-inflammatory properties of fluticasone have shown clear dose-dependent effects, yet the data derived from clinical trials has produced less convincing evidence for dose–response relationships between fluticasone and clinical efficacy.[9–12]

A group of 304 patients with moderately severe asthma (mean 65% of the predicted FEV_1) were switched from their current inhaled corticosteroid therapy to fluticasone (100, 250 or 500 μg twice daily), or placebo, for 12 weeks.[9] In patients receiving placebo, the mean FEV_1 decreased by 0.31 L from baseline. This contrasted with increases in mean FEV_1 of 0.39, 0.30 and 0.43 L in patients receiving fluticasone, 100, 250 and 500 μg twice daily, respectively (all comparisons $p<0.001$ *vs* placebo; no difference between doses). Mean PEF was also improved in fluticasone-treated patients (an increase of 16–31 L/minute) compared with placebo (PEF fell by 9 L/minute, $p<0.05$). Greater improvements in morning PEF were observed with the 100 μg dose of fluticasone (25 L/minute) compared with fluticasone 250 μg (16 L/minute; $p<0.05$). No other dose-related differences were reported with respect to any of the other parameters examined, including physician-rated efficacy, symptom scores, rescue medication and night-time awakenings. The doses of fluticasone examined in this study were not associated with any suppression of the hypothalamic–pituitary–adrenal axis, as assessed by morning cortisol measurements.[9] Thus, in conclusion, there were no dose-related therapeutic or adverse safety effects of fluticasone in the treatment of moderate asthma when administered over 12 weeks. A lack of a dose effect was reported in a further study of similar design, which examined lower doses of fluticasone (50, 100 and 250 μg, twice daily) in 342 moderately asthmatic patients.[13]

Two meta-analyses have been performed, which have specifically examined the dose–response relationship of inhaled fluticasone in patients over 12 years with asthma ranging from mild to severe.[11,12] The earliest of these analyses comprised eight placebo-controlled, randomised clinical trials conducted in 2324 patients who were taking fluticasone twice daily at doses ranging from 50 to 1000 μg/day.[12] From these combined data, the authors determined that 80% of the benefit derived from the maximum daily dose of fluticasone (1000 μg) was achieved at doses between 70 and 170 μg/day, with 90% of maximum benefit achieved with doses between 100 and 250 μg/day, depending on the outcome measure evaluated (Table 2). Thus, the effects of fluticasone appear to plateau around the 100–200 μg/day dose range, whilst there is no evidence for further clinical benefit with doses above 200 μg/day.

Fluticasone doses greater than 200 μg provided little additional clinical benefit.

A later meta-analysis was performed with the objective of providing further data on higher doses of fluticasone (>500 μg/day) and was conducted in 2431 patients with moderate-to-severe asthma enrolled into seven controlled clinical studies.[11] The conclusions from this analysis were in accord with those previously reported, with fluticasone doses greater than 200 μg/day providing little additional clinical benefit. There were a number of non-significant trends towards increases in PEF, FEV_1, decreases in rescue bronchodilator therapy, and a decrease in discontinuations from treatment amongst patients treated with fluticasone doses above 500 μg/day, though these trends were not statistically different from the lower dose (200 μg/day).[11]

Table 2. Doses of fluticasone at which 80 and 90% of the maximum effect was achieved in dose-ranging studies.[12] NB. The effect obtained with fluticasone, 1000 μg/day was taken as the 'maximum effect'.

Outcome measure	Dose at which 80% of the maximum effect was achieved (μg/day)	Dose at which 90% of the maximum effect was achieved (μg/day)
FEV_1	146	209
Morning PEF	172	247
Evening PEF	175	251
Use of rescue medication	71	102
Major exacerbations	108	155
Night-time awakenings	135	193

FEV_1, forced expiratory volume in 1 second; PEF, peak expiratory flow.

In patients with mild or moderate asthma it is likely that a lower dose of fluticasone is sufficient for complete control of symptoms and thus no dose effect is evident. The maximal recommended dose of fluticasone is 2000 μg/day and it is possible that a dose effect of fluticasone will be more apparent in those with more severe disease. Several clinical trials have evaluated higher doses of fluticasone, particularly in comparison with other inhaled corticosteroids in those with severe asthma.[14–16] One of these studies compared two doses of fluticasone (1000 and 2000 μg/day, given twice-daily via an MDI; n=450) and indicated an enhanced effect of fluticasone, 2000 μg, in increasing morning and evening PEF (24 and 18 L/minute, respectively) compared with the lower dose (21 and 11 L/minute, respectively).[14] This pattern was also repeated with regard to FEV_1 and FVC, though differences in symptom scores or the use of rescue medication were not consistently observed between the two doses.

In summary, despite isolated reports to the contrary,[10] the balance of evidence does not indicate any consistent dose-dependency of fluticasone, particularly in mild-to-moderate asthma.[9,11–13,17,18] In addition, the majority of the effects of fluticasone are achieved at doses between 150 and 250 μg/day (administered twice daily) with higher doses conferring minimal additional clinical benefit. These data are also consistent with British Thoracic Society (BTS) guidelines for the control of asthma that remains uncontrolled with low-dose inhaled corticosteroids (i.e. fluticasone at 200–500 μg/day). Thus, these data suggest that, in patients with moderate-to-severe asthma, it is probably more beneficial to add a long-acting β_2-agonist to a patient's treatment regimen than it is to adjust the dose of fluticasone above 500 μg/day.[11] However, there is some evidence suggesting that the maximal dose of fluticasone (2000 μg/day) may be of benefit in patients suffering from more severe asthma.[14,16,19]

The balance of evidence does not indicate any consistent dose-dependency of fluticasone, particularly in mild-to-moderate asthma.

Dose frequency

A number of studies have been performed to determine whether fluticasone is equally effective when administered once daily, rather than twice daily.[20,21] Given the relatively long elimination half-life of fluticasone (11–15 hours), it is perhaps not unreasonable to suggest that a simpler, once-daily dosing regimen may be more appropriate for patients with asthma.[8] Fluticasone, 250 μg, administered twice daily, was compared with a 500 μg once-daily dose in a group of moderately asthmatic patients (n=256, aged >12 years; mean FEV_1 67% of the predicted normal).[21] Patients were randomised to active treatment or placebo for an initial 12-week double-blind treatment phase. Following this, all patients were then re-randomised to receive either once- or twice-daily fluticasone for a subsequent 54-week open-label extension.[21]

During the initial 12-week phase, both fluticasone treatment regimens resulted in significant improvements in FEV_1 and morning and evening PEF, together with decreases in asthma symptom scores, frequency of salbutamol use and night-time awakenings, compared with placebo (all comparisons $p<0.001$ *vs* placebo). Comparison of different dosing regimens demonstrated that twice-daily administration was superior to once-daily dosing, with significantly greater improvements observed in FEV_1 together with significant decreases in salbutamol use and treatment discontinuations due to lack of efficacy. The percentage of patients with at least a 0.25 L improvement in FEV_1 was 45% in the once-daily, and 64% in the twice-daily fluticasone groups ($p<0.05$). The efficacy of fluticasone compared with placebo was maintained in the 54-week open-label phase, but the differences between the two dosing regimens of fluticasone did not persist. In fact, the only significant difference between the two doses that remained was the number of symptom-free days, which was actually lowest in patients treated with the once-daily regimen.[21]

A study of similar design was conducted in 252 children (aged 4–11 years with mild-to-moderate asthma; mean FEV_1 71% of the predicted normal) who were given either 100 μg twice-daily or 200 μg once-daily doses of fluticasone, or placebo.[22] Patients receiving placebo, fluticasone once daily, and fluticasone twice daily in the double-blind phase were then switched to either fluticasone once- or twice-daily to provide six distinct treatment groups over the 52-week open-label phase of the study. During double-blind treatment, both fluticasone treatment regimens improved lung function compared with placebo ($p<0.05$). However, twice-daily fluticasone provided consistently greater improvements than once-daily treatment, though statistical significance was achieved between groups only in terms of the percentage predicted FEV_1 (change of 12.2 *vs* 6.5% for twice- and once daily treatment, respectively; $p<0.05$). Data from the open-label phase of this study revealed that the patients who were switched from placebo to fluticasone demonstrated greater improvements when they were switched to twice-daily rather than once-daily treatment (improvements over 1 year: FEV_1 40 *vs* 30%; morning PEF 37 *vs* 30%). However, no statistical analysis was performed on data from the open-label phase of this trial due to the small patient numbers (19–34) in each group. The mean change in FEV_1 was also greater in those patients switched from once-daily to twice-daily fluticasone (24%) compared with those switched from twice daily to once-daily fluticasone (10%) during the open-label phase. Mean change in morning clinic PEF was also slightly greater in the twice-daily group (25%) compared with the once-daily group (20%).

Thus, in conclusion, the balance of data would appear to support a greater efficacy of twice-daily dosing, rather than a once-daily dose of fluticasone in moderately asthmatic children and adults.[20–22]

The balance of data supports a greater efficacy of twice-daily dosing, rather than a once-daily dose of fluticasone in moderately asthmatic children and adults.

Onset of action

A large-scale, randomised, double-blind, placebo-controlled, 8–12-week long study was performed in 1461 corticosteroid-naïve adults (aged >12 years) with an FEV_1 of 40–90% of the predicted normal value at baseline.[18] The primary objective of this study was to determine the time to onset of fluticasone's effect (25–500 μg twice daily).

Fluticasone has a rapid onset of action, and patients should begin to experience improvement in symptoms and lung function between 1 and 7 days from the start of treatment.

A significant improvement in both PEF and FEV_1 from baseline was observed as early as the first day of treatment. The time to reach 50% of the maximum observed effect in PEF and FEV_1 was 5–7 days, whilst the time to reach 90% of the maximum observed effect was approximately 3 weeks. Symptom scores and use of rescue salbutamol reached 50% of their maximum observed effect in 1 and 2 days, respectively, whilst 90% of the greatest observed effect was reached within 2 weeks.[18] It should be noted that although the greatest improvement in most efficacy parameters is observed within the first few weeks of treatment, smaller improvements often continue over the course of several months. This is illustrated in longer term studies where morning PEF continues to improve through weeks 4 to 24 in one study (Figure 3) and from weeks 16 to 52 in another (Figure 4), whilst in a budesonide study airway hyper-responsiveness continued to improve until study end at 72 weeks.[23–25] In summary, fluticasone has a rapid onset of action, and patients should begin to experience improvement in symptoms and lung function between 1 and 7 days from the start of treatment, with smaller improvements continuing to occur with long-term regular treatment.

Asthma severity

A secondary objective of the aforementioned study[18] was to examine if there were any differential effects of fluticasone in subgroups of patients stratified according to the severity of their asthma, defined as follows:

- mild (PEF/FEV_1 >80% predicted best; diurnal variation in PEF <20%)
- moderate (PEF/FEV_1 60–80% predicted best; diurnal variation PEF 20–30%)
- severe (PEF/FEV_1 ≤60% predicted best; diurnal variation in PEF >30%).

The predicted best values of PEF or FEV_1 are either based on expected normal values for a healthy subject of similar age, gender and height, or on percentage personal best scores.

When analysed by disease severity, those patients with severe asthma (mean baseline: PEF 290 L/minute, 55% predicted; FEV_1 2.1 L, 61% predicted; n=127) demonstrated the greatest change in morning PEF, whilst those with mild asthma (mean baseline: PEF 494 L/minute, 89% predicted; FEV_1 2.8 L, 70% predicted, n=390) demonstrated the smallest change (Figure 5). Despite the fact that patients with severe asthma experienced the greatest change in PEF from baseline, their maximum predicted PEF (65%) still remained lower than in the moderate (79%) and mild groups (93%) at all time points, although it is possible that this group may simply take longer to reach maximum benefit. Thus, the mild asthma group consistently displayed the greatest predicted PEF (Figure 5). Improvements from baseline in PEF were observed amongst all severity groups (mild, moderate and severe) from day 1 of treatment ($p<0.001$). However, the most rapid improvement in PEF was observed in patients with the most severe disease. This is perhaps intuitive since patients with the more severe airway obstruction

Improvements from baseline in PEF were observed amongst all severity groups (mild, moderate and severe) from day 1 of treatment ($p<0.001$).

Figure 3. Mean change from baseline in FEV_1 (top) and morning PEF (bottom) in patients receiving fluticasone (88 µg twice daily) or montelukast (10 µg four-times daily) over 24 weeks. BL, baseline; EP, endpoint.

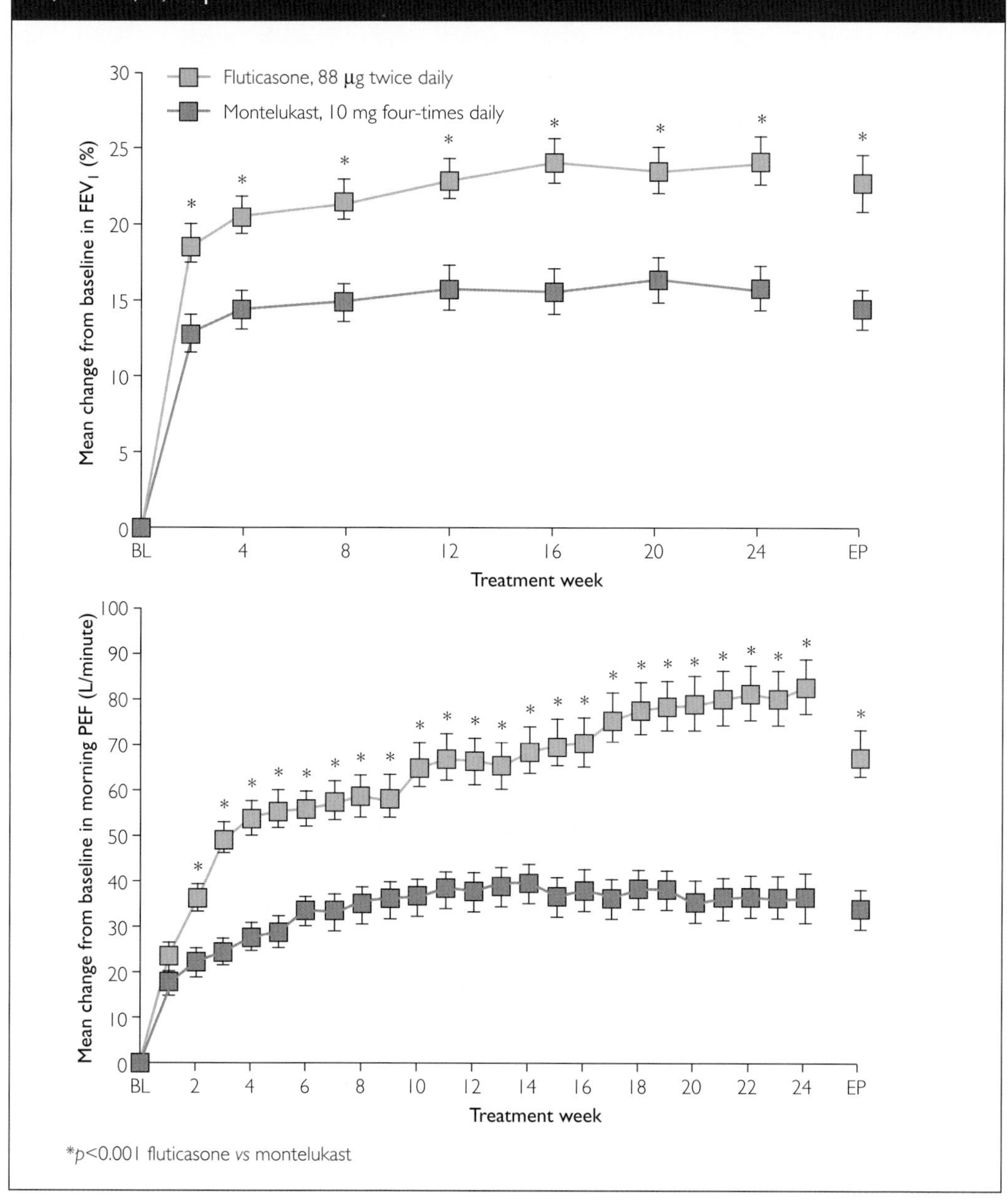

have the greatest capacity for improvement. This group took 3 days to reach 50% of their maximum observed response compared with 5 and 7 days in patients with moderate and mild asthma, respectively. In addition, the time to reach 90% of the best observed response in PEF was approximately 3 weeks in patients with moderate or severe asthma but was approximately 4 weeks in those with mild asthma.[18]

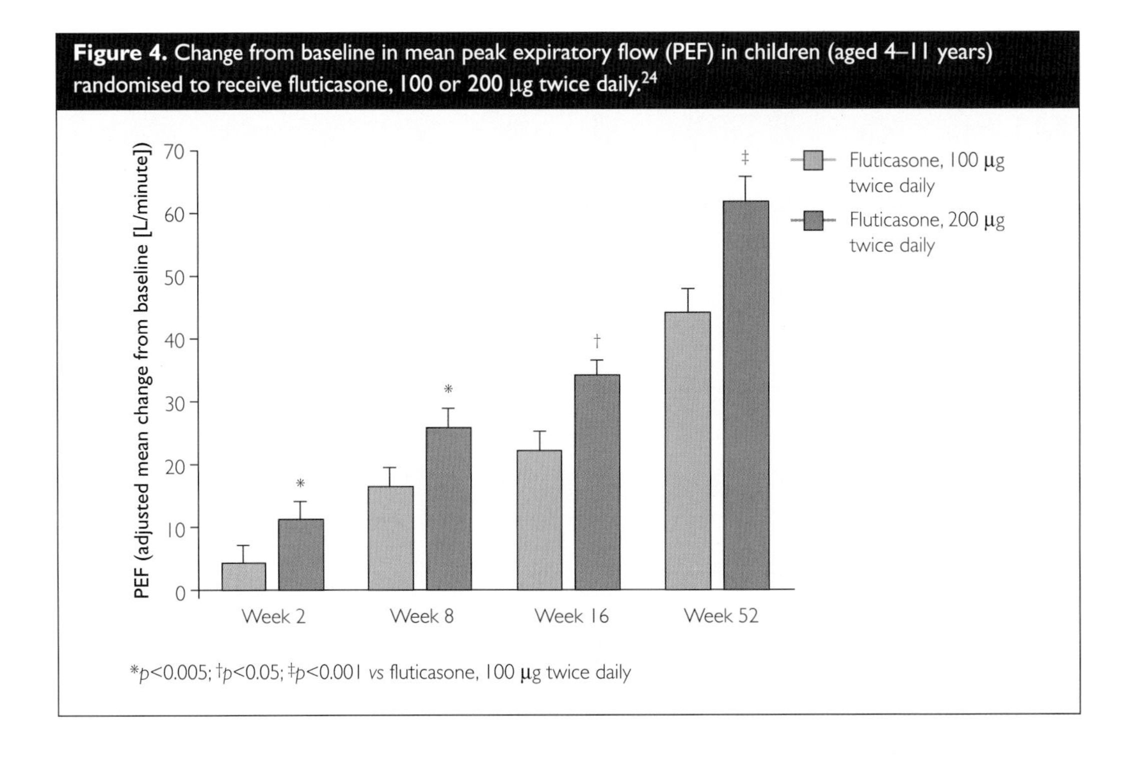

Figure 4. Change from baseline in mean peak expiratory flow (PEF) in children (aged 4–11 years) randomised to receive fluticasone, 100 or 200 µg twice daily.[24]

Fluticasone mediated the greatest change from baseline in PEF, over a relatively short period, in those with severe asthma.

Thus, in summary, patients with milder forms of asthma appear to take longer to achieve maximum improvements in lung function with fluticasone treatment, and these changes were generally of a smaller magnitude than in those with more severe airway obstruction. Fluticasone mediated the greatest change from baseline in PEF, over a relatively short period, in those with severe asthma. However, the maximum PEF achieved was lower at all time points in those with severe asthma than in those with mild or moderate asthma.

Formulation

Fluticasone is available in MDI (Evohaler®) and in DPI forms (Accuhaler®and Diskhaler®).The Evohaler utilises a pressurised inhalation system where a suspension of fluticasone is delivered to the lungs with each actuation. This type of inhaler device requires a degree of co-ordination between inspiration and operation of the device, which may be problematic in the very young, the elderly or those with chronic asthma. DPIs were developed to provide an alternative inhaler system characterised by reliable administration and a simpler mode of operation. Both the Accuhaler and the Diskhaler are breath actuated and administer a fixed dose of drug in micronised powder form.

Several studies have been conducted to determine whether the pharmacokinetics and the efficacy and safety of fluticasone are affected by the formulation and/or the type of inhaler used.[7,26,27] The two powder formulations of fluticasone (Diskus® [the US trademark for the Accuhaler device] and Diskhaler) have been compared in a large

Figure 5. Change from baseline in peak expiratory flow (PEF) and per cent of predicted PEF in patients with mild, moderate or severe asthma treated with fluticasone. Change from baseline, $p<0.001$ for all time points and for all levels of severity.[18]

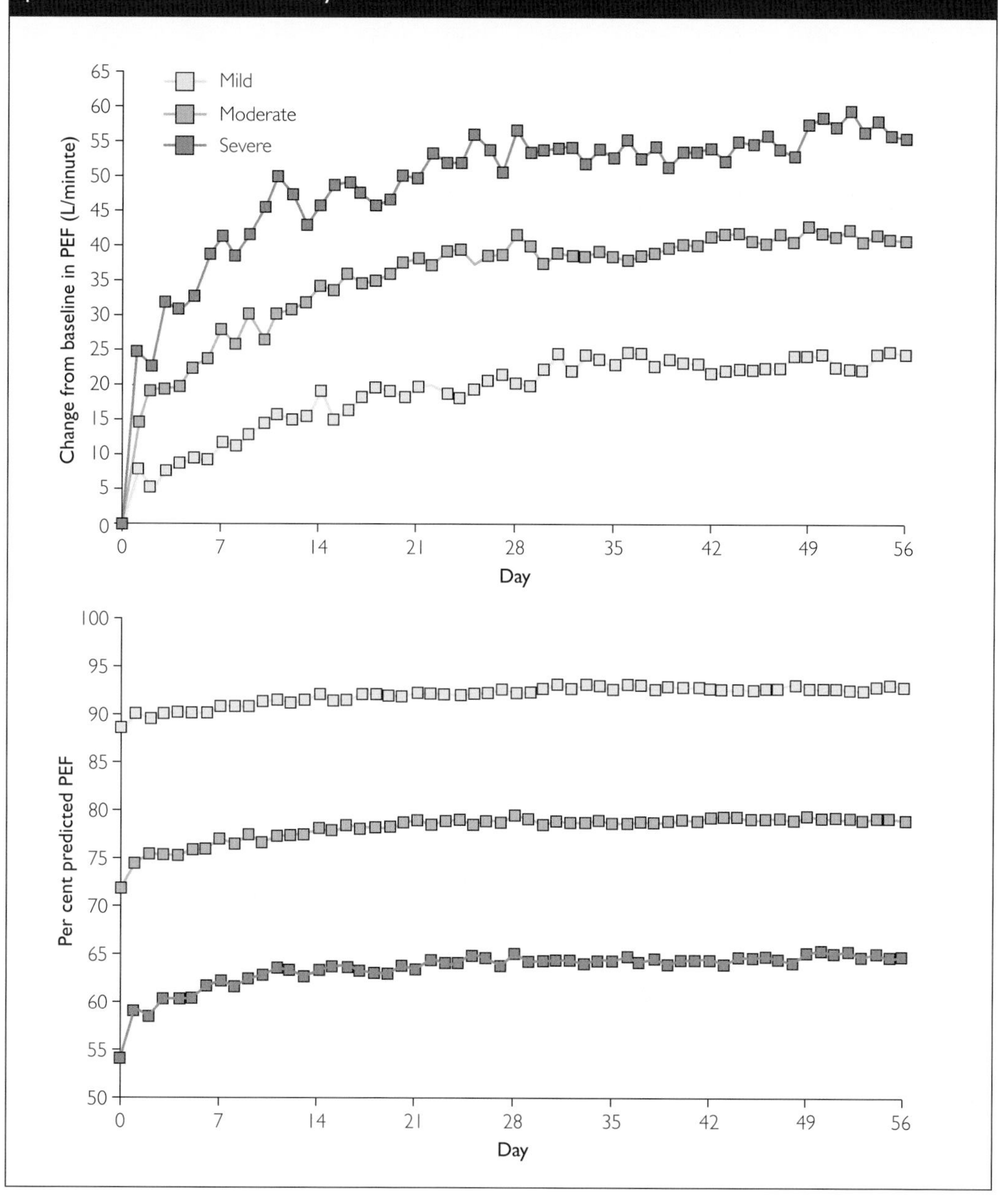

paediatric 12-week study performed in the US in 437 children (aged 4–11 years) with a history of chronic asthma.[26] Two doses of fluticasone (50 µg and 100 µg twice daily) were evaluated in this study, each delivered by both devices, and compared with placebo in a double-dummy design. Fluticasone, at both doses and administered by both devices, mediated improvements from baseline in both FEV_1

(Diskus 50 and 100 µg: 16 and 18%; Diskhaler 50 and 100 µg: 18 and 19%) and morning PEF (Diskus 50 and 100 µg: 26 and 27%; Diskhaler 50 and 100 µg: 30 and 33%) compared with placebo (7 and 14%, respectively; $p<0.05$). However, no differences were observed between doses or between inhaler devices. Similarly, no differences were reported between either the dose or the delivery device used in terms of asthma symptoms, salbutamol use, night-time awakenings, adverse events, or the effects upon the hypothalamic–pituitary–adrenal axis. The performance and ease of use of both devices was rated highly by 80% of the parents or guardians of the children enrolled in the study.[26] A common criticism invoked by studies of this type is that the rigid entry requirements to many of these trials (such as the ability to demonstrate good inhaler technique, compliance and specific reversibility of FEV_1) precludes accurate extrapolation to the general population, in whom inhaler technique is often poor and use of medication frequently haphazard. These issues may be clarified by the use of large-scale retrospective naturalistic studies.[28]

The pharmacokinetic parameters of fluticasone delivered at higher doses (100 µg and 500 µg twice daily) administered either by the Diskus or Diskhaler were examined in adults with mild-to-moderate asthma (18–72 years; n=444).[7] This study found no notable differences in the pharmacokinetic properties of fluticasone delivered by either of the two DPI devices.

No differences have been reported in either the efficacy or tolerability of differing formulations of fluticasone delivered by either DPIs or MDIs.

DPIs have also been compared with MDIs and were found to have equal efficacy.[29,30] The move away from chlorofluorocarbon (CFC) propellants has led to the development of inhalers utilising newer propellants, such as hydrofluoroalkane (HFA) 134a, which are not reported to be associated with ozone-depleting properties.[27] A 1-year, multinational, double-blind, randomised study compared the effects of fluticasone (500 µg twice daily) formulated with two different propellants (HFA 134a or CFC propellants 11 and 12) in 412 patients with moderate-to-severe asthma.[27] At doses up to 1000 µg/day, both formulations provided equally effective control of lung function and asthma symptomology in patients with moderate-to-severe asthma.

In summary, no differences have been reported in either the efficacy or tolerability of differing formulations of fluticasone delivered by either DPIs or MDIs.

Comparison with other inhaled corticosteroids

The most informative data concerning the efficacy and safety of fluticasone has come from clinical studies that have directly compared its performance with the other inhaled corticosteroids in common clinical use. Several studies have compared the effects of fluticasone with inhaled beclometasone, budesonide or triamcinolone in sufferers of chronic asthma.[14–16,19,31–34] As we have seen, *in vitro* and *in vivo* studies have shown that fluticasone is significantly more potent, at an equivalent dose, than either budesonide or beclometasone, and also exhibits much lower oral bioavailability than either.[31]

Fluticasone *vs* beclometasone

Comparisons of fluticasone with beclometasone have been performed with a variety of daily doses ranging from 200 to 1500 μg of fluticasone and from 200 to 2000 μg of beclometasone.[15,32,34] In general, these studies have reported that fluticasone appears to be twice as potent as beclometasone, with half the dose of fluticasone providing equivalent efficacy to, or in some cases, greater efficacy than, beclometasone.

The effects of high dosages of fluticasone and beclometasone (1500 μg/day) were compared in a long-term study of 274 adults with moderate-to-severe asthma.[15] This study demonstrated the superior performance of fluticasone over beclometasone at these higher dosages and also showed that this superiority was maintained over 1 year of treatment. At month 12, the increase in PEF was 20 L/minute greater with fluticasone than with beclometasone, with an additional 0.15 L greater increase in FEV_1 (p<0.05 for both comparisons).[15]

Other studies have compared fluticasone to a doubling in the dose of beclometasone, as this is more representative of clinical practice, and also reflects the greater potency of fluticasone.[32,34] Raphael *et al.* conducted a randomised, double-blind, parallel group comparison of fluticasone (88 or 220 μg twice daily) with beclometasone (168 or 336 μg twice daily) in 399 subjects with moderate-to-severe asthma administered over 12 weeks.[34] The efficacy outcomes of this trial, presented in Table 3, indicate that fluticasone was superior to beclometasone (at both doses) with regard to measures of pulmonary function (FEV_1, $FEF_{25-75\%}$,[a] FVC and morning PEF) and in decreasing asthma symptoms and the use of rescue salbutamol. A further study comparing fluticasone, 500 μg twice daily, with beclometasone, 1000 μg twice daily, also demonstrated equivalent potency of fluticasone and a double dose of beclometasone in the control of severe asthma.[32]

Fluticasone *vs* budesonide

A number of other studies have also reported superior efficacy of fluticasone compared with higher doses of budesonide in patients with asthma of varying severity.[14,16,19,31] A meta-analysis examined data from seven studies conducted in patients with asthma, which ranged in severity from mild to moderately severe (and excluded any patients taking oral corticosteroids), in order to compare the efficacy and safety of fluticasone (200–800 μg/day) with budesonide (400–1600 μg/day).[31] Morning PEF was the only efficacy endpoint that was monitored in this meta-analysis, whilst serum cortisol levels were analysed as part of the safety evaluation. Of the seven studies included in this meta-analysis, one was conducted in a paediatric population (patient ages not reported), whilst the remaining studies were in adult asthmatic populations exclusively. The pooled analysis revealed a greater improvement in morning PEF with fluticasone than with budesonide, with a mean difference between the two of 11 L/minute. In addition,

A number of studies have reported superior efficacy of fluticasone compared with higher doses of budesonide in patients with asthma of varying severity.

[a]$FEF_{25-75\%}$, forced expiratory flow over 25–75% of the FVC.

Table 3. Efficacy outcomes of fluticasone (88 and 220 µg twice daily) compared with beclometasone (168 and 336 µg twice daily) in moderate-to-severe asthma.[34]

Efficacy evaluation	Mean changes from baseline at endpoint				
	Fluticasone, 88 µg (n=99)	Fluticasone, 220 µg (n=101)	Beclometasone, 168 µg (n=104)	Beclometasone, 36 µg (n=95)	Fluticasone *vs* beclometasone[a] *p*-value
FEV_1 (L)	0.31	0.36	0.18	0.21	0.006
$FEF_{25-75\%}$ (L/second)	0.27	0.41	0.14	0.22	0.0150
FVC (L)	0.33	0.39	0.23	0.24	0.0034
Morning PEF (L/minute)	15.8	22.8	0.7	7.2	≤0.001
Evening PEF (L/minute)	7.8	14.2	2.1	9.7	0.06
Salbutamol use (puffs/day)	–0.9	–0.5	0.0	–0.3	0.004
Days with no salbutamol use (%)	15.8	11.0	5.0	7.7	0.01
Night-time awakenings	–0.03	–0.12	–0.03	–0.07	0.458
Symptom score (0–3 scale)	–0.24	–0.26	–0.05	–0.15	0.024
Days with no symptoms (%)	14.0	8.7	4.9	4.4	0.027

$FEF_{25-75\%}$, forced expiratory flow over 25–75% of the FVC; FEV_1, forced expiratory volume in 1 second; FVC, forced vital capacity; PEF, peak expiratory flow.
[a]Comparison of the combined drug effect of fluticasone *vs* beclometasone.

higher doses of fluticasone (≥500 µg/day) mediated less suppression of cortisol than high-dose budesonide (≥1200 µg/day).[31]

Fluticasone is commonly used at higher doses in patients suffering from more severe asthma, up to its licensed maximum dose of 1000 µg twice daily in adults, and 200 µg twice daily in children, aged 4–16 years.[3,14,16,19] A double-blind, double-dummy, parallel-group, randomised study (stratified according to the use of oral corticosteroids at baseline) compared two doses of fluticasone (500 µg or 1000 µg twice daily) with budesonide (800 µg twice daily) in 671 patients with severe asthma.[14] Fluticasone at both the 1000 and 2000 µg daily doses mediated greater improvements in morning PEF than did budesonide (change in morning PEF: 21 and 24 L/minute, respectively, *vs* 13 L/minute with budesonide; $p<0.05$) and also led to greater reductions in diurnal variation in PEF ($p<0.05$). Fluticasone also mediated greater improvements in FEV_1 (1000 µg: 0.21 L; 2000 µg: 0.26 L) compared with budesonide (0.12 L; $p<0.05$), but the improvement in FVC was only significantly greater with the 2000 µg dose of fluticasone compared with budesonide. The use of rescue medication, frequency of asthma exacerbations and symptom scores were all similar between the different groups. However, a greater percentage of patients who received fluticasone, 1000 and 2000 µg (48 and 50%, respectively), reported a reduction in the night-time use of rescue therapy, compared with budesonide (38%; $p<0.05$). The proportion of patients experiencing adverse events was 61% in the fluticasone, 1000 μg group, 49% in the fluticasone, 2000 μg group, and 51% in the budesonide group. The most common adverse effect was asthma and related events which occurred in 18% of budesonide-treated patients, and 12–13% of the fluticasone, 1000 or 2000 μg groups. The remaining side-effects were not different between the groups and comprised (in decreasing order of frequency) upper respiratory tract infections, hoarseness, headache, musculoskeletal pain, respiratory infections, sore throat, influenza, rhinitis, candidiasis of the mouth and cough.[14]

A comparison of fluticasone and budesonide administered at equivalent doses (fluticasone, 1000 μg twice daily, and budesonide, 1200 μg in the morning and 800 μg in the evening) in 395 adults with severe asthma also reported a greater efficacy for fluticasone.[16] A greater number of patients treated with fluticasone experienced a greater than 10% improvement in morning PEF compared with those who received budesonide (38.8 *vs* 29.1%; $p<0.05$). Likewise, a greater percentage of symptom-free days (31.5 *vs* 22.8%; $p<0.05$) and a higher percentage of salbutamol rescue-therapy-free days (42.7 *vs* 33.7%; $p<0.05$) was observed in the fluticasone group compared with budesonide. Whilst the frequency of asthma exacerbations was not different between the two groups, the mean time to resolution of exacerbations was significantly shorter with fluticasone treatment (11.0 *vs* 14.7 days; $p<0.05$). These studies confirm the conclusions that were made previously in patients with more moderate asthma and extend them to more severely affected patients, and demonstrate that fluticasone is more effective than the same dose of budesonide in these patients.

A greater percentage of symptom-free days and a higher percentage of salbutamol rescue-therapy-free days was observed in the fluticasone group compared with budesonide.

Fluticasone *vs* triamcinolone

An additional study has compared fluticasone (250 μg twice daily) with triamcinolone (200 μg four-times daily) in patients with moderate severe asthma, and also reported superior efficacy of fluticasone.[33] Specifically, fluticasone mediated greater improvement in FEV_1 ($p<0.01$), greater improvement in PEF (rather than decreases that were observed with triamcinolone; $p<0.001$) and greater reductions in supplemental salbutamol use ($p<0.05$) compared with triamcinolone.

Comparison with theophylline

There are very few data available reporting on the relative effectiveness of fluticasone and theophylline (an orally administered bronchodilator). This may be due to the narrow therapeutic range of theophylline, which must be carefully titrated to achieve plasma concentrations of 10–20 μg/mL. One study has determined that inhaled fluticasone, 50 or 100 μg twice daily, was more effective than theophylline in improving pulmonary function and in controlling asthma symptoms over a 12-week period in patients (n=353) with mild-to-moderate asthma.[35]

Comparison with leukotriene receptor antagonists

Fluticasone provides greater efficacy as a first-line treatment of persistent asthma compared with either montelukast or zafirlukast.

The leukotriene receptor antagonists (montelukast and zafirlukast) are another class of anti-asthma medications indicated for the maintenance treatment of asthma. These orally administered agents have been shown to provide improvements in lung function and asthma symptoms in placebo-controlled trials, whilst comparator studies have sought to determine their efficacy relative to fluticasone.[23,36–39] These studies concur with current UK guidelines, in that inhaled corticosteroid (in this case fluticasone) provides greater efficacy as a first-line treatment of persistent asthma compared with either montelukast or zafirlukast.[1]

Two multicentre, randomised, double-blind, double-dummy studies of similar design have compared fluticasone (88 µg twice daily) with montelukast (10 mg once daily) given over a 24-week period.[23,38] Inclusion criteria included a baseline FEV_1 of between 50 and 80% of the predicted normal (mean FEV_1 65% of predicted normal) and no inhaled corticosteroids for the previous 30 days. The first of these studies reported a significantly greater improvement in all measures of lung function (PEF, FEV_1, FVC and $FEF_{25–75\%}$) in fluticasone-treated patients compared with montelukast-treated patients (all comparisons $p<0.005$ at study endpoint).[23] The superior improvements in FEV_1 associated with fluticasone treatment were observed as early as week 2 and remained consistent over the entire treatment period (Figure 3). The improvement in morning PEF was also significantly greater in the fluticasone group, whilst differences between the two treatment groups were apparent as early as day 2 of treatment ($p<0.05$) and continued to increase over the 24-week treatment period, and remained significantly different at the study endpoint (Figure 3). Fluticasone was also superior to montelukast in terms of improvements in asthma symptom scores and the percentage of symptom-free days, and also in reducing the use of rescue salbutamol and the number of nights disturbed by asthma symptoms. However, the incidence of asthma exacerbations was not significantly different between the two groups (4 and 8% for fluticasone and montelukast, respectively). Both physicians and patients rated fluticasone more highly than montelukast. For example, 71% of physicians rated fluticasone effective or very effective compared with 53% for montelukast, whilst 85% of patients were satisfied with fluticasone in contrast to 65% for montelukast ($p<0.001$ at endpoint). The incidence of adverse events was similar between the groups (71% of fluticasone-treated and 68% of montelukast-treated patients reporting side-effects) with very few of these considered by the investigators to be drug related.

Fluticasone provides better control of lung function and asthma symptoms than montelukast in patients with moderate asthma.

These data have demonstrated that 24-week treatment with fluticasone provides better control of lung function and asthma symptoms than montelukast in patients with moderate asthma.[23] These conclusions were corroborated in a second study of similar design.[38]

The efficacy of fluticasone was also compared to zafirlukast in three randomised, double-blind, double-dummy studies.[36,37,39] Greater efficacy of fluticasone compared with zafirlukast was reported across all measured endpoints (FEV_1, morning and evening PEF, asthma symptom scores, symptom-free days, salbutamol use, salbutamol-free days, nights undisturbed by asthma symptoms) in two of the three studies.[36,37] The first of these studies was of 440 patients with mild-to-moderate asthma (FEV_1 60–85% of predicted normal) who were previously receiving inhaled corticosteroids (principally triamcinolone up to 800 μg, or beclometasone up to 336 μg daily). Patients were randomised to treatment with either fluticasone (88 μg twice daily) or zafirlukast (20 mg twice daily).[37] Fluticasone was shown to be consistently superior to zafirlukast for all parameters of asthma measured (FEV_1, morning and evening PEF, symptom-free days, rescue-free days, undisturbed nights and asthma exacerbations). Therefore, the authors concluded that switching patients already receiving inhaled corticosteroids to fluticasone resulted in better control of mild-to-moderate asthma than switching to zafirlukast.

Switching patients already receiving inhaled corticosteroids to fluticasone resulted in better control of mild-to-moderate asthma than switching to zafirlukast.

A second placebo-controlled, 12-week study was conducted in 338 patients with baseline FEV_1 ranging from 50 to 80% of the predicted normal.[36] Greater improvements with fluticasone were observed relative to zafirlukast as early as day 4 of treatment with regard to both FEV_1 and morning and evening PEF. These differences persisted until the end of the study (FEV_1: 23, 15 and 10%; morning PEF: 47, 15, and 7L/minute; for fluticasone, zafirlukast and placebo, respectively; all comparisons $p<0.05$ *vs* placebo and between treatments).[36]

A further comparative study comprised a 4-week, double-blind treatment phase (fluticasone, 88 μg twice daily, and zafirlukast, 20 mg twice daily) followed by a 4-week open-label phase, where all patients received fluticasone (88 μg twice daily).[39] Again, patients had asthma of moderate severity (baseline FEV_1 50 to 80% of predicted normal [mean FEV_1 69%]). In addition to a greater effect of fluticasone compared with zafirlukast on the morning PEF over the 4-week double-blind treatment phase, this study demonstrated further improvements in patients who switched from zafirlukast to fluticasone during the open-label period (Figure 6). Patients who switched from zafirlukast to fluticasone after 4 weeks also demonstrated additional improvements in morning and evening PEF and FEV_1, and further reductions in daily salbutamol use, during the open-label treatment period.[39]

In conclusion, fluticasone is consistently superior to either montelukast or zafirlukast in improving lung function and symptom control in patients with asthma of mild-to-moderate or moderate severity. To our knowledge, there are as yet no published studies comparing fluticasone with either montelukast or zafirlukast in populations with mild asthma.

Fluticasone is consistently superior to either montelukast or zafirlukast in improving lung function and symptom control in patients with asthma of mild-to-moderate or moderate severity.

Treatment in children

The efficacy and safety of fluticasone has been evaluated in younger sufferers of asthma. Fluticasone is currently licensed in the UK for treatment of children (aged 4–16 years) at doses between 50 and 100 μg twice daily, with a maximal dose of 200 μg twice daily. Fluticasone is also included amongst the options for regular inhaled preventer therapy (along with beclometasone, budesonide and mometasone) in British

Figure 6. Mean change from baseline in morning PEF after a 4-week double-blind treatment period with zafirlukast (20 mg twice daily) or fluticasone (88 μg twice daily), followed by a 4-week open-label phase with fluticasone (88 μg twice daily).[39]

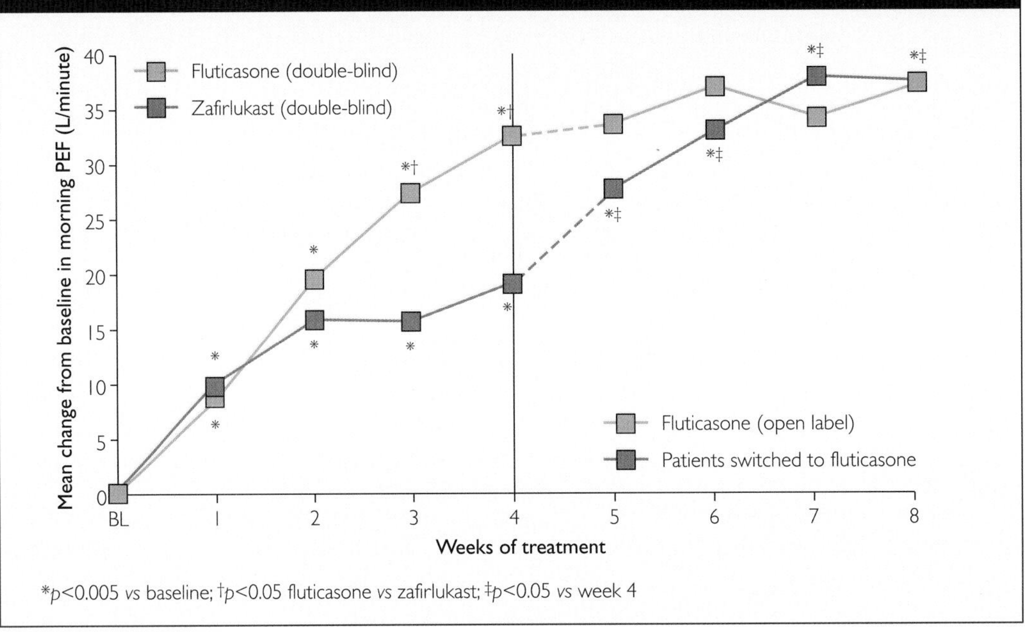

guidelines on the treatment of asthma in children younger than 5 years.[1] Asthma management and research in children younger than 5 years presents a great challenge to clinicians and investigators since both the diagnosis and evaluation of the efficacy of anti-asthma treatments must be achieved in the absence of objective data derived from spirometric lung function tests, which are inappropriate in young children.[40] As such, PEF is the only lung function test which is consistently used in this age group.

Children aged under 4 years

There are many uncertainties regarding the diagnosis and treatment of asthma in young children, largely due to the reliance on subjective assessment of symptoms to determine the presence and severity of asthma. This represents a significant problem since it has been estimated that up to 40% of children younger than 4 years of age experience recurrent cough, wheeze or breathlessness. Thus, a diagnosis of asthma in this age group is rarely definitive.

The present UK licenced indication for fluticasone in children is for those aged 4–16 years. However, two studies have examined the effects of 12 weeks of inhaled fluticasone (50–100 μg twice daily) in children aged 12 to 47 months using symptom scores, frequency of asthma exacerbations and the use of rescue salbutamol treatment as outcome measures.[41,42] Inclusion criteria were the presence of wheeze, cough or shortness of breath, or symptomatic use of salbutamol, on at least 7 of the last 14 days of the 4-week run-in period. In a study of 305 children, fluticasone (100 µg twice daily) increased the percentage of days and nights with no overall symptoms from 11% at baseline to 54% at the end of the study. This contrasted with corresponding increases of 8 and 36% with placebo ($p<0.005$).[41] The proportion of children free from asthma exacerbations also increased from 64% with placebo to 75% with fluticasone treatment ($p<0.05$). This study also reported that young children with frequent symptoms of asthma and with a family history of asthma were likely to benefit most from early prophylactic fluticasone treatment.

A second study involved 237 children with moderately severe and recurrent asthma symptoms, and reported significant improvements in symptom scores, rates of asthma exacerbation and use of rescue salbutamol treatment with fluticasone (50 or 100 µg twice daily), with the higher dose providing greater efficacy.[42] Thus, both studies have demonstrated good efficacy of fluticasone for control of asthma-like symptoms in children aged between 1 and 3 years.

A further study examined the long-term safety and efficacy of fluticasone (100 µg twice daily) compared with sodium cromoglicate (5 mg, four-times daily) each administered via an MDI with a spacer device, in 625 children aged between 12 and 47 months.[43] This study was a randomised, multicentre, open-label study conducted over 12 months, and demonstrated the superior efficacy of fluticasone over sodium cromoglicate. Specifically, fluticasone treatment resulted in fewer cases of mild or severe exacerbations of asthma, a reduced requirement for oral corticosteroid treatment and a greater number of symptom-free days and days with no requirement for rescue therapy.[43] Both treatments were well tolerated, with no difference in growth rates reported between the groups. Furthermore, although serum cortisol levels were significantly lower with fluticasone compared with sodium cromoglicate, they remained within normal limits.

In summary, fluticasone appears to be a viable option for the treatment of young children with asthmatic symptoms of recurrent wheeze, cough or breathlessness. Moreover, fluticasone demonstrates good safety and tolerability in this population over 1 year of treatment.

Fluticasone appears to be a viable option for the treatment of young children with asthmatic symptoms of recurrent wheeze, cough or breathlessness.

Children aged 4–11 years

Several studies have examined the effects of fluticasone in children aged between 4 and 11 years, with the particular objective of determining the most appropriate dose and dosing schedule.[22,24,26,44] A meta-analysis evaluated four studies in an investigation of the efficacy of fluticasone (50–200 µg twice daily) in this age group of children.[44] The studies ranged from 12 to 52 weeks in duration, with the children previously receiving other inhaled corticosteroids (principally triamcinolone, beclometasone or flunisolide). Patients were recruited into the study on the basis of pre-study FEV_1 values of 50–85% of the predicted normal (for children aged 6–11 years) or a baseline PEF of less than 85% of the predicted normal (for children aged 4–5 years). This analysis demonstrated a significantly greater improvement in all efficacy parameters evaluated in children treated with fluticasone at doses from

100 μg twice daily, compared with their baseline inhaled corticosteroid therapy. The improvements mediated by fluticasone included a 13% increase in FEV_1, increases of 16 and 14% in morning and evening PEF respectively, a 29% decrease in asthma symptom scores, a 38% decrease in rescue salbutamol use and an 18% increase in symptom-free days (all evaluations $p<0.005$ from baseline).

A further study of 437 children (aged 4–11 years; mean FEV_1 73% of predicted normal [measured in >5 year age group only]) also reported the efficacy of fluticasone, at both 50 and 100 μg twice daily, compared with placebo with regard to all efficacy parameters examined.[26] Two dry powder formulations of fluticasone were also compared in this study and neither the dose nor the formulation of fluticasone was found to differ, in either efficacy or tolerability.

A further two studies examined the long-term effects of fluticasone given over 1 year in children aged 4–11 years.[22,24] The first of these examined a cohort of children (n=252) with mild-to-moderate asthma (recruited using the guidelines described above and with a mean FEV_1 of 71% of the predicted normal) and has been described in detail in the 'Dose frequency' section (page 106).[22] To reiterate, this study demonstrated the efficacy and safety of both once-daily and twice-daily dosing with fluticasone at 200 μg/day for up to 64 weeks (12 week double-blind period plus a 52 week open-label phase). The twice-daily dosing regimen also appeared to provide the greatest efficacy. The second study was a year-long, randomised, double-blind, dose-comparison study conducted in 528 children, aged 4–11 years, with moderate-to-severe asthma previously being treated with high-dose inhaled corticosteroids (i.e. beclometasone 800–1600 μg/day or equivalent).[24] The study compared the maximal licensed dose of fluticasone (200 μg twice daily) with a 100 μg twice-daily dose, with the primary outcome being the time to exacerbation. The risk of asthma exacerbation was not different between the two fluticasone groups although a subgroup analysis (which separated the group according to the dose of inhaled corticosteroids at baseline: 800 μg/day or >800 μg/day for the 'severe' group) indicated that the higher dose of fluticasone significantly decreased the risk of exacerbation in the severe group, compared with the lower dose of fluticasone. However, this somewhat nebulous distinction was poorly backed up by baseline data and thus the conclusions drawn regarding severe asthma are perhaps less than convincing. Thus, fluticasone at both doses improved clinic PEF from baseline, with the 200 μg fluticasone dose mediating greater improvements in PEF than the 100 μg dose (Figure 4).

The maximal licensed dose of fluticasone may be of use in the treatment of children with moderate-to-severe asthma.

In summary, the maximal licensed dose of fluticasone may be of use in the treatment of children with moderate-to-severe asthma.

The effects of inhaled fluticasone have been compared with oral prednisolone in the acute treatment of severe asthma in children in a double-blind, randomised trial.[45] This study demonstrated that oral prednisolone, 2 mg, was superior to inhaled fluticasone, 2000 μg, in the treatment of 100 children aged over 5 years with severe acute asthma (FEV_1 <60% of predicted). Prednisolone mediated greater improvements in FEV_1, FVC and PEF, and also resulted in lower rates of hospitalisation than children treated with inhaled fluticasone (10 *vs* 31%; $p<0.01$). It is likely that the drastically narrowed airways characteristic of acute severe asthma results in suboptimal delivery of inhaled therapy ensuring that oral corticosteroid treatment is far more effective in these cases.[45] Once more, these data are consistent with current UK guidelines, which do not advocate doses of inhaled fluticasone greater than 400 µg/day in children.

In summary, children aged 4–11 years may be treated effectively with inhaled fluticasone (50–200 µg twice daily). Doses from 100 µg twice daily appear to provide optimal improvements in lung function to children with mild-to-moderate asthma, whilst the higher dose (200 µg twice daily) may be more appropriate in the treatment of moderate-to-severe asthma. Children with acute severe asthma, on the other hand, are more likely to benefit from oral corticosteroid therapy.

Children aged 4–11 years may be treated effectively with inhaled fluticasone (50–200 µg twice daily).

Safety and tolerability

Systemic adverse events

The increasing use of high doses of inhaled corticosteroids over long periods has led to concern over possible adverse systemic affects.[31] The most clinically important of these include the suppression of the hypothalamic–pituitary–adrenal axis, effects on bone metabolism and effects on growth in children.[31] Glaucoma and an increased risk of cataract are also potential systemic adverse effects associated with corticosteroids.[46]

Adrenal insufficiency

High levels of exogenous inhaled corticosteroids, such as fluticasone, will decrease expression of glucocorticoid receptors in the anterior pituitary gland and hypothalamus, via a negative-feedback mechanism. As a consequence of this downregulation, the release of corticotropin-releasing hormone and corticotropin is suppressed, leading to a reduction in cortisol secretion from the adrenal cortex which may, over time, result in atrophy of the adrenal cortex.[46] Adrenal insufficiency has the potential to be fatal in situations of high stress, such as surgery, trauma, infection or myocardial infarction, when the atrophied adrenal cortex may be unable to mount a sufficient endogenous cortisol response.[46] Clinical manifestation of adrenal insuffiency include a decrease in the rate of linear growth, anorexia nervosa, weight loss, vomiting, diarrhoea, fatigue, headache, dizziness, hypoglycaemia and convulsions.[2] In order to avoid adrenal insuffiency, it is recommended that all inhaled corticosteroids are titrated downwards to achieve the lowest effective maintenance dose.[2,47] The insulin tolerance test is said to be the gold standard for assessment of adrenal function but frequently, basal cortisol levels (either urinary free cortisol or plasma cortisol) are measured, or alternatively dynamic stimulation tests (e.g. cosyntropin to test adrenal cortical reserve) are conducted, in order to determine

In order to avoid adrenal insuffiency, it is recommended that all inhaled corticosteroids are titrated downwards to achieve the lowest effective maintenance dose.

adrenocortical activity. Unstimulated cortisol levels of less than 150 nmol/L are considered to be abnormally low.[2,46]

A meta-analysis has reported that fluticasone, at doses above 800μg/day, caused greater suppression of both urinary and plasma cortisol than the equivalent doses of triamcinolone, beclometasone and budesonide.[46] In contrast, fluticasone, 2000 μg/day (the maximal recommended dose), had little effect on serum cortisol in two studies where levels remained within the normal range, though there were decreases from baseline (357 nmol/L at baseline falling to 286 nmol/L after 24 weeks of treatment in one study; 276 nmol/L at baseline falling to 243 nmol/L after 6 weeks' treatment).[14,16] Moreover, the majority of studies that have examined lower doses of inhaled fluticasone (up to 1500 μg/day) have reported no changes, and even slight increases, in plasma cortisol levels.[9,10,13–15,21,27,32] For example, a study performed over 2 years in mildly asthmatic patients (n=160) demonstrated transient decreases in cosyntropin-stimulated plasma cortisol levels after 6 months ($p<0.005$) and 1 year ($p<0.05$) of treatment with fluticasone, 440 μg twice daily, though no differences were reported when treated patients were compared with placebo patients at week 104.[48]

When fluticasone is used in paediatric populations, it is generally used at lower doses that have no reported effects upon adrenal function, as demonstrated in several studies using doses of up to 200 μg/day.[22,24,26] A comprehensive safety profile has also been conducted in 625 children aged from 12 to 47 months, and showed that the proportion of children with abnormally low serum cortisol levels (<150 nmol/L) was actually reduced by fluticasone when administered at 100 μg twice daily (from 3% at baseline to <1% at week 52).[43] A small study from the US investigating cortisol levels in children given fluticasone (176–1320 μg/day; mean age 12 years; n=62) reported an increased percentage of children with abnormally low plasma cortisol (<140 nmol/L) after treatment with higher doses of fluticasone (≥440 μg/day).[49] Additionally, an observational UK report describes the cases of six children with severe asthma who were treated with high doses of inhaled fluticasone (≥1000 μg/day) who experienced growth retardation and adrenal suppression.[50] These data underline the need for adherence to UK guidelines, which recommend a maximum of 400 μg fluticasone per day in children aged 4 to 16 years.[3]

Thus, the balance of data indicate that the use of low-dose inhaled fluticasone (<800 μg/day in adults and <200 μg/day in children) has no clinically significant effect on the hypothalamic–pituitary–adrenal axis and also offers a good ratio of efficacy to safety. However, at doses above 800 μg/day there is evidence, albeit inconsistent, for adrenal suppression and thus, as is recommended by current guidelines, the lowest effective dose of inhaled corticosteroid is always recommended.

The use of low-dose inhaled fluticasone has no clinically significant effect on the hypothalamic–pituitary–adrenal axis and also offers a good ratio of efficacy to safety.

Bone density and osteoporosis

Another concern regarding long-term use of high doses of inhaled corticosteroids is the potential for a reduction in bone mineral density, which may result in a heightened risk of osteoporosis and bone fracture.[46] The gold-standard method for assessment of bone mineral density is dual energy x-ray absorptiometry (DXA) scanning, but biochemical markers of bone formation (e.g. osteocalcin) and bone resorption (e.g. collagen) are commonly used as surrogate markers of bone density.[46]

Fluticasone was reported to have little effect on skeletal function in several dedicated studies, conducted over 6 months to 2 years, in both children and adults. In a group of severely asthmatic patients (n=198) treated with inhaled fluticasone, 2000 µg/day for 24 weeks, no clinically significant changes were observed in markers of bone turnover (calcium: 42 ng/mL; collagen: increased slightly from 92 to 107 ng/mL; osteocalcin: fell slightly from 4.9 to 4.2 ng/mL).[16] Two further studies conducted over 2 years found no effect of fluticasone (100 µg twice daily for children [n=174] or 440 µg twice daily for adults [n=160]) on bone mineral density as assessed by DXA scan.[48,51] Thus, these studies indicate that fluticasone, when administered up to its maximal recommended dose (1000 µg twice daily), does not appear to have detrimental effects on bone density or metabolism.

Fluticasone, when administered up to its maximal recommended dose does not appear to have detrimental effects on bone density or metabolism.

Linear growth in children

Long-term therapy with oral corticosteroids is known to suppress growth in children. Therefore, it is also vitally important to evaluate the effects of inhaled corticosteroid on growth rates in paediatric populations.[46] Where comparison with placebo was considered unethical, fluticasone treatment was compared with chromone therapy (i.e. sodium cromoglicate or nedocromil sodium), which have no known effects on either bone mineral density or childhood growth, and also provide control of asthma symptoms.[51]

In children aged 12–47 months, no difference in mean adjusted growth rate was observed between children treated with fluticasone (100 µg twice daily) and sodium cromoglicate (5 mg four-times daily) when administered over 1 year.[43] Similarly, children (aged 6–14 years) treated for 2 years with fluticasone (100 µg twice daily) had growth rates that were similar to that of children treated with nedocromil sodium (6.1 cm/year *vs* 5.8 cm/year).[51] Finally, a double-blind randomised study of 325 pre-pubescent children with persistent asthma, treated for 1 year with fluticasone (50 or 100 µg twice daily) displayed no differences in mean height or mean growth velocity between any of the treatment groups at any time.[52] These findings therefore demonstrate that there is no apparent association of fluticasone with suppression of childhood growth when used at the current recommended doses.

There is no apparent association of fluticasone with suppression of childhood growth at the current recommended doses.

Ocular effects

An increased risk of cataracts and glaucoma has been reported with prolonged exposure to high doses of inhaled corticosteroids.[46] It is, therefore, surprising that very few studies have investigated the effect of fluticasone on ocular health. A randomised, double-blind, placebo-controlled trial of fluticasone (440 µg twice daily) in mildly asthmatic adults reported that no clinically important ocular changes occurred over the 2-year study period.[48] A year-long comparative study of fluticasone with sodium cromoglicate in children (aged 12–47 months) reported one incidence of cataracts (out of 358 children examined at week 52) in a 44-month old child treated with fluticasone, 100 µg twice daily.[43] However, a retrospective observational study has reported no association between fluticasone and the risk of cataracts in asthma sufferers under 40 years of age.[53]

General adverse event profile

The most commonly reported side-effects of inhaled fluticasone in asthmatic adults are illustrated in Table 4.[27] Respiratory infections and asthma symptoms were the most commonly reported adverse events associated with fluticasone treatment. Headache, influenza, hoarseness, cough, rhinitis and sore throat comprise the majority of remaining side-effects.[27] Hypersensitivity reactions (including rash and angioedema) are also reported rarely. A similar adverse event profile was reported in a year-long study, which randomised patients with moderate-to-severe asthma to fluticasone, 1500 µg/day.[15] Pharmacologically predictable side-effects of inhaled corticosteroids (including fluticasone) include hoarseness and candidiasis of the mouth or throat. However, the incidence of these side-effects may be reduced by rinsing the mouth with water after each dose. Paradoxical bronchospasm is another potential adverse event with fluticasone treatment and evidence of its occurrence should be met with immediate discontinuation of fluticasone and its replacement with a short-acting bronchodilator.[3]

Table 4. The most frequently reported (>5% of patients) and pharmacologically predictable adverse events in 203 patients with moderate-to-severe asthma treated with fluticasone, 500 µg twice daily, for 1 year.[27]

Adverse event	Number of patients (%)
Common adverse events (>5% of patients)	
Upper respiratory tract infection	61 (30)
Asthma and related events	59 (29)
Headache	38 (19)
Influenza	25 (12)
Respiratory infection	20 (10)
Hoarseness	20 (10)
Rhinitis	20 (10)
Cough	14 (7)
Predictable adverse events	
Hoarseness	20 (10)
Candidiasis	11 (5)
Rash/skin eruption	6 (3)
Allergic skin reactions	2 (<1)
Overall incidence	**166 (82)**

Cautions, contra-indications and drug interactions

All inhaled corticosteroids should be used cautiously in active or quiescent tuberculosis.[3] Treatment with either oral corticosteroids or high doses of inhaled corticosteroids should not be stopped abruptly due to the risk of triggering acute adrenal crisis. Instead, patients should be weaned slowly from their habitual systemic dose, particularly in the case of patients transferring from oral to inhaled corticosteroids.[3] Interactions between fluticasone and potent inhibitors of the CYP 3A4 isoenzyme (e.g. ketoconazole and protease inhibitors such as ritonavir) may result in increased exposure to fluticasone.[3]

Treatment with either oral or high doses of inhaled corticosteroids should not be stopped abruptly due to the risk of triggering acute adrenal crisis.

Pregnancy and lactation

There is little safety evidence available regarding the use of fluticasone in human pregnancy and in breast-feeding mothers. However, there is evidence that corticosteroids may cause foetal abnormalities when administered to pregnant animals and thus, the use of fluticasone during pregnancy and lactation should only be considered if the expected benefit to the mother is greater than any possible risk to the foetus or child.[3]

Pharmacoeconomics

A UK-based economic analysis was performed to compare the cost-effectiveness of fluticasone with budesonide, where fluticasone was administered at half the milligram dosage of budesonide.[54] This analysis examined four measures of effectiveness including total increase in morning PEF, number of successfully treated weeks (in terms of >5% improvement in PEF from baseline), symptom-free days and exacerbation-free days. These efficacy measures were correlated to cost, which included direct cost of the corticosteroids and relief medications, together with the incidence and duration of hospitalisations. Drug costs were taken from the British National Formulary as of March 1995. This study showed that the mean weekly cost of fluticasone treatment was £7.78 whilst for budesonide the calculated cost was £12.33. In all, fluticasone was both cheaper and more effective than budesonide in the treatment of both children and adults with asthma (of unspecified severity).[54]

Fluticasone was both cheaper and more effective than budesonide in the treatment of both children and adults with asthma.

Other analyses conducted in the US have also reported a greater cost-effectiveness of fluticasone compared with budesonide, oral zafirlukast, triamcinolone, flunisolide and sodium cromoglicate.[55,56]

Key points

- Fluticasone is a potent corticosteroid with a high therapeutic index and low systemic bioavailability, which is currently used as an inhaled asthma preventer therapy for both children and adults.
- Fluticasone has a high affinity for the glucocorticoid receptor and a high degree of lipophilicity rendering it highly retained within lung tissue.
- Studies performed *in vitro* and *in vivo* have shown that fluticasone is a more potent anti-inflammatory agent than beclometasone, triamcinolone, budesonide or mometasone.
- In patients with mild-to-moderate asthma, maximal clinical benefit from fluticasone appears to be achieved with doses up to 200 µg/day but the maximum recommended dose of fluticasone (2000 µg/day) may be of benefit for patients suffering with more severe asthma.
- Fluticasone treatment improves lung function (including increases in morning and evening PEF, FEV_1 and FVC) and reduces asthma symptoms and the use of rescue bronchodilator therapy.
- Fluticasone tends to be more effective when administered twice daily rather than once daily, whilst improvements occur rapidly and within 7 days of treatment.
- Greater efficacy of fluticasone has been reported when compared with other inhaled asthma therapies including budesonide, beclometasone, triamcinolone, theophylline or leukotriene receptor antagonists.
- At current recommended doses, fluticasone appears to be well tolerated with little or no effect on adrenal function, bone mineral density or childhood growth rates.

References

A list of the published evidence which has been reviewed in compiling the preceding section of *BESTMEDICINE*.

1. BTS/SIGN. British guideline on the management of asthma. British Thoracic Society Scottish Intercollegiate Guidelines Network, 2004. *www.sign.ac.uk*
2. Crowley S. Inhaled glucocorticoids and adrenal function: an update. *Paediatr Respir Rev* 2003; **4**: 153–61.
3. Allen and Hanburys Ltd. Flixotide® (fluticasone). *Summary of product characteristics*: Uxbridge, Middlesex, 2003.
4. Johnson M. Development of fluticasone propionate and comparison with other inhaled corticosteroids. *J Allergy Clin Immunol* 1998; **101**: S434–9.
5. Crim C, Pierre LN, Daley-Yates PT. A review of the pharmacology and pharmacokinetics of inhaled fluticasone propionate and mometasone furoate. *Clin Ther* 2001; **23**: 1339–54.
6. Fuller R, Johnson M, Bye A. Fluticasone propionate–an update on preclinical and clinical experience. *Respir Med* 1995; **89(Suppl A)**: 3–18.
7. Falcoz C, Horton J, Mackie AE, Harding SM, Daley-Yates PT. Pharmacokinetics of fluticasone propionate inhaled via the Diskhaler and Diskus powder devices in patients with mild-to-moderate asthma. *Clin Pharmacokinet* 2000; **39(Suppl 1)**: 31–7.
8. Jarvis B, Faulds D. Inhaled fluticasone propionate: a review of its therapeutic efficacy at dosages < or = 500 microg/day in adults and adolescents with mild to moderate asthma. *Drugs* 1999; **57**: 769–803.
9. Wolfe JD, Selner JC, Mendelson LM, Hampel F, Jr., Schaberg A. Effectiveness of fluticasone propionate in patients with moderate asthma: a dose-ranging study. *Clin Ther* 1996; **18**: 635–46.
10. Nathan RA, Li JT, Finn A *et al.* A dose-ranging study of fluticasone propionate administered once daily via multidose powder inhaler to patients with moderate asthma. *Chest* 2000; **118**: 296–302.
11. Masoli M, Weatherall M, Holt S, Beasley R. Clinical dose-response relationship of fluticasone propionate in adults with asthma. *Thorax* 2004; **59**: 16–20.
12. Holt S, Suder A, Weatherall M *et al.* Dose-response relation of inhaled fluticasone propionate in adolescents and adults with asthma: meta-analysis. *BMJ* 2001; **323**: 253–6.
13. Pearlman DS, Noonan MJ, Tashkin DP *et al.* Comparative efficacy and safety of twice daily fluticasone propionate powder versus placebo in the treatment of moderate asthma. *Ann Allergy Asthma Immunol* 1997; **78**: 356–62.
14. Ayres JG, Bateman ED, Lundback B, Harris TA. High dose fluticasone propionate, 1 mg daily, versus fluticasone propionate, 2 mg daily, or budesonide, 1.6 mg daily, in patients with chronic severe asthma. International Study Group. *Eur Respir J* 1995; **8**: 579–86.
15. Fabbri L, Burge PS, Croonenborgh L *et al.* Comparison of fluticasone propionate with beclomethasone dipropionate in moderate to severe asthma treated for one year. International Study Group. *Thorax* 1993; **48**: 817–23.
16. Heinig JH, Boulet LP, Croonenborghs L, Mollers MJ. The effect of high-dose fluticasone propionate and budesonide on lung function and asthma exacerbations in patients with severe asthma. *Respir Med* 1999; **93**: 613–20.
17. Chervinsky P, van As A, Bronsky EA *et al.* Fluticasone propionate aerosol for the treatment of adults with mild to moderate asthma. The Fluticasone Propionate Asthma Study Group. *J Allergy Clin Immunol* 1994; **94**: 676–83.
18. Szefler SJ, Boushey HA, Pearlman DS *et al.* Time to onset of effect of fluticasone propionate in patients with asthma. *J Allergy Clin Immunol* 1999; **103**: 780–8.
19. Rutherford C, Mills R, Gibson PG, Price MJ. Improvement in health-related quality of life with fluticasone propionate compared with budesonide or beclomethasone dipropionate in adults with severe asthma. *Respirology* 2003; **8**: 371–5.
20. Purucker ME, Rosebraugh CJ, Zhou F, Meyer RJ. Inhaled fluticasone propionate by diskus in the treatment of asthma: a comparison of the efficacy of the same nominal dose given either once or twice a day. *Chest* 2003; **124**: 1584–93.
21. ZuWallack R, Adelglass J, Clifford DP *et al.* Long-term efficacy and safety of fluticasone propionate powder administered once or twice daily via inhaler to patients with moderate asthma. *Chest* 2000; **118**: 303–12.
22. LaForce CF, Pearlman DS, Ruff ME *et al.* Efficacy and safety of dry powder fluticasone propionate in children with persistent asthma. *Ann Allergy Asthma Immunol* 2000; **85**: 407–15.
23. Busse W, Raphael GD, Galant S *et al.* Low-dose fluticasone propionate compared with montelukast for first-line treatment of persistent asthma: a randomized clinical trial. *J Allergy Clin Immunol* 2001; **107**: 461–8.
24. Verona E, Petrov D, Cserhati E *et al.* Fluticasone propionate in asthma: a long term dose comparison study. *Arch Dis Child* 2003; **88**: 503–9.
25. Reddel HK, Jenkins CR, Marks GB *et al.* Optimal asthma control, starting with high doses of inhaled budesonide. *Eur Respir J* 2000; **16**: 226–35.
26. Peden DB, Berger WE, Noonan MJ *et al.* Inhaled fluticasone propionate delivered by means of two different multidose powder inhalers is effective and safe in a large pediatric population with persistent asthma. *J Allergy Clin Immunol* 1998; **102**: 32–8.

27 Perruchoud AP, Lundback B, Yigla M, Sykes AP. Clinical efficacy and safety of fluticasone propionate 1 mg per day administered via a HFA 134a pressurized metered dose inhaler to patients with moderate to severe asthma. International study group. *Respir Med* 2000; **94(Suppl B)**: S35–41.

28 Price D, Thomas M, Mitchell G, Niziol C, Featherstone R. Improvement of asthma control with a breath-actuated pressurised metred dose inhaler (BAI): a prescribing claims study of 5556 patients using a traditional pressurised metred dose inhaler (MDI) or a breath-actuated device. *Respir Med* 2003; **91**: 12–19.

29 Lundback B, Alexander M, Day J *et al.* Evaluation of fluticasone propionate (500 micrograms day^{-1}) administered either as dry powder via a Diskhaler inhaler or pressurized inhaler and compared with beclomethasone dipropionate (1000 micrograms day^{-1}) administered by pressurized inhaler. *Respir Med* 1993; **87**: 609–20.

30 Lodha R, Gupta G, Baruah BP, Nagpal R, Kabra SK. Metered doseinhaler with spacer versus dry powder inhaler for delivery of salbutamol in acute exacerbations of asthma: a randomized controlled trial. *Indian Pediatr* 2004; **41**: 15–20.

31 Barnes NC, Hallett C, Harris TA. Clinical experience with fluticasone propionate in asthma: a meta-analysis of efficacy and systemic activity compared with budesonide and beclomethasone dipropionate at half the microgram dose or less. *Respir Med* 1998; **92**: 95–104.

32 Barnes NC, Marone G, Di Maria GU *et al.* A comparison of fluticasone propionate, 1 mg daily, with beclomethasone dipropionate, 2 mg daily, in the treatment of severe asthma. International Study Group. *Eur Respir J* 1993; **6**: 877–85.

33 Condemi JJ, Chervinsky P, Goldstein MF *et al.* Fluticasone propionate powder administered through Diskhaler versus triamcinolone acetonide aerosol administered through metered-dose inhaler in patients with persistent asthma. *J Allergy Clin Immunol* 1997; **100**: 467–74.

34 Raphael GD, Lanier RQ, Baker J *et al.* A comparison of multiple doses of fluticasone propionate and beclomethasone dipropionate in subjects with persistent asthma. *J Allergy Clin Immunol* 1999; **103**: 796–803.

35 Galant SP, Lawrence M, Meltzer EO *et al.* Fluticasone propionate compared with theophylline for mild-to-moderate asthma. *Ann Allergy Asthma Immunol* 1996; **77**: 112–18.

36 Busse W, Wolfe J, Storms W *et al.* Fluticasone propionate compared with zafirlukast in controlling persistent asthma: a randomized double-blind, placebo-controlled trial. *J Fam Pract* 2001; **50**: 595–602.

37 Brabson JH, Clifford D, Kerwin E *et al.* Efficacy and safety of low-dose fluticasone propionate compared with zafirlukast in patients with persistent asthma. *Am J Med* 2002; **113**: 15–21.

38 Meltzer EO, Lockey RF, Friedman BF *et al.* Efficacy and safety of low-dose fluticasone propionate compared with montelukast for maintenance treatment of persistent asthma. *Mayo Clin Proc* 2002; **77**: 437–45.

39 Nathan RA, Bleecker ER, Kalberg C. A comparison of short-term treatment with inhaled fluticasone propionate and zafirlukast for patients with persistent asthma. *Am J Med* 2001; **111**: 195–202.

40 Asthma in children under five years of age. The General Practitioner in Asthma Group, the British Association of Accident and Emergency Medicine, the British Paediatric Respiratory Society and the Royal College of Paediatrics and Child Health. *Thorax* 1997; **52(Suppl 1)**: S9–10, S18–21.

41 Roorda RJ, Mezei G, Bisgaard H, Maden C. Response of preschool children with asthma symptoms to fluticasone propionate. *J Allergy Clin Immunol* 2001; **108**: 540–6.

42 Bisgaard H, Gillies J, Groenewald M, Maden C. The effect of inhaled fluticasone propionate in the treatment of young asthmatic children: a dose comparison study. *Am J Respir Crit Care Med* 1999; **160**: 126–31.

43 Bisgaard H, Allen D, Milanowski J *et al.* Twelve-month safety and efficacy of inhaled fluticasone propionate in children aged 1 to 3 years with recurrent wheezing. *Pediatrics* 2004; **113**: e87–94.

44 Stoloff SW, Srebro SH, Edwards LD, Johnson MC, Rickard KA. Improved asthma control after changing from low-to-medium doses of other inhaled corticosteroids to low-dose fluticasone propionate. *MedGenMed* 2001; **3**: 2.

45 Schuh S, Reisman J, Alshehri M *et al.* A comparison of inhaled fluticasone and oral prednisone for children with severe acute asthma. *N Engl J Med* 2000; **343**: 689–94.

46 Lipworth BJ. Systemic adverse effects of inhaled corticosteroid therapy: A systematic review and meta-analysis. *Arch Intern Med* 1999; **159**: 941–55.

47 Todd GR, Acerini CL, Ross-Russell R *et al.* Survey of adrenal crisis associated with inhaled corticosteroids in the United Kingdom. *Arch Dis Child* 2002; **87**: 457–61.

48 Kemp JP, Osur S, Shrewsbury SB *et al.* Potential effects of fluticasone propionate on bone mineral density in patients with asthma: a 2-year randomized, double-blind, placebo-controlled trial. *Mayo Clin Proc* 2004; **79**: 458–66.

49 Eid N, Morton R, Olds B *et al.* Decreased morning serum cortisol levels in children with asthma treated with inhaled fluticasone propionate. *Pediatrics* 2002; **109**: 217–21.

50 Todd G, Dunlop K, McNaboe J *et al.* Growth and adrenal suppression in asthmatic children treated with high-dose fluticasone propionate. *Lancet* 1996; **348**: 27–9.

51 Roux C, Kolta S, Desfougeres JL, Minini P, Bidat E. Long-term safety of fluticasone propionate and nedocromil sodium on bone in children with asthma. *Pediatrics* 2003; **111**: e706–13.

52 Allen DB, Bronsky EA, LaForce CF *et al.* Growth in asthmatic children treated with fluticasone propionate. Fluticasone Propionate Asthma Study Group. *J Pediatr* 1998; **132**: 472–7.

53 Jick SS, Vasilakis-Scaramozza C, Maier WC. The risk of cataract among users of inhaled steroids. *Epidemiology* 2001; **12**: 229–34.

54 Barnes NC, Thwaites RM, Price MJ. The cost-effectiveness of inhaled fluticasone propionate and budesonide in the treatment of asthma in adults and children. *Respir Med* 1999; **93**: 402–7.

55 Lamb HM, Culy CR, Faulds D. Inhaled fluticasone propionate. A pharmacoeconomic review of its use in the management of asthma. *Pharmacoeconomics* 2000; **18**: 487–510.

56 Stempel DA, Stanford RH, Thwaites R, Price MJ. Cost-efficacy comparison of inhaled fluticasone propionate and budesonide in the treatment of asthma. *Clin Ther* 2000; **22**: 1562–74.

Acknowledgements

Figure 2 is adapted from Crowley, 2003.[2]
Figure 3 is adapted from Szefler *et al.*, 1999.[18]
Figure 4 is adapted from Busse *et al.*, 2001.[23]
Figure 5 is adapted from Nathan *et al.*, 2001.[39]
Figure 6 is adapted from Verona *et al.*, 2003.[24]

6. Drug review – Formoterol (Foradil® Oxis®)

Dr Eleanor Bull
CSF Medical Communications Ltd

You are strongly urged to consult your doctor before taking, stopping or changing any of the products reviewed or referred to in *BESTMEDICINE* or any other medication that has been prescribed or recommended by your doctor.

Summary

Formoterol is a potent, long-acting β_2-adrenoceptor-selective agonist (β_2-agonist) that relaxes bronchial smooth muscle and thereby elicits bronchodilation in patients with asthma. Recommended for use in combination with inhaled corticosteroids, formoterol provides additional benefits to those patients inadequately controlled with corticosteroids alone and may ultimately permit tapering of the dose of inhaled steroid. However, formoterol should not be used as monotherapy nor is it licensed for use in children under the age of 6 years. Formoterol has a rapid onset of action (1–3 minutes), which is comparable with that of the short-acting β_2-agonists (e.g. salbutamol and terbutaline), and a mean duration of action of 12 hours following inhalation of a single dose. Thus, patients can experience prolonged bronchodilation with formoterol, together with a reduction in day- and night-time symptoms and night-time awakenings. In clinical studies, treatment with formoterol was associated with sustained dose-dependent improvements in morning and evening peak expiratory flow (PEF), increased forced expiratory volume in 1 second (FEV_1), reduced day- and night-time asthma symptoms and a reduced need for rescue medication with short-acting β_2-agonists. Efficacy was comparable with that of another long-acting β_2-agonist, salmeterol, and was consistently equal or superior to that of salbutamol and terbutaline. Children with asthma experienced similar improvements to adults, whilst tolerability was considered to be good across both age categories. However, there is a marginal increased risk of QTc interval prolongation, paradoxical bronchospasm and hypokalaemia associated with formoterol treatment, which may necessitate careful use in some patients.

Introduction

Long-acting β_2-agonists have many advantages over the short-acting β_2-agonists, such as prolonged bronchodilation, reduced day- and night-time symptoms and reduced night-time awakenings.

The use of long-acting β_2-adrenoceptor agonists (β_2-agonists) is now well established in asthma management as the preferred second-line controller therapy in addition to inhaled corticosteroids. Long-acting β_2-agonists (e.g. salmeterol and formoterol) have many advantages over the short-acting β_2-agonists (e.g. salbutamol and terbutaline), such as prolonged bronchodilation, reduced day- and night-time symptoms and reduced night-time awakenings.[1] Guidelines issued jointly by the Scottish Intercollegiate Guidelines Network (SIGN) and the British Thoracic Society (BTS) in 2004, recommend the use of long-acting β_2-agonists as add-on therapy if moderate doses of inhaled steroids (200–800 μg/day in adults and 200–400 μg/day in children up to 12 years of age) are failing to adequately control asthma in adults and children over the age of 5 years.[2] When administered alone, long-acting β_2-agonists are less effective than inhaled corticosteroids, and, therefore, they should not be used as monotherapy in clinical practice.

In the past, there has been some controversy surrounding a reported increase in asthma morbidity and mortality associated with β_2-agonist use in general.[3] The withdrawal of the short-acting β_2-agonist, fenoterol, in New Zealand in 1990, was associated with a substantial decline in asthma morbidity and mortality.[3] The potential worsening of asthma control associated with β_2-agonists may be related to the development of tolerance (tachyphylaxis), reduced protection against provoking stimuli, an increased allergen load, or masking of the symptoms of deteriorating asthma.[4] Although long-acting β_2-agonists have, in general, not been associated with worsening of asthma control, the potential for tachyphylaxis should not be ignored, and it is important to consider the possibility of reduced asthma control and increased bronchial hyper-responsiveness with regular or longer-term use.[5,6]

Formoterol is a β_2-adrenoceptor selective agonist that combines a rapid onset with a prolonged duration of effect.

Formoterol is a β_2-adrenoceptor selective agonist that combines a rapid onset (1–3 minutes) with a prolonged duration of action. The patient experiences significant bronchodilation within minutes of inhaling formoterol, and this is maintained for a mean duration of 12 hours.[7] Indicated for reversible airways obstruction – including nocturnal asthma and the prevention of exercise-induced bronchospasm – in patients requiring long-term regular bronchodilator therapy, formoterol may be added to an asthma management regimen when corticosteroid monotherapy has failed to control the condition effectively.[7,8] If necessary, formoterol may also be used for the relief of symptoms up to a maximum total daily dose of 12 actuations (including the maintenance dose).[7] Initially marketed as an oral short-acting β_2-agonist in Japan, the sustained duration of action of inhaled formoterol was discovered serendipitously.[1,9,10] Within Europe, formoterol is licensed for use in adults and children aged over 6 years age, at daily doses of up to 48 and 24 μg, respectively.[8] The use of formoterol for the short-term relief of symptoms (but not for the treatment of acute asthma) is also permitted.[8]

This review discusses the pharmacological properties of formoterol and its efficacy in controlled clinical trials in both adults and children with asthma. In line with other reviews of anti-asthma drugs previously published in the journal *Drugs in Context*, clinical trials of formoterol in patients with Chronic Obstructive Pulmonary Disease (COPD) are beyond the scope of the review and are not discussed herein. Formoterol is available as an inhalation powder that is administered via a number of devices, including the Oxis® Turbohaler® and the Foradil® Aerolizer®.[7,11,12] Throughout this review, we have commented on data pertaining specifically to the Oxis Turbohaler, though references to other formulations have been included where appropriate. Symbicort® – the combination of formoterol with the inhaled corticosteroid, budesonide – is discussed later in this edition of *BESTMEDICINE.*

Pharmacology

Chemistry

The chemical structure of formoterol (or eformoterol), a phenylethanolamine derivative, is illustrated in Figure 1.[13] The formulation of formoterol used clinically is a pure diastereomer of the RR and SS enantiomers of the fumarate dihydrate salt. The RR enantiomer binds to the β_2-adrenoceptor and inhibits bronchial contraction in response to spasmogens, whilst the SS enantiomer may antagonise the therapeutic effects of RR formoterol to some extent.[14]

The chemistry of formoterol is of essentially academic interest and most healthcare professionals will, like you, skip this section.

The unique pharmacological profile of formoterol, which combines rapid onset with a long duration of action, can be attributed to its intermediate physiochemical properties.[15] Formoterol is less hydrophilic than salbutamol and less lipophilic than salmeterol, which consequently produces a compound that shares the most valuable pharmacological attributes of these short- and long-acting β_2-compounds.[15]

Mechanism of action

Formoterol is a potent and selective β_2-adrenoceptor agonist that relieves bronchoconstriction by relaxing airway smooth muscle.[13] In humans, bronchodilation occurs within 1–3 minutes of inhalation and is

Figure 1. The chemical structure of formoterol.

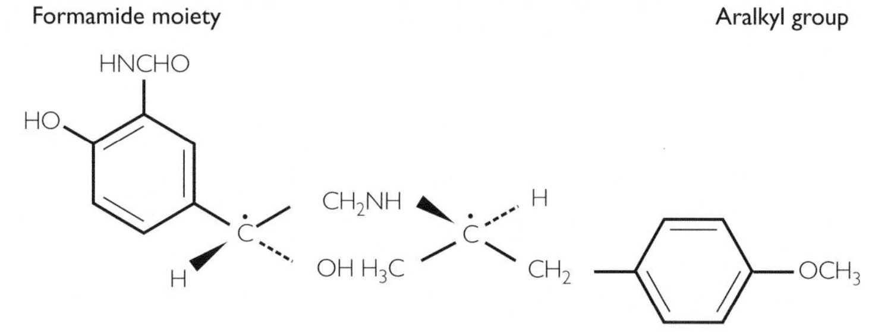

Formoterol displays very high binding affinity and selectivity for the β_2-adrenoceptor in lung preparations.

maintained for a mean duration of 12 hours.[7] Table 1 shows the relative potency and efficacy (intrinsic activity) of formoterol compared with the non-selective β-agonist, isoprenaline, salbutamol and salmeterol on human isolated bronchi at resting tone or when pre-contracted with acetylcholine.[13] Formoterol displays very high binding affinity and selectivity for the β_2-adrenoceptor in lung preparations (dissociation constant [K_D] 8.12 *vs* 6.44 and 7.10 for formoterol, salbutamol and isoprenaline, respectively).[13] In humans with or without asthma, the dose potency of formoterol was 28–109-times greater than that of salbutamol, depending on the systemic effect variable evaluated (e.g. cardiovascular or metabolic).[16]

Bronchoprotective effects

Both short- and long-acting β_2-agonists afford protection against bronchoconstrictive stimuli such as methacholine and adenosine monophosphate. Regular treatment with both long- and short-acting β_2-agonists may ultimately result in the development of tolerance to these bronchoprotective effects, though the implications of this, in terms of long-term asthma control, remain unclear.[6,17]

A double-blind placebo-controlled study of 72 patients with stable mild-to-moderate asthma examined the magnitude of bronchoprotection against methacholine challenge afforded by pre-treatment with formoterol or terbutaline.[18] Patients received either formoterol (6 or 24 µg twice daily, or 12 µg once daily) or terbutaline (500 µg four-times daily) via a dry powder inhaler (DPI) over a 2-week treatment period. The provocative dose of methacholine that elicited a 20% decrease in FEV_1 (PD_{20}) was measured at baseline, 1 hour after the first dose of active treatment and again after 2 hours, 7 days and 2 weeks. The protection afforded by the first dose of formoterol (24 µg) was three-times greater than that for terbutaline. Significant tachyphylaxis to protection against methacholine-induced bronchoconstriction was observed for all active treatments, such that

Table 1. The potency and efficacy of selected agonists in human bronchus *in vitro*.[13]

Agonist	Basal tone			Acetylcholine (1 mM)		
	EC_{50}	E_{max}	IA	EC_{50}	E_{max}	IA
Isoprenaline	7.31	98	1.00	6.56	85	1.00
Adrenaline	6.85	95	0.97	6.29*	87*	1.02
Formoterol	9.63	94†	0.96	8.74*	71*	0.84
Salbutamol	7.12	83†	0.85	–	55*,†	0.64
Salmeterol	7.96	70†	0.71	–	53*,†	0.62

*$p<0.05$, *vs* baseline, †$p<0.05$ *vs* isoprenaline

EC_{50}, the dose necessary to produce a half-maximal response; E_{max}, maximal percentage relaxation of the maximal effect elicited by theophylline (3 nM); IA, intrinsic activity (defined as E_{max}[drug]/E_{max} [isoprenaline]).

the percentage loss of protection between the first and last dose after 14 days of dosing was 87, 76, 71 and 47% for formoterol 24 μg twice daily, 12 μg once daily, 6 μg twice daily and terbutaline, respectively.

β_2-adrenoceptor polymorphism

There is some evidence to suggest that the development of tolerance to long-acting β_2-agonists may be influenced by a polymorphism in the gene encoding the β_2-adrenoceptor, which affects agonist-induced down-regulation and de-sensitisation of β_2-adrenoceptors.[19] The exact influence of such polymorphisms (e.g. arginine-16, glycine-16) on the bronchoprotective effects of long-acting β_2-agonists have yet to be determined.

A retrospective analysis of six placebo-controlled studies in patients with mild-to-moderate asthma who were already receiving corticosteroids, examined the effects of formoterol or salmeterol on the PD_{20} of methacholine or adenosine monophosphate, and further stratified patients according to their genotype.[20] Those patients who had homozygous or heterozygous genotypes containing the arginine-16 polymorphism showed greater bronchoprotective subsensitivity to bronchoconstrictive challenge, compared with those patients with a homozygous glycine-16 genotype. The difference between genotypes amounted to a mean PD_{20} doubling dose difference of 1.49 after the last dose. This subsensitivity was greater for formoterol than salmeterol for all genotypes, in particular the arginine-16 polymorphism, and amounted to a doubling dose (dd) shift from the respective baselines of 3.00 between the two drugs.

Patients who had homozygous or heterozygous genotypes containing the arginine-16 polymorphism showed greater bronchoprotective subsensitivity to bronchoconstrictive challenge.

Pharmacokinetics

The pharmacokinetic properties of formoterol are presented in Table 2.[7,11,12,15,21] Absorbed rapidly following inhalation, peak plasma concentrations (C_{max}) of formoterol are reached approximately

The pharmacokinetics of a drug are of interest to healthcare professionals because it is important for them to understand the action of a drug on the body over a period of time.

Table 2. The pharmacokinetic properties of formoterol.[7,11,12,15,21]

Pharmacokinetic parameter	
Total systemic availability (%)	61
t_{max} (minutes)	15
Volume of distribution (L/kg)	4
Mean lung deposition	28–49% of delivered dose
Plasma protein binding (%)	50
Total clearance (L/minute)	1.4
$t_{1/2}$ (hours)	8–17
Excretion (%)	8–13 of delivered dose (urine)

t_{max}, time to reach maximum drug plasma concentration (C_{max}); $t_{1/2}$, elimination half-life.

15 minutes after administration.[7] The total plasma clearance and volume of distribution of formoterol have not been directly determined in pharmacokinetic studies.[7] Formoterol is extensively metabolised via direct glucuronidation and O-demethylation followed by further glucuronidation. Although the precise enzyme responsible for O-demethylation has not been identified, it is likely that the cytochrome P450 (CYP) isoenzymes 2D6, 2C19, 2C9 and 2A6 are involved.[7,12] The potential for clinically significant drug–drug interactions associated with formoterol is lessened by the observation that it shows limited inhibition of CYP enzymes at therapeutic concentrations, although as a CYP substrate, it may be affected by other compounds which are inhibitors/inducers of the enzyme.[21]

Delivery device

The Turbohaler was developed as an alternative to the pMDI and combines convenience for the user with efficient drug deposition.

Formoterol may be inhaled via a number of delivery devices, which differ in terms of their deposition characteristics. The pressurised metered dose inhaler (pMDI) is propellant driven and delivers only approximately 10–15% of the metered dose, even if inhalation technique is optimal.[15] However, many patients experience difficulties using these devices properly, particularly children.[21] The more recently introduced DPIs – Turbohaler and Aerolizer – deliver 20–35% of a metered dose.[15] The Turbohaler – an inspiratory flow driven DPI – was developed as an alternative to the pMDI and combines convenience for the user with efficient drug deposition.[7,11] By delivering approximately twice as much drug directly to the lungs, effective bronchodilation is achieved with lower doses of formoterol than those necessary when using pMDIs.[9]

Dosage

As mentioned previously, inhaled formoterol should be administered as an adjunct to an existing regimen of inhaled or oral corticosteroids, in order to improve asthma control without increasing the dose of steroid administered.[2,8] It is essential that patients do not discontinue their use of corticosteroids during formoterol treatment, though downwards adjustment of corticosteroid dosage is permitted.

When administering formoterol using the Turbohaler, the recommended dose in adults and children over the age of 6 years is 6–12 μg, 1–2 times daily, increasing to 24 μg twice daily in more severe cases of airways obstruction.[8] It should be noted that there are two strengths of Turbohaler currently available, corresponding to a delivered dose of 4.5 or 9 μg per administration or actuation.[7,11] The recommended daily dose of formoterol administered via the Aerolizer is 12 μg twice daily, which can be increased to 24 μg twice daily during more severe airways obstruction.[8] Formoterol may also be used for short-term symptom relief (but not for the treatment of acute asthma), up to a daily maximum of 72 μg in adults, as administered using the Turbohaler. When used for the prevention of exercise-induced bronchospasm, two actuations of formoterol should be administered before exercise.

Special patient groups

Formoterol is not indicated for use by children aged 6 years of age or under, and to date, there are no pharmacokinetic data available that relate specifically to children in this age category.[7] There is no need for dosage adjustment when administering formoterol to elderly patients or patients with renal or hepatic impairment.[7] However, since formoterol is primarily eliminated by metabolism, increased exposure can be expected in patients with severe liver cirrhosis and appropriate caution should therefore be observed.[7]

Clinical efficacy

Onset and duration of action

Data pertaining to the onset and duration of action of formoterol, administered via the Turbohaler, in adult patients with asthma are summarised in Table 3.[22–25] In general, these studies have demonstrated that formoterol possesses a rapid onset of action that is comparable with that of the short-acting β_2-agonist, salbutamol, but has a duration of action that more closely resembles that of the long-acting β_2-agonist, salmeterol.

Placebo-controlled studies

The lowest effective dose of inhaled formoterol was determined in a 4-week, double-blind, placebo-controlled study in 221 adult patients with moderate asthma – defined according to criteria set out by the American Thoracic Society – and who had a basal FEV_1 of 1 L or more and between 40–80% of predicted values.[26] Following a 1-week run-in phase, patients received formoterol, 6, 12 or 24 μg twice daily, or placebo, for 4 weeks, administered using the Turbohaler. Morning PEF was recorded immediately prior to and 15 minutes after drug inhalation. At baseline, the mean FEV_1 was 2.01 L, 58% of the predicted normal, with a mean bronchodilator reversibility of 27%. The changes in morning and evening PEF from run-in to post-treatment are illustrated in Figure 2. The lowest effective dose of formoterol, in terms of eliciting a significant improvement in morning and evening PEF, was 6 μg twice daily (mean treatment difference: 22 and 23 L/minute for morning and evening PEF respectively; p=0.008 and p=0.004 *vs* placebo). The mean additional effect of increasing the formoterol dose to 24 μg twice daily was an improvement of 15 and 18 L/minute, for morning and evening PEF, respectively (p>0.05 and p=0.035 *vs* placebo). There was no significant difference in terms of PEF between the 6 and 12 μg doses of formoterol, and diurnal variation was very low, ranging from 3.4–5.5%. Overall, the immediate change in morning PEF following formoterol was greater than 40 L/minute for all doses of formoterol, compared with 9 L/minute for placebo (42 L/minute for formoterol, 6 μg; p<0.0001). The incidence of day and night-time asthma symptoms was significantly reduced following all doses of formoterol. Again, the lowest effective dose of formoterol was 6 μg twice daily (change in symptom score:

The lowest effective dose of formoterol, in terms of eliciting a significant improvement in morning and evening PEF, was 6 μg twice daily.

Table 3. Summary of clinical trials investigating the onset and duration of action of formoterol, administered via Turbohaler.[22–25]

Study	Asthma severity at baseline	Dosage regimen	Main outcomes
Palmqvist *et al.*, 1997[22] Double-blind Crossover n=28	FEV_1 >40% of predicted normal Reversibility ≥10%	Formoterol, 6, 12 or 24 μg or Salmeterol, 50 μg or Placebo	• Percentage of patients responding with FEV_1 ≥15% over baseline within 1 hour of dosing 43, 68 and 64% for formoterol, 6, 12 and 24 μg, *vs* 61% for salmeterol, 50 μg, and 4% for placebo (*p*-values not reported). • Median time to onset was 12.4 and 3.6 minutes for formoterol, 12 and 24 μg, respectively, and 31.0 minutes for salmeterol, 50 μg ($p<0.05$ *vs* salmeterol). • The mean duration of ≥15% increases in FEV_1 was 244, 337 and 459 minutes for formoterol, 6, 12 and 24 μg, respectively, *vs* 345 minutes for salmeterol, 50 μg ($p>0.05$ *vs* salmeterol). • Formoterol, 24 μg, was significantly more potent than salmeterol, 50 μg ($p<0.05$, calculated using Fieller's method). Formoterol 9 μg was estimated to be equipotent with salmeterol 50 μg.
Ringdal *et al.*, 1998[23] Double-blind Crossover n=31	Mean FEV_1 of 1.97 L Mean reversibility 31% of baseline	Formoterol, 6, 12, 24 or 48 μg or Placebo	• Maximum increase in FEV_1 over placebo was dose-dependent (12, 18, 19, 26% for formoterol, 6, 12, 24 and 48 μg, respectively; $p<0.001$ *vs* placebo). • Mean increases in FEV_1 over placebo after 12 hours were 7, 15, 18 and 27% for formoterol, 6, 12, 24 and 48 μg, respectively. • Headache was the most frequently reported adverse event.
Sill and Ortland, 1998[24] Open-label n=99	Median FEV_1 69% of predicted normal Median reversibility 29% of baseline	Formoterol, 9 μg or Salmeterol, 50 μg, via Diskus	• sRAW decreased significantly by 29% within 2 minutes of formoterol inhalation (*vs* no change following salmeterol, +1%;, $p<0.0001$) • 49% of salmeterol-treated patients showed a mean increase in sRAW of 16% immediately following inhalation. • The onset of action of formoterol was more rapid than that of salmeterol, which actually elicited an increase in airways resistance immediately following inhalation.

FEV_1, forced expiratory volume in 1 second; PEF, peak expiratory flow; pMDI, pressurised metered dose inhaler; sRAW, specific airway resistance.

Table 3. Continued

Study	Asthma severity at baseline	Dosage regimen	Main outcomes
Seberova and Andersson, 2000[25] Double-blind Crossover n=36	Mean FEV_1 73.8% of predicted normal Mean reversibility 24.2% of baseline	Formoterol, 4.5 or 9 µg or Salbutamol, 100 or 200 µg via pMDI or Placebo	• All drugs caused significantly greater bronchodilation than placebo (11.7 and 11.8% for formoterol, 4.5 and 9 µg, and 10.0 and 11.4% for salbutamol, 100 and 200 µg, respectively; $p<0.001$ *vs* placebo for all comparisons). • Median time to response ranged between 2.8 and 5.3 minutes, for formoterol, 9 µg, and salbutamol, 200 µg, respectively. • All treatments were well tolerated.

FEV_1, forced expiratory volume in 1 second; PEF, peak expiratory flow; pMDI, pressurised metered dose inhaler; sRAW, specific airway resistance.

–0.21 *vs* 0.15 and –0.24 *vs* 0.12 for day and night-time symptoms, respectively; p=0.001 and p<0.001 *vs* placebo). The need for rescue medication (terbutaline, 0.25 mg, by inhalation as-needed) was significantly reduced during the daytime by formoterol, 12 µg twice daily (–1.30 *vs* –0.64 inhalations; p=0.019 *vs* placebo), whilst the lowest effective dose that significantly reduced night-time rescue medication was 6 µg twice daily (–0.72 *vs* –0.32 inhalations; p=0.034 *vs* placebo). All doses of formoterol were well tolerated in this study with headache and tremor the most frequently reported adverse events.

A longer-term, placebo-controlled study in 239 patients with mild-to-moderate asthma, evaluated the efficacy of formoterol (24 µg twice daily via Turbohaler) over a period of 24 weeks.[27] All study participants were already receiving regular inhaled corticosteroids (100–3200 µg daily) but their asthma was not completely controlled and, as such, they still required at least five inhalations of a short-acting β_2-agonist per week to control asthma symptoms. At baseline, mean FEV_1 was 67.1% of the predicted normal, mean reversibility was 25.7% and the mean total asthma symptom score was 3.6 (out of 21). The rate of premature treatment discontinuations was comparable between treatment groups (14 *vs* 11% for formoterol and placebo, respectively). Overall, treatment with formoterol elicited a modest but significant reduction in asthma symptom scores compared with placebo (mean difference of 0.64 *vs* placebo; p=0.039). Over the course of the study, the mean difference between formoterol- and placebo-treated patients in terms of morning and evening PEF, was 28 and 27.1 L/minute, respectively (p<0.001 *vs* placebo for both comparisons). Compared with placebo, formoterol treatment elicited a significant reduction in the use of rescue medication, both during the day and at night-time (mean difference: –1.1 and –0.8 inhalations for day- and night-time use, respectively; p<0.001 *vs* placebo for both comparisons). The number of asthma exacerbations

Figure 2. Daily means of pre-medication morning (upper) and evening (lower) peak expiratory flow (PEF) following the run-in, formoterol (6–24 μg, twice daily) and placebo treatment periods.[26]

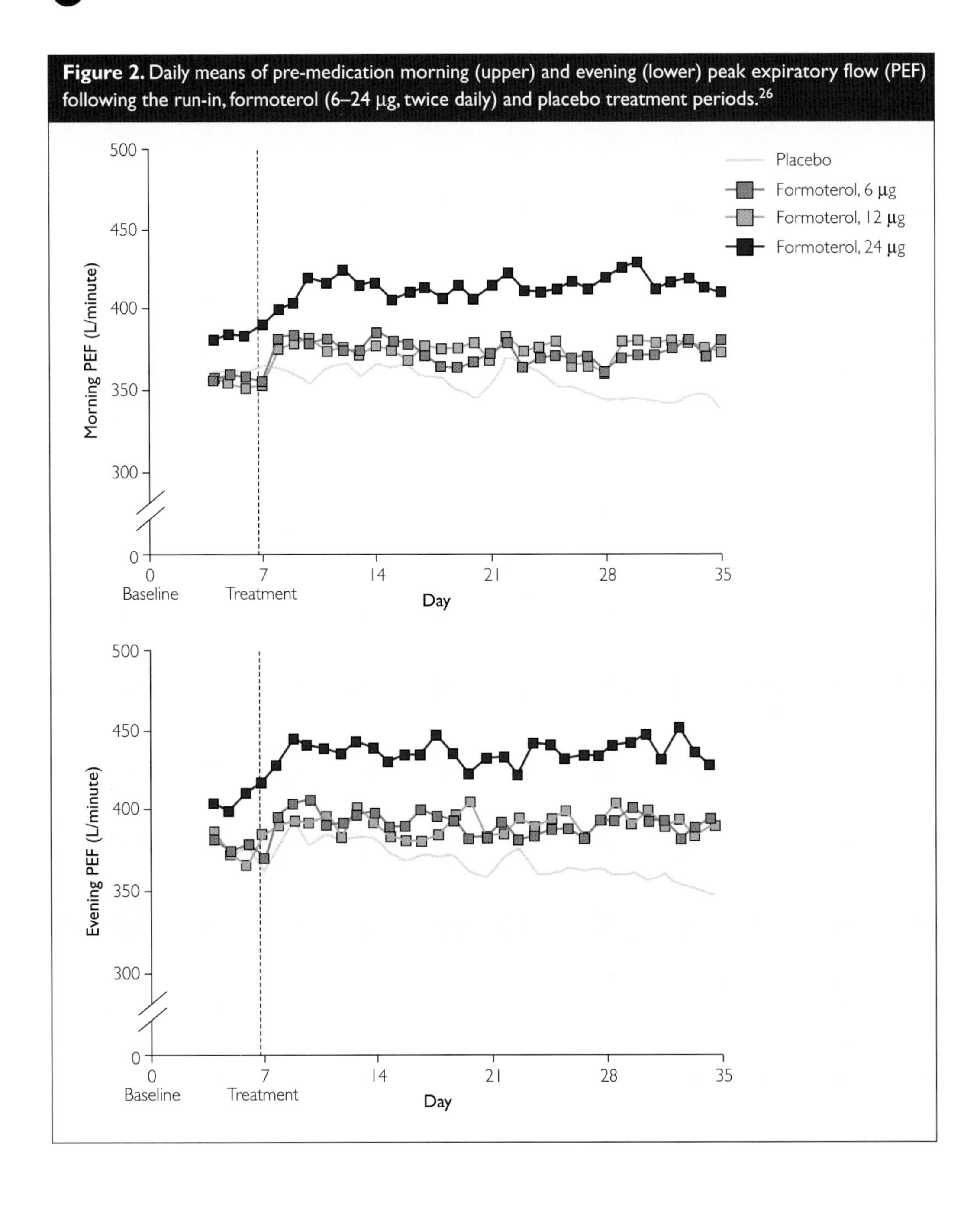

experienced by patients over the course of the study, as determined by the number of courses of oral prednisolone taken, was similar between treatment groups (26.4 *vs* 28.1% for formoterol and placebo treatment groups, respectively; $p>0.05$). The improvements in PEF and asthma symptom scores associated with formoterol treatment were reversed following cessation of therapy.

Comparative studies

Formoterol *vs* salbutamol

Clinical studies that have compared the efficacy of formoterol with that of the short-acting β_2-agonist, salbutamol, are summarised in Table 4.[28–33] In general, the overall efficacy of formoterol was at least equal to that of salbutamol and in many instances was superior. The duration of action of formoterol was sustained longer than that of salbutamol, and formoterol was associated with less night-time symptoms and awakenings, as well as a reduced need for rescue medication.

Formoterol *vs* terbutaline

A placebo-controlled study of 397 adults with mild-to-moderate asthma (baseline FEV_1 40–80% of predicted normal) compared the relative effectiveness of formoterol, 6 μg twice daily, with that of terbutaline, 0.5 mg four-times daily, administered via the Turbohaler over a 12-week treatment period.[34] At baseline, the mean FEV_1 was 62% of predicted normal and mean reversibility was 25%. The improvement in mean morning PEF was significantly greater following treatment with formoterol than with terbutaline or placebo (20 *vs* 9 and 2 L/minute, respectively; p=0.014 and p=0.001 *vs* terbutaline and placebo). Improvement in evening PEF was also significant following formoterol treatment compared with placebo (17 *vs* 2 L/minute; p=0.0001), though the difference between formoterol and terbutaline did not reach significance with reference to this parameter (17 *vs* 9 L/minute; p=0.061). Formoterol also elicited a significant reduction in day- and night-time asthma symptoms compared with both terbutaline and placebo treatment (differences in daytime symptom score of –0.14 and –0.09 from placebo and terbutaline, respectively; p=0.003 and p=0.038; differences in night-time score of –0.10 and –0.11; p=0.029 and p=0.015, respectively). The use of rescue medication, terbutaline 0.25 mg via Turbohaler, was significantly reduced following both formoterol and terbutaline treatment compared with placebo (difference in daytime inhalations of –0.37 and –0.15 for formoterol and terbutaline, respectively, p=0.001 and p=0.043 *vs* placebo).

Formoterol elicited a significant reduction in day- and night-time asthma symptoms compared with both terbutaline and placebo treatment.

A similarly designed double-blind study compared the efficacy of formoterol with terbutaline over a 12-week period in 362 adult patients with moderate-to-severe asthma (mean FEV_1 74% of predicted normal) who required an inhaled short-acting β_2-agonist between three- and eight-times daily during a 2-week run-in period.[35] Patients self-administered either formoterol (4.5 μg) or terbutaline (0.5 mg) as-needed via Turbohaler, up to maximum daily doses of 54 μg or 6 mg, respectively. The time to the first severe asthma exacerbation was significantly longer amongst those patients receiving formoterol than those receiving terbutaline (relative risk ratio 0.55; p=0.013). Formoterol treatment was also associated with greater improvements in morning and evening PEF than terbutaline (mean difference in change of 11 and 8 L/minute for morning and evening PEF, respectively; p=0.009 and p=0.043). Pre-medication FEV_1 (i.e. measured immediately before

Table 4. Summary of controlled clinical trials comparing the efficacy of formoterol with that of the short-acting β_2-agonist, salbutamol.[28–33]

Study	Asthma severity at baseline	Dosage regimen	Main outcomes
Hekking *et al.*, 1990[28] Double-blind 12 weeks n=301	Mean FEV_1 56% of predicted normal Mean reversibility 33% of baseline	Formoterol, 12 µg, twice daily or Salbutamol, 200 µg, four-times daily Given via a metered dose inhaler	• Formoterol had a significantly longer duration of action than salbutamol (morning PEF 341 *vs* 304 L/minute, taken 14 and 9 hours after the last dose of formoterol and salbutamol respectively; p=0.0004). • Formoterol-treated patients had significantly less weekly asthma attacks (1 *vs* 2 night-time attacks for formoterol and salbutamol, respectively; p=0.002). • Formoterol-treated patients required significantly less rescue medication (4.9 *vs* 7.9 daytime puffs for formoterol and salbutamol, respectively; p=0.001). • 10% of formoterol-treated patients discontinued treatment prematurely compared with 20% of salbutamol patients (p-value not reported).
Kesten *et al.*, 1991 and 1992[29,30] Double-blind 12 weeks n=145 Open-label, 9-month extension n=112	Initial FEV_1 at least 40% of predicted normal Mean pre-medication FEV_1 2.1 L	Formoterol, 12 µg, twice daily or Salbutamol, 200 µg, four-times daily Follow-up: Formoterol only, 12 µg, twice daily	• Morning pre-medication FEV_1 was significantly higher following formoterol at week 8 (2.4 *vs* 1.92 L for formoterol and salbutamol, respectively; p<0.001). • The diurnal variation in PEF was significantly reduced by formoterol at week 12 (17 *vs* 42 L/minute for formoterol and salbutamol, respectively; p<0.001). Follow-up: • Efficacy of formoterol was sustained in the long-term (FEV_1: 2.31 *vs* 2.42 L, at study endpoint *vs* baseline; p<0.05. PEFR: 413 *vs* 421 L/minute; p<0.05 *vs* baseline). • Patients switching from salbutamol to formoterol experienced improvements in flow rate and asthma symptoms. • No evidence of tachyphylaxis was reported.

FEV_1, forced expiratory volume in 1 second; PEF(R), peak expiratory flow (rate).

Table 4. Continued

Study	Asthma severity at baseline	Dosage regimen	Main outcomes
Steffensen *et al.*, 1995[31] Placebo-controlled Double-blind 12 weeks n=304 Open-label, 12-month extension n=116	Mean pre-medication FEV_1 2.1 L Mean reversibility 27%	Formoterol, 12 µg, twice daily or Salbutamol, 400 µg, four-times daily Follow-up: Formoterol only, 12 µg twice daily	• Morning pre-medication PEFR was significantly improved by formoterol treatment (mean difference of 32 L/minute *vs* salbutamol and 28 L/minute *vs* placebo (p<0.001 for both comparisons). • The efficacy of formoterol was sustained during the 12-month extension period with no signs of tachyphylaxis. • Night-time symptom score was significantly lower following treatment with formoterol (0.4 *vs* 0.54 and 0.66 for formoterol, salbutamol and placebo, respectively; p<0.05 *vs* salbutamol and p<0.001 *vs* placebo). • Use of rescue medication was significantly lower following formoterol than salbutamol or placebo treatment (p<0.005 for both comparisons). • Tolerability was comparable between the treatment groups.
Bensch *et al.*, 2001[32] Placebo-controlled Double-blind 12 weeks n=541	Mean FEV_1 66.5% of predicted normal	Formoterol, 12 or 24 µg, twice daily or Salbutamol, 180 µg, four-times daily	• Morning and evening PEF were improved by a greater extent in the formoterol treatment groups compared with salbutamol (p<0.001) and placebo (p≤0.003) treatment groups. • Percentage of days free of asthma symptoms were significantly greater for 12 and 24 µg formoterol-treatment groups (52 and 53% *vs* 42 and 33%, for salbutamol and placebo groups, respectively; p<0.016 and p<0.001). • Percentage of days free of nocturnal awakenings was significantly greater for 12 and 24 µg formoterol-treatment groups (72 and 73% *vs* 59 and 53%, for salbutamol and placebo groups, respectively; p≤0.001 for both comparisons). • Adverse events were comparable between the treatment groups.

FEV_1, forced expiratory volume in 1 second; PEF(R), peak expiratory flow (rate).

Table 4. Continued

Study	Asthma severity at baseline	Dosage regimen	Main outcomes
Pleskow *et al.*, 2003[33] Placebo-controlled Double-blind 12 weeks n=554	Mean FEV_1 66.5% of predicted normal	Formoterol, 12 or 24 µg, twice daily or Salbutamol, 180 µg, four-times daily	• FEV_1 in 12 and 24 µg formoterol treatment groups was superior to placebo on all test days ($p \leq 0.017$). • FEV_1 in 12 and 24 µg formoterol treatment groups was superior to salbutamol for the majority of time-points on all test days ($p \leq 0.001$). • The percentage of patients experiencing a 15% increase in FEV_1 within 5 minutes of administration was 57, 71 and 65%, for formoterol, 12 and 24 µg, and salbutamol, respectively (*p*-values not reported). • The use of rescue medication was significantly reduced compared with placebo in formoterol and salbutamol treatment groups (*p*-values not reported).

FEV_1, forced expiratory volume in 1 second; PEF(R), peak expiratory flow (rate).

The use of rescue medication was significantly less frequent following treatment with formoterol than terbutaline.

administration of the respective study bronchodilators) increased in the formoterol treatment group compared with the terbutaline group (mean ratio 105%) but there was no difference between the two drugs in terms of post-medication FEV_1 values (Figure 3). The use of rescue medication was significantly less frequent following treatment with formoterol than terbutaline (difference in total use of 0.76 inhalations per day, p=0.0005).

The quality of life of patients from the above study was assessed using the Asthma Quality of Life Questionnaire (AQLQ), which was completed by 341 patients at 4, 8 and 12 weeks after randomisation.[36] Although overall quality of life was significantly improved by both treatments, the level of improvement was greatest amongst those receiving formoterol (overall AQLQ score improvements of 0.41 and 0.17, respectively; p=0.0003). The greatest improvements were observed in the symptom domain of the AQLQ (change of 0.49 *vs* 0.21 following formoterol and terbutaline, respectively; p=0.002).

Formoterol *vs* salmeterol

The relative efficacy of formoterol and salmeterol was compared in an 8-week single-blinded study with a 4-week crossover period.[37] Adult patients (n=469), with a history of mild-to-moderate asthma and who had received at least 200 µg of inhaled steroid per day during the 4 weeks preceding the study, were randomised to receive either

Figure 3. Mean forced expiratory volume in 1 second (FEV_1) before and after inhalation of bronchodilator (terbutaline, 1.5 mg), following as-needed treatment with formoterol or terbutaline.[35]

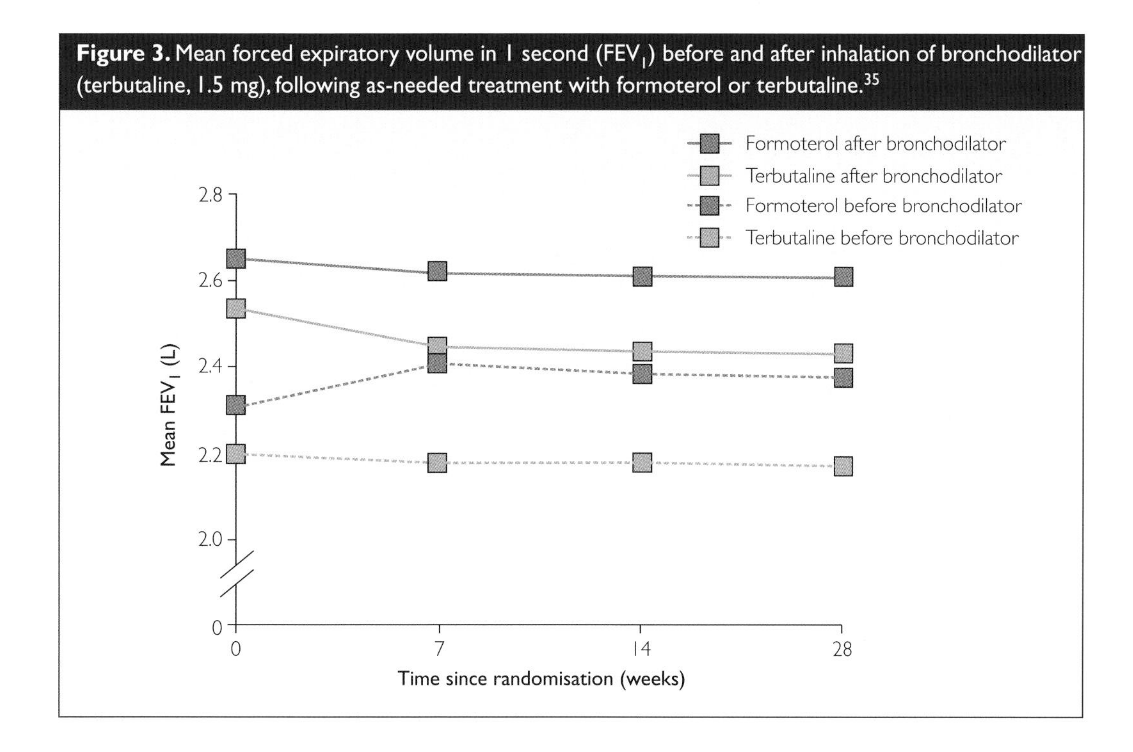

formoterol via Turbohaler (12 µg, twice daily) or salmeterol (50 µg, twice daily) via Accuhaler® or pMDI. Over the 8 weeks of the treatment period, morning PEF was similarly improved by all treatment regimens (increases of 29.7, 27.8 and 32.1 L/minute for formoterol, salmeterol Accuhaler and salmeterol pMDI, respectively; p=0.0001 from baseline for all treatments, with no between-group differences). Following 4 weeks' treatment, the improvement in morning PEF was most pronounced in the formoterol and salmeterol pMDI treatment groups (28.9, 19.9 and 26.1 L/min, respectively; p=0.0001 from baseline with no between-group differences). Formoterol treatment elicited superior improvements in daytime asthma symptoms over 4 weeks than the salmeterol Accuhaler group (–0.54 *vs* –0.35; p=0.014), though there was no difference between the formoterol and salmeterol pMDI treatment groups. The number of symptom-free days reported during treatment was higher amongst formoterol- than salmeterol-treated patients, though this did not reach significance (32.8, 24.1 and 28.0%, for formoterol, salmeterol Accuhaler and salmeterol pMDI, respectively). Out of all treatment regimens, formoterol was rated most highly in terms of patient preference and was significantly more convenient to carry than the salmeterol Accuhaler (p<0.0001). If given the choice, significantly more patients stated that they would rather use the Turbohaler than the pMDI (p=0.0168). All treatments were well tolerated and the rate of treatment discontinuation was comparable between groups (15, 14 and 17% for formoterol, salmeterol Accuhaler and salmeterol pMDI, respectively).

Formoterol was rated most highly in terms of patient preference and was significantly more convenient to carry than the salmeterol Accuhaler.

Efficacy in paediatric asthma

A double-blind, placebo-controlled study conducted in 302 children (aged 6–11 years) with asthma not optimally managed with inhaled corticosteroids alone, examined the effectiveness of inhaled formoterol as add-on therapy.[38] Participants continued with their existing dose of corticosteroid and in addition, received either formoterol (4.5 or 9 μg, twice daily, given via Turbohaler) or placebo, for a period of 12 weeks. At baseline, the mean FEV_1 was 78% of the predicted normal and mean reversibility was 15%, with no significant demographic differences between treatment groups. The rate of premature treatment discontinuation was significantly higher amongst placebo-treated patients than those receiving formoterol, 4.5 μg (7 *vs* 16%; $p=0.02$). However, the rate of treatment discontinuation amongst children receiving formoterol, 9 μg, was not significantly different to those receiving placebo (12 *vs* 16%, respectively; $p>0.05$). Following 12 weeks of treatment, morning PEF was improved significantly by both doses of formoterol (treatment differences of 7.8 and 10.8 L/minute for formoterol, 4.5 and 9 μg, respectively; $p=0.035$ and $p=0.0045$ *vs* placebo). Evening PEF was similarly improved (treatment differences of 9.2 and 9.2 L/minute for formoterol, 4.5 and 9 μg, respectively; $p=0.011$ and $p=0.014$ *vs* placebo). Likewise, FEV_1 (% predicted normal) was also increased by formoterol treatment (treatment differences of 4.01 and 3.63% for formoterol, 4.5 and 9 μg, respectively; $p=0.0051$ and $p=0.015$ *vs* placebo). For all parameters, there was no significant difference between formoterol, 4.5 and 9 μg. There was no significant difference between any of the treatment groups in terms of total symptom score and the use of rescue medication (mean change from baseline –0.37, –0.28 and –0.27 for total symptom score and –0.13, –0.27 and –0.21 for daily inhalations of rescue medication for formoterol, 4.5 and 9 μg, and placebo, respectively; $p>0.05$). The incidence of severe asthma exacerbations was lower in the formoterol treatment groups than in the placebo group (hazard ratios: 0.529 and 0.747 for formoterol, 4.5 and 9 μg, *vs* placebo). All treatments were well tolerated and there was no evidence of tachyphylaxis.

The incidence of severe asthma exacerbations was lower in the formoterol treatment groups than in the placebo group.

An additional placebo-controlled study, identical in design and duration to the previous study, evaluated the efficacy of formoterol (4.5 or 9 μg, twice daily, given via Turbohaler) in 248 children aged 6–17 years.[39] Participants had a diagnosis of asthma in agreement with American Thoracic Society criteria and an FEV_1 of at least 40% of the predicted normal value. At baseline, mean FEV_1 was 81% of the predicted normal and mean reversibility was 11%, with no significant demographic differences between treatment groups. The incidence of treatment discontinuations over the course of the study was low and comparable between each treatment group. Treatment with formoterol, 9 μg twice daily, elicited significant improvement in morning PEF over the 12 weeks of the study (mean change of 13.0 L/minute; $p=0.02$ *vs* placebo). The change in morning PEF following treatment with formoterol, 4.5 μg, approached significance (11.1 L/minute; $p=0.051$ *vs* placebo). However, the change in evening PEF following treatment with formoterol, although positive, did not reach significance (8.4 and 10.4 L/minute for formoterol, 4.5 and 9 μg, respectively; *p*-value not reported). Overall, both doses of formoterol elicited a significant increase in pre-bronchodilator FEV_1 values (5.2 and 6.7% for formoterol, 4.5 and 9 μg, respectively; $p<0.05$). In addition, the use of rescue medication and the number of night-time awakenings was significantly reduced following treatment with formoterol ($p\leq0.05$; Figure 4).

Overall, both doses of formoterol elicited a significant increase in pre-medication FEV_1 values.

Use of formoterol as reliever medication

The rapid onset of action of formoterol has sparked investigation into its potential use as a reliever medication. Although current treatment guidelines do not endorse the use of formoterol as first-line relief therapy, it is licensed for such an application. The use of a single inhaler for both maintenance and as-needed therapy may also enhance patient compliance.[40] Whilst formoterol would appear in principal to be an effective reliever medication, there are some concerns regarding the development of tolerance to long-acting β_2-agonists when used on a regular basis, as well as the risk of adrenergic and metabolic effects that may ultimately lead to worsening asthma control and increased exacerbations.[41]

The RELIEF study was a large, open-label investigation into the safety and efficacy of formoterol and salbutamol in both adults and children with asthma, enrolling over 18,000 patients.[42] Patients were randomised to treatment with either formoterol (4.5 μg, given via Turbohaler) or salbutamol (200 μg, given via pMDI or equivalent), as-needed, for a 6-month period in a 'real-life' setting. The rate of treatment discontinuation was 7.3% amongst formoterol- and 5.8% amongst salbutamol-treated patients ($p<0.001$). Clinical efficacy was measured as the time to the first asthma exacerbation and this was significantly longer for patients receiving formoterol than those receiving salbutamol ($p<0.001$; Figure 5). The hazard ratios between treatment groups showed a 14% reduction in the relative risk for a first exacerbation and a 12% reduction in the relative risk for a first severe exacerbation in the formoterol treatment group ($p<0.001$ and $p=0.0013$; respectively). The safety data pertaining to this study are reviewed in detail in the subsequent Safety and Tolerability section.

The time to the first asthma exacerbation was significantly longer for patients receiving formoterol than for those receiving salbutamol.

Overall, these data suggest that formoterol is at least as effective as salbutamol at relieving the acute symptoms of asthma and is associated with fewer exacerbations. However, the subjective evaluation of exacerbations, with no measurements of daily peak flow and spirometry does detract slightly from the study design.[41] Taken together with the safety data derived from this study, formoterol would appear to be an effective alternative to short-acting β_2-agonists in the treatment of the acute symptoms of asthma.

Figure 4. The mean number of day- and night-time rescue inhalations (top and middle) and the mean number of awakenings (bottom) following administration of formoterol (4.5 or 9 μg, twice daily) or placebo, to children over a 12-week period.[39]

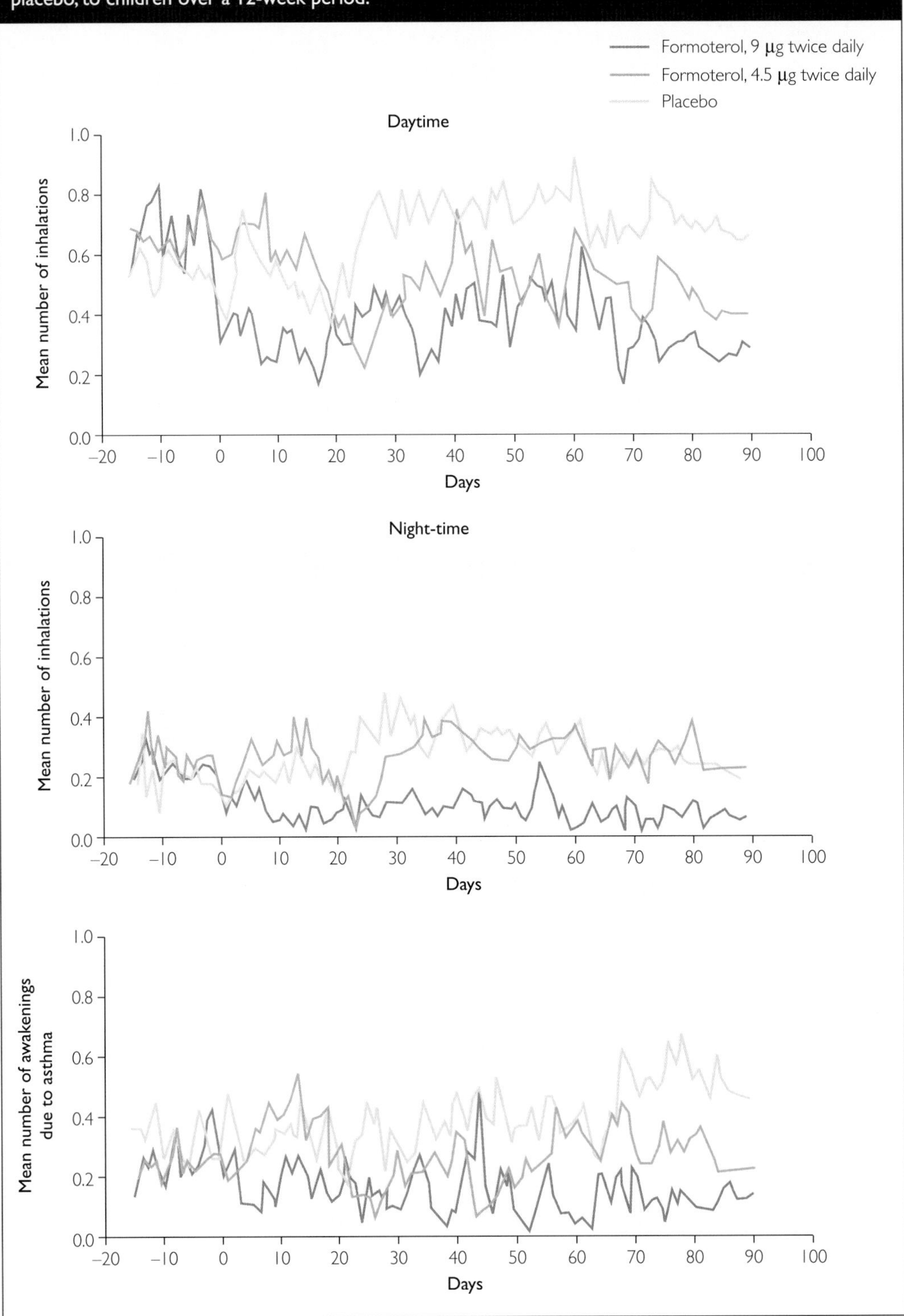

Figure 5. Kaplan–Meier survival curve showing the percentage of formoterol- and salbutamol-treated patients who did not experience an asthma exacerbation of any severity (top) and the reduction in relative risk with respect to the first exacerbation, formoterol *vs* salbutamol (bottom), over the course of 6 months open-label treatment.[42]

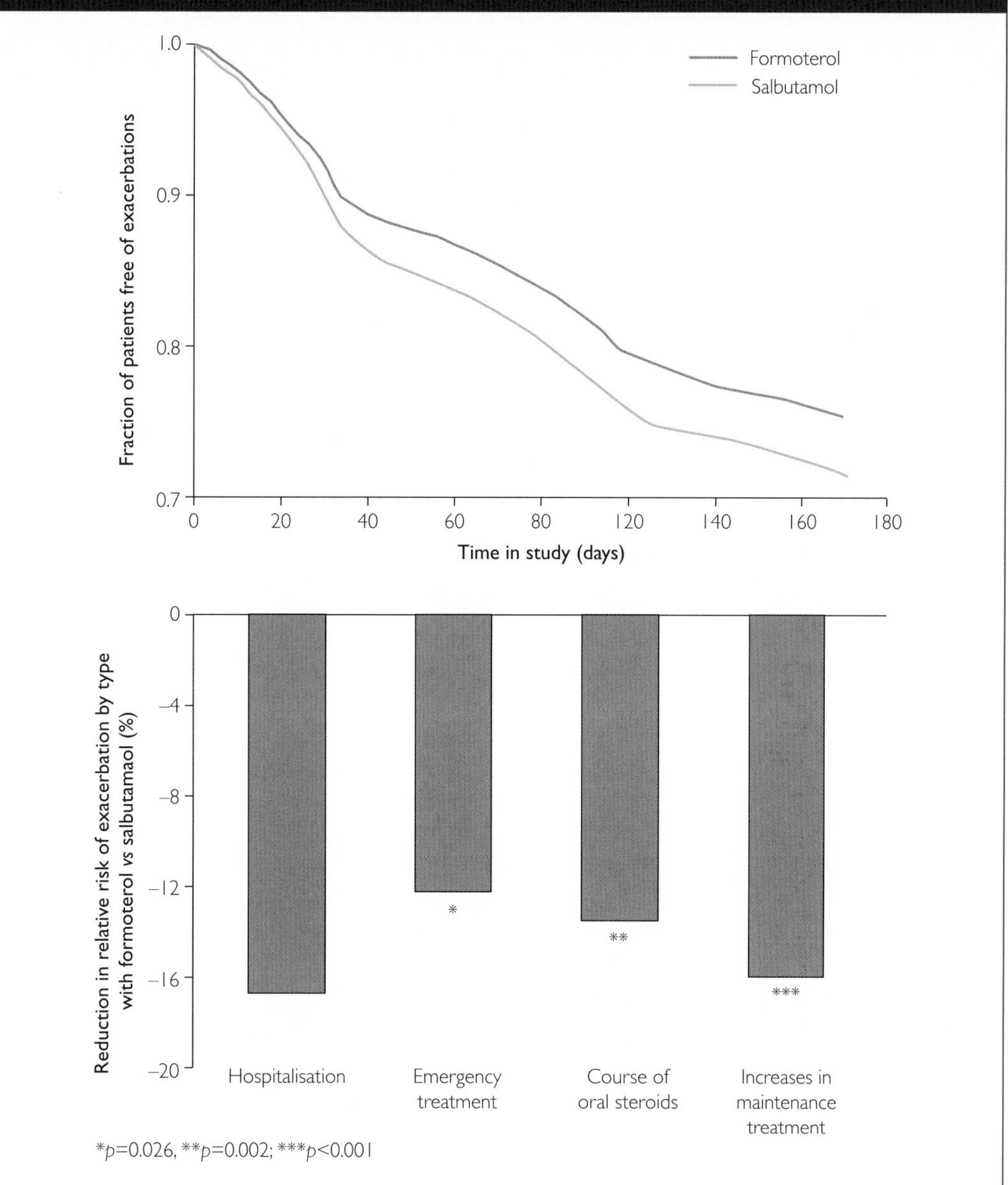

You are strongly urged to consult your doctor before taking, stopping or changing any of the products reviewed or referred to in *BESTMEDICINE* or any other medication that has been prescribed or recommended by your doctor.

Safety and tolerability

In general, β_2-agonists are commonly associated with fine tremor (particularly of the hands), nervous tension, headache, peripheral dilatation, anxiety and palpitations.[8] Tachycardia and arrhythmias, and disturbances of sleep and behaviour in children have also been reported following the regular use of β_2-agonists.[8] However, these side-effects are usually mild in severity and tend to resolve within a few days of treatment.[7,8] Clinical experience drawn from trials conducted in a large number of adults and children have shown that whilst the use of formoterol may be accompanied by these adverse events, it is generally well tolerated.[15,21] Oropharyngeal irritation, taste disturbances, rash, insomnia, nausea and pruritus have all been reported, albeit rarely, following formoterol treatment.[8] It should also be noted that treatment with formoterol may cause prolongation of the corrected QT interval (QTc) of the electrocardiogram (ECG), and as with all inhalation therapies, there is a potential risk of paradoxical bronchospasm.[7,8] The risk of potentially serious hypokalaemia following treatment with formoterol, and β_2-agonists in general, merits the monitoring of serum potassium levels in some patients. Concomitant treatment with xanthine derivatives, steroids and diuretics may potentiate the risk of hypokalaemia.[7]

As outlined earlier in this review, formoterol should not be used as an alternative to short-acting β_2-agonists in the event of an acute asthma attack, but it may be used for the relief of broncho-obstructive symptoms.[7] In addition, corticosteroid therapy should not be discontinued after initiating formoterol.[7] Physicians should also be aware that regular high doses of formoterol (e.g. 24 μg, twice daily) may rarely be associated with an increase in severe asthma exacerbations. As such, the use of initial lower doses is advocated unless unavoidable.[8]

Precautions for use

Caution should be observed when administering formoterol to patients with:

- thyrotoxicosis
- phaeochromocytoma
- hypertrophic obstructive cardiomyopathy
- idiopathic subvalvular aortic stenosis
- severe hypertension
- aneurysm
- severe cardiovascular disorders (e.g. ischaemic heart disease, tachyarrhythmias, severe heart failure)
- prolongation of the QTc interval
- diabetes (additional blood glucose monitoring is recommended initially).[7,11,12]

Drug interactions

Although to date, no specific drug interaction studies have been conducted, the co-administration of formoterol with the following substances merits caution:

- other sympathomimetic substances (may potentiate adverse events associated with formoterol)
- xanthine derivatives, steroids or diuretics (may potentiate the possible hypokalaemic effect of formoterol)
- L-dopa, L-thyroxine, oxytocin and alcohol (may impair cardiac tolerance towards β_2-agonists)
- monoamine oxidase inhibitors, including agents with similar properties such as furazolidone and procarbazine (may cause hypertensive reactions)
- β-adrenoceptor antagonists (may weaken the effect of formoterol).[7,11,12]

Comparative safety trials

Formoterol *vs* salbutamol

As mentioned previously, the RELIEF study was a large open-label, international comparison of formoterol and salbutamol as reliever medications in 18,124 adults and children with asthma conducted over a 6-month period.[42] The incidence of adverse events associated with the long-term use of formoterol and salbutamol is illustrated in Figure 6. Overall, adverse events were comparable between treatment groups, with 42% of patients from both groups experiencing at least one event. The occurrence of asthma-related adverse events (e.g. asthma aggravated symptoms or asthma not otherwise specified) was significantly lower amongst formoterol- than salbutamol-treated patients (12.3 *vs* 13.5%, for formoterol and salbutamol, respectively; p=0.018).

The occurrence of asthma-related adverse events was significantly lower amongst formoterol- than salbutamol-treated patients.

Formoterol *vs* terbutaline

A double-blind study of 357 patients with moderate asthma taking moderate-to-high dose of inhaled corticosteroids, compared the relative safety of formoterol or terbutaline, taken as needed, in addition to formoterol, 9 µg twice daily via Turbohaler, over a 12-week period.[43] The rate of premature treatment discontinuation as a result of asthma deterioration was identical for each treatment (6%). No significant differences were detected between treatments in terms of a number of safety variables, and the distribution of adverse events was similar and of comparable intensity, with aggravated asthma, respiratory infection and headache being the most common side-effects. Compared with formoterol-treated patients, terbutaline-treated patients showed a modest but significant increase in cardiac frequency (2.6 beats/minute; p=0.03). Although formoterol treatment was associated with significant prolongation of the QT interval (6.7 msecs; p=0.02 *vs* terbutaline), comparison of cardiac frequency-adjusted QTc showed no significant differences between formoterol and terbutaline treatment groups (p=0.82).

Figure 6. Safety and tolerability of formoterol and salbutamol in the RELIEF study: the most frequent adverse events (top) and the most frequent serious adverse events (bottom) reported in patients using formoterol or salbutamol as reliever medication.[42]

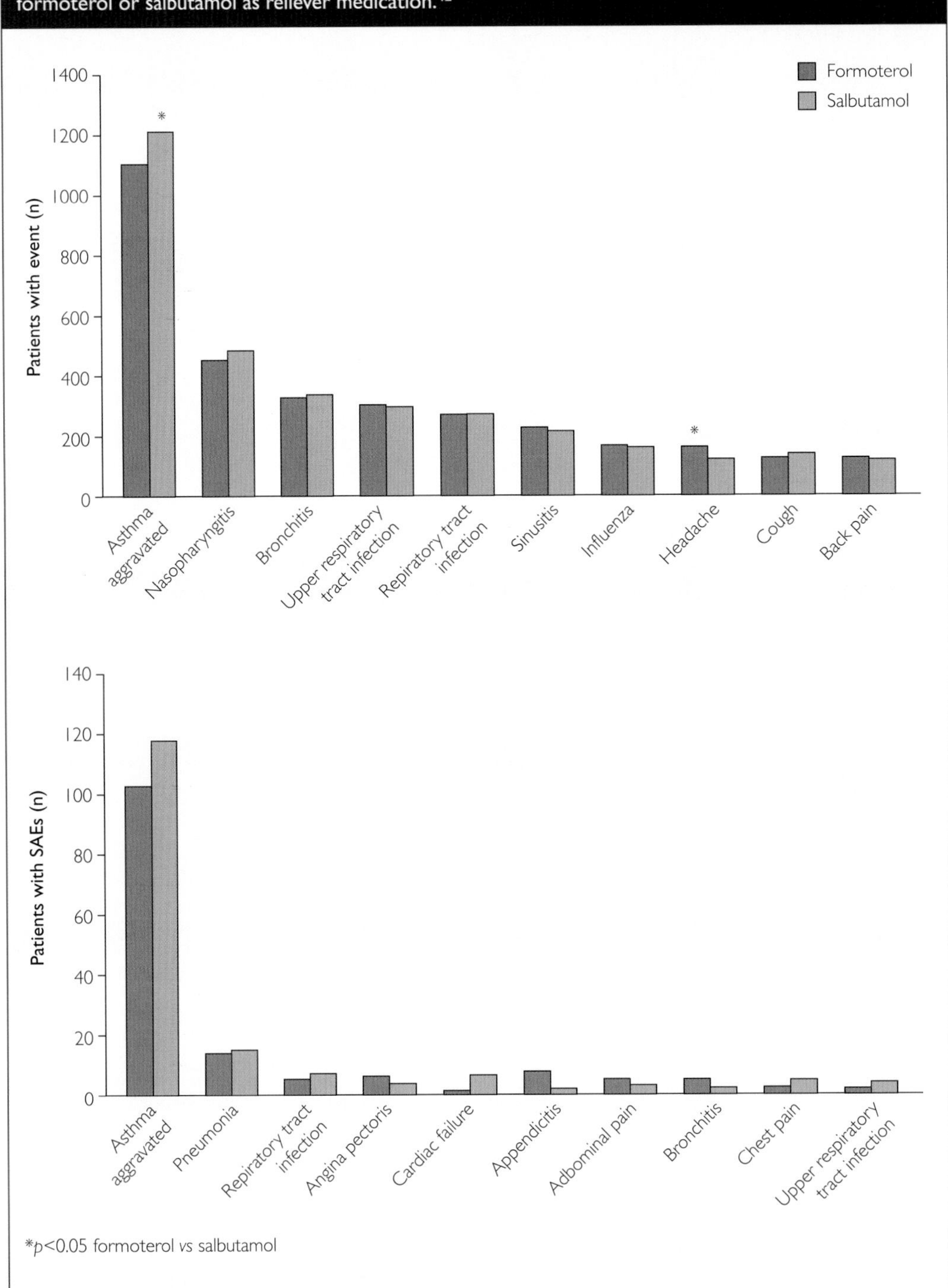

*$p<0.05$ formoterol *vs* salbutamol

Key points

- Formoterol is a long-acting β_2-adrenoceptor agonist, indicated for the relief of reversible airways obstruction – including nocturnal asthma and the prevention of exercise-induced bronchospasm.
- Current guidelines recommend that formoterol is administered when corticosteroid therapy alone fails to effectively control asthma. The use of formoterol as monotherapy is not recommended.
- The rapid onset of action of formoterol resembles that of the short-acting β_2-agonists (e.g. salbutamol), but its sustained duration of action of approximately 12 hours, is similar to that of the long-acting β_2-agonist, salmeterol.
- Although regular treatment with formoterol is associated with the development of tachyphylaxis to protection against methacholine-induced bronchoconstriction, the clinical implications of this are unclear.
- Formoterol can be administered via a number of inhalation devices (e.g. pMDI, Turbohaler and Aerolizer), which differ in terms of their deposition characteristics.
- Compared with placebo, formoterol elicited significant and sustained improvements in PEF that showed low diurnal variation. Additionally, formoterol was associated with a lower incidence of day- and night-time symptoms and a reduced need for rescue medication.
- Studies conducted in children with asthma over the age of 5 years, showed similar outcomes to adult studies, both in terms of clinical efficacy, and safety and tolerability.
- When compared with salbutamol or terbutaline, the overall efficacy of formoterol as reliever medication was at least equal and was in many instances superior.
- Formoterol demonstrated similar efficacy to salmeterol in terms of PEF and symptom improvements, and in one study, was rated more highly in terms of patient preference.
- Well tolerated, both in controlled studies and in clinical practice, adverse events associated with formoterol treatment are mild in severity and transient in nature. A slight risk of QTc interval prolongation, paradoxical bronchospasm or hypokalaemia, may necessitate caution when used by some patients.

References

A list of the published evidence which has been reviewed in compiling the preceding section of *BESTMEDICINE.*

1 Waldeck B. Beta-adrenoceptor agonists and asthma – 100 years of development. *Eur J Pharmacol* 2002; **445**: 1–12.

2 Scottish Intercollegiate Guidelines Network & the British Thoracic Society. British Guidelines on the Management of Asthma. SIGN, Edinburgh, 2004.

3 Spitzer W, Suissa S, Ernst P *et al.* The use of beta-agonists and the risk of death and near death from asthma. *New Engl J Med* 1992; **326**: 501–6.

4 Beasley R, Pearce N, Crane J, Burgess C. Beta-agonists: what is the evidence that their use increases the risk of asthma morbidity and mortality? *J Allergy Clin Immunol* 1999; **104**: S18–30.

5 Abramson M, Walters J, Walters E. Adverse effects of beta-agonists: are they clinically relevant? *Am J Respir Med* 2003; **2**: 287–97.

6 Bjermer L, Larsson L. Long-acting beta(2)-agonists: how are they used in an optimal way? *Respir Med* 1997; **91**: 587–91.

7 AstraZeneca UK Limited. Oxis Turbohaler 12. *Summary of product characteristics.* Luton, 2004.

8 *British National Formulary (BNF) 48.* London: British Medical Association and Royal Pharmaceutical Society of Great Britain. September, 2004.

9 Selroos O, Ekstrom T. Formoterol Turbuhaler 4.5 microg (delivered dose) has a rapid onset and 12-h duration of bronchodilation. *Pulm Pharmacol Ther* 2002; **15**: 175–83.

10 Lofdahl C, Svedmyr M. Effect duration of inhaled formoterol, a new beta2-adrenoceptor agonist, compared to salbutamol in asthmatic patients. *Acta Pharmacol Toxicol* 1986; **5**: 229.

11 AstraZeneca UK Limited. Oxis Turbohaler 6. *Summary of product characteristics.* Luton, 2004.

12 Novartis Pharmaceuticals UK Ltd. Foradil. *Summary of product characteristics.* Camberley, 2004.

13 Anderson G. Formoterol: pharmacology, molecular basis of agonism, and mechanism of long duration of a highly potent and selective beta 2-adrenoceptor agonist bronchodilator. *Life Sci* 1993; **52**: 2145–60.

14 Handley D, Senanayake C, Dutczak W *et al.* Biological actions of formoterol isomers. *Pulm Pharmacol Ther* 2002; **15**: 135–45.

15 Bartow R, Brogden R. Formoterol. An update of its pharmacological properties and therapeutic efficacy in the management of asthma. *Drugs* 1998; **55**: 303–22.

16 Rosenborg J, Bengtsson T, Larsson P *et al.* Relative systemic dose potency and tolerability of inhaled formoterol and salbutamol in healthy subjects and asthmatics. *Eur J Clin Pharmacol* 2000; **56**: 363–70.

17 Lipworth B. Airway subsensitivity with long-acting beta 2-agonists. Is there cause for concern? *Drug Saf* 1997; **16**: 295–308.

18 Lipworth B, Tan S, Devlin M *et al.* Effects of treatment with formoterol on bronchoprotection against methacholine. *Am J Med* 1998; **104**: 431–8.

19 Jackson C, Lipworth B. Benefit-risk assessment of long-acting beta2-agonists in asthma. *Drug Saf* 2004; **27**: 243–70.

20 Lee D, Currie G, Hall I, Lima J, Lipworth B. The arginine-16 beta2-adrenoceptor polymorphism predisposes to bronchoprotective subsensitivity in patients treated with formoterol and salmeterol. *Br J Clin Pharmacol* 2004; **57**: 68–75.

21 Cheer S, Warner G, Easthope S. Formoterol delivered by Turbuhaler: in pediatric asthma. *Paediatr Drugs* 2003; **5**: 63–8.

22 Palmqvist M, Persson G, Lazer L *et al.* Inhaled dry-powder formoterol and salmeterol in asthmatic patients: onset of action, duration of effect and potency. *Eur Respir J* 1997; **10**: 2484–9.

23 Ringdal N, Derom E, Wahlin-Boll E, Pauwels R. Onset and duration of action of single doses of formoterol inhaled via Turbuhaler. *Respir Med* 1998; **92**: 1017–21.

24 Sill V, Ortland C. Specific airway resistance (sRAW) measurements to compare the onset of action of formoterol turbuhaler and salmeterol Diskus. *Eur Respir J* 1998; **12**: S40.

25 Seberova E, Andersson A. Oxis (formoterol given by Turbuhaler) showed as rapid an onset of action as salbutamol given by a pMDI. *Respir Med* 2000; **94**: 607–11.

26 Schreurs A, Sinninghe Damste H, de Graaff C, Greefhorst A. A dose-response study with formoterol Turbuhaler as maintenance therapy in asthmatic patients. *Eur Respir J* 1996; **9**: 1678–83.

27 van der Molen T, Postma D, Turner M *et al.* Effects of the long acting beta-agonist formoterol on asthma control in asthmatic patients using inhaled corticosteroids. The Netherlands and Canadian Formoterol Study Investigators. *Thorax* 1997; **52**: 535–9.

28 Hekking P, Maesen F, Greefhorst A *et al.* Long-term efficacy of formoterol compared to salbutamol. *Lung* 1990; **168**: 76–82.

29 Kesten S, Chapman K, Broder I *et al.* A three-month comparison of twice daily inhaled formoterol versus four times daily inhaled albuterol in the management of stable asthma. *Am Rev Respir Dis* 1991; **144**: 622–5.

30 Kesten S, Chapman K, Broder I *et al.* Sustained improvement in asthma with long-term use of formoterol fumarate. *Ann Allergy* 1992; **69**: 415–20.

31 Steffensen I, Faurschou P, Riska H, Rostrup J, Wegener T. Inhaled formoterol dry powder in the treatment of patients with reversible obstructive airway disease. A 3-month, placebo-controlled comparison of the efficacy and safety of formoterol and salbutamol, followed by a 12-month trial with formoterol. *Allergy* 1995; **50**: 657–63.

32 Bensch G, Lapidus R, Levine B *et al.* A randomized, 12-week, double-blind, placebo-controlled study comparing formoterol dry powder inhaler with albuterol metered-dose inhaler. *Ann Allergy Asthma Immunol* 2001; **86**: 19–27.

33 Pleskow W, LaForce C, Yegen U, Matos D, Della Cioppa G. Formoterol delivered via the dry powder Aerolizer inhaler versus albuterol MDI and placebo in mild-to-moderate asthma: a randomized, double-blind, double-dummy trial. *J Asthma* 2003; **40**: 505–14.

34 Ekstrom T, Ringdal N, Sobradillo V, Runnerstrom E, Soliman S. Low-dose formoterol Turbuhaler (Oxis) b.i.d., a 3-month placebo-controlled comparison with terbutaline (q.i.d.). *Respir Med* 1998; **92**: 1040–5.

35 Tattersfield A, Lofdahl C, Postma D *et al.* Comparison of formoterol and terbutaline for as-needed treatment of asthma: a randomised trial. *Lancet* 2001; **357**: 257–61.

36 Stahl E, Postma D, Svensson K *et al.* Formoterol used as needed improves health-related quality of life in asthmatic patients uncontrolled with inhaled corticosteroids. *Respir Med* 2003; **97**: 1061–6.

37 Campbell L, Anderson T, Parashchak M *et al.* A comparison of the efficacy of long-acting beta 2-agonists: eformoterol via Turbohaler and salmeterol via pressurized metered dose inhaler or Accuhaler, in mild to moderate asthmatics. Force Research Group. *Respir Med* 1999; **93**: 236–44.

38 Zimmerman B, D'Urzo A, Berube D. Efficacy and safety of formoterol Turbuhaler when added to inhaled corticosteroid treatment in children with asthma. *Pediatr Pulmonol* 2004; **37**: 122–7.

39 Von Berg A, Papageorgiou Saxoni F, Wille S *et al.* Efficacy and tolerability of formoterol Turbuhaler in children. *Int J Clin Pract.* 2003; **57**: 852–6.

40 Pauwels R. Formoterol – where does it fit in the current guidelines? *Respir Med* 2001; **95**: S30–4.

41 Jenkins C. Formoterol as relief medication in asthma: the jury is still out. *Eur Respir J* 2003; **22**: 723–4.

42 Pauwels R, Sears M, Campbell M *et al.* Formoterol as relief medication in asthma: a worldwide safety and effectiveness trial. *Eur Respir J* 2003; **22**: 787–94.

43 Ind P, Villasante C, Shiner R *et al.* Safety of formoterol by Turbuhaler as reliever medication compared with terbutaline in moderate asthma. *Eur Respir J* 2002; **20**: 859–66.

Acknowledgements

Figure 2 is adapted from Schreurs *et al.*, 1996.[26]
Figure 3 is adapted from Tattersfield *et al.*, 2001.[35]
Figure 4 is adapted from Von Berg *et al.*, 2003.[39]
Figures 5 and 6 are adapted from Pauwels *et al.*, 2003.[42]

7. Drug review – Mometasone (Asmanex®)

Dr Susan Chambers and Dr Scott Chambers
CSF Medical Communications Ltd

You are strongly urged to consult your doctor before taking, stopping or changing any of the products reviewed or referred to in *BESTMEDICINE* or any other medication that has been prescribed or recommended by your doctor.

Summary

Mometasone fuorate (hereafter referred to as mometasone) is one of the newer and more potent inhaled corticosteroids used in the management of persistent mild-to-moderate asthma in adults and adolescents. Mometasone is available as a dry-powder formulation in two dosage forms (200 µg and 400 µg) and is delivered by a breath-actuated dry-powder inhaler (DPI) called the Twisthaler®. The optimum daily dose of mometasone in patients with mild-to-moderate persistent asthma has been determined to be 400 µg, although current guidelines suggest using the lowest possible effective dose initially, followed by dose escalation as necessary. Once-daily administration of mometasone appears to be as effective as twice-daily dosing, which in combination with the greater acceptability of the inhaler device compared with metered dose inhalers (MDIs), may promote patient compliance by simplifying treatment. Dose-ranging comparative studies reveal that mometasone has comparable efficacy to fluticasone propionate in the management of asthma, and appears to be more potent than budesonide. In addition, mometasone appears to be at least as effective as beclometasone dipropionate. However, the dose equivalence of mometasone and these other inhaled corticosteroids requires further evaluation. The use of mometasone can also result in a decreased requirement for oral corticosteroids in patients with severe persistent asthma. Mometasone has been shown to be well tolerated in clinical trials, with a similar incidence of adverse events as placebo and other inhaled corticosteroids. As with other inhaled corticosteroids, additional studies are still required to clarify the dose-dependent and long-term treatment effects of the drug on the hypothalamic–pituitary–adrenal (HPA) axis.

Introduction

Inhaled corticosteroids have revolutionised the treatment of asthma, and are generally considered to be the most effective agents for long-term control of this condition. They have a variety of beneficial anti-inflammatory effects, although the precise mechanisms by which these agents exert their effects are not yet fully understood. Clinically, treatment with inhaled corticosteroids results in a variety of positive outcomes. They are generally effective in reducing asthma-related morbidity and mortality, by reducing respiratory symptoms and optimising pulmonary function.[1] Inhaled corticosteroids may also reduce airway hyper-responsiveness, though this is dependent on the dose and duration of therapy. Airway inflammation is reduced with inhaled corticosteroids, though there is a less striking effect on airway remodelling.

Inhaled corticosteroids exert their anti-inflammatory effects by reducing the proliferation of inflammatory cells (e.g. eosinophils, macrophages, mast cells, T lymphocytes) and by inhibiting the activation of these cells in the airways. In addition, corticosteroids inhibit airway mucus secretion, inhibit the production of pro-inflammatory cytokines (e.g. interleukins [ILs], tumour necrosis factor [TNF] and chemokines) by various cell types (e.g. macrophages, T lymphocytes and mast cells) and reduce the expression of cytokine receptors.[2]

Mometasone is one of the newer and more potent inhaled corticosteroids. It was originally licensed as a topical treatment for psoriasis and atopic dermatitis, and then as an intranasal formulation for the relief of allergic rhinitis. However, an inhaled formulation for the treatment of persistent asthma was introduced in the UK in 2003. This formulation employs a DPI, the Twisthaler, that enables precise drug delivery with a simple operating technique, which may contribute to greater patient concordance with treatment compared with MDI devices.

This section focuses on the pharmacology, clinical efficacy and safety of inhaled mometasone in the management of persistent asthma in adults and children over the age of 12 years. We discuss the evidence that has accumulated for the drug in the context of data obtained from studies with other inhaled corticosteroids, including fluticasone propionate, budesonide and beclometasone dipropionate.

Pharmacology

Chemistry

Mometasone is a synthetic corticosteroid and its chemical structure is illustrated in Figure 1. It is available for the treatment of mild-to-moderate persistent asthma as a dry powder. This is formulated as stabilised agglomerates of spherical clusters approximately 0.5 mm in diameter comprised of micronised particles of mometasone and lactose (one part mometasone to 5.8 parts lactose) and is delivered via a breath-acutated DPI device called the Twisthaler.[3]

The chemistry of mometasone is of essentially academic interest and most healthcare professionals will, like you, skip this section.

Pharmacokinetics

In a study of healthy volunteers (n=24), the systemic bioavailability of mometasone after inhalation of a single 400 μg dose was shown to be below 1%, with mean plasma concentrations below the limit of detection (0.05 μg/L) in the majority of subjects. This indicates that mometasone is not significantly absorbed systemically after inhalation of a single dose.[4] Peak plasma concentrations (C_{max}) after inhalation were 0.05 μg/L, the time to peak plasma concentrations (t_{max}) was 2.09 hours and the mean area under the plasma concentration–time curve (AUC) from zero hours to the final measurable sampling time was 0.09 μg/L.hour. Other pharmacokinetic parameters could not be determined because plasma concentrations were too low for reliable estimates. The low systemic absorption of mometasone was further confirmed in a study determining the lung deposition of radioactively labelled mometasone, 200 μg, given by an MDI.[5] In this study, plasma concentrations of mometasone were below the limit of quantification in all patients immediately after inhalation and during the subsequent 12 hours.

The pharmacokinetics of a drug are of interest to healthcare professionals because it is important for them to understand the action of a drug on the body over a period of time.

However, the bioavailability of mometasone after multiple dosing (400 μg twice daily for 15 days) has been reported as 11%.[6] This is similar to that reported with fluticasone propionate administered by

Figure 1. The chemical structure of mometasone.

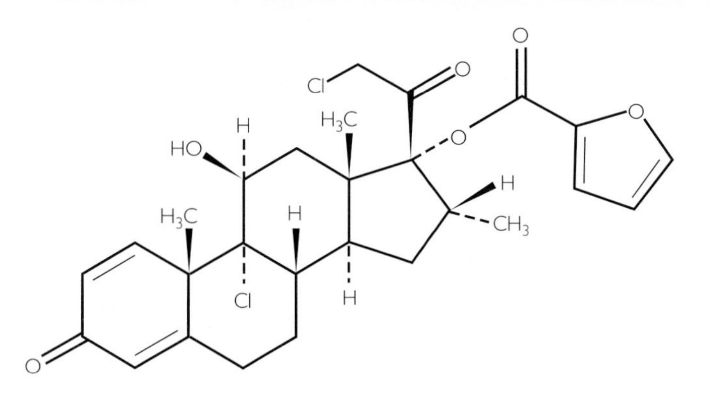

DPI, and indicates that inhaled mometasone, like other inhaled corticosteroids may accumulate with repeated dosing.[7,8] As such, the single-dose pharmacokinetic studies may underestimate the actual bioavailability of mometasone when used clinically, indicating that the single-dose studies are not particularly informative in this regard. Indeed, there has been some criticism of the methodology employed in some of the pharmacokinetic studies of mometasone.[7–9] Thus, further evaluation of the systemic bioavailability of mometasone after repeated inhaled administration appears to be warranted.

Other pharmacokinetic studies have shown that the majority of an inhaled dose of mometasone is deposited in the oropharynx, swallowed and then excreted unchanged in the faeces (mean 74% of the total dose, range 50–87%).[4,5] Any drug that is systemically absorbed is metabolised in the liver and subsequently excreted in the urine and/or bile (mean 8% of the total dose, range 6–10%). The remainder of the total drug dose is exhaled. In a study evaluating the deposition of mometasone in the respiratory tract after inhalation via an MDI, 13.9% of the metered dose was shown to be deposited in the lungs, 79.1% in the oropharynx, 6.3% in the mouthpiece of the MDI and 0.7% was exhaled.[5] The lung deposition value of around 14% was comparable to the 10–20% observed with other corticosteroid suspensions delivered via an MDI. The systemic clearance of mometasone after intravenous administration (400 μg) is 53.5 L/hour, which is similar to that observed with other inhaled corticosteroids (Table 1).[10]

Mometasone possesses a higher binding affinity for the glucocorticosteroid receptor than fluticasone propionate, budesonide, triamcinolone acetonide and dexamethasone.

In vitro *receptor affinity*

The anti-inflammatory effects of corticosteroids are mediated by their interactions with corticosteroid receptors. These receptors are found in the cytoplasm of most cells, but are particularly abundant in the respiratory tract epithelium and in the endothelium of the lung vascular system.[10] *In vitro* receptor affinity studies using African green monkey kidney cells have demonstrated that mometasone possesses a higher binding affinity for the glucocorticosteroid receptor than fluticasone propionate, budesonide, triamcinolone acetonide and dexamethasone (1.5-, 4.8-, 7.5- and 12.4-times greater binding affinity, respectively; Table 2).[11] However, the greater *in vitro* potency of mometasone demonstrated in this study does not necessarily indicate greater clinical efficacy, which can be influenced by a variety of other factors including

Table 1. Systemic clearance of inhaled corticosteroids.[4,10]

Corticosteroid	Systemic clearance (L/hour)
Mometasone	53.5
Budesonide	51.6
Fluticasone propionate	62.4
Triamcinolone acetonide	69.5

Table 2. Relative *in vitro* binding affinities of various corticosteroids for the glucocorticosteroid receptor in African green monkey kidney cells.[11]

Corticosteroid	Relative binding affinity
Mometasone	1235
Fluticasone propionate	813
Budesonide	258
Triamcinolone acetonide	164
Dexamethasone	100

pharmacokinetic parameters and the nature of the delivery system employed.[12]

In vitro *anti-inflammatory activity*

In vitro studies have shown that mometasone exerts a variety of anti-inflammatory effects including the inhibition of:

- cytokine release by T-helper cells (interferon β, IL-4 and IL-5)
- histamine and cysteinyl leukotriene release by basophils
- peripheral blood mononuclear cell proliferation
- adhesion molecule expression on epithelial cells.[7,10]

Mometasone also has a negative effect on eosinophil survival. These anti-inflammatory effects appear to be comparable to those observed with fluticasone propionate but are more potent than those associated with budesonide, beclometasone dipropionate and triamcinolone acetonide.[7,10]

In one study, pre-treatment with topical mometasone inhibited rhinovirus-induced expression of intercellular adhesion molecule-1 (ICAM-1) in a dose-dependent manner (IC_{50}[a]: 10^{-11} mol/L).[13] ICAM-1 plays a central role in the recruitment of inflammatory cells in asthmatic airways and is the receptor for 90% of rhinoviruses, which, in turn, are associated with the majority of asthma exacerbations. The inhibition of ICAM-1 associated with mometasone administration was similar to that observed with hydrocortisone and dexamethasone. Mometasone also inhibited rhinovirus-induced ICAM-1 up-regulation on primary bronchial epithelial cells, and rhinovirus-induced ICAM-1 mRNA induction and promoter activation on A549 cells.[13]

In another study, mometasone was shown to enhance human eosinophil apoptosis in a dose-dependent manner.[14] The maximum enhancement of apoptosis was 2.1-fold, and the concentration required to produce 50% of this effect (EC_{50}) was 5.63 nM. Enhancement of apoptosis was reversed by the corticosteroid receptor antagonist, mifepristone. By contrast, mometasone inhibited neutrophil apoptosis in

[a]IC_{50} represents the concentration required to inhibit ICAM-1 expression by 50%.

Mometasone exerts opposite effects on eosinophil and neutrophil apoptosis, and these effects are mediated by the corticosteroid receptor.

a dose-dependent manner. The maximum inhibitory effect was 50%, the EC_{50} value was 0.17 nM and the inhibitory effect was partially reversed by mifepristone. Thus, mometasone exerts opposite effects on eosinophil and neutrophil apoptosis, and these effects are mediated by the corticosteroid receptor.

Clinical efficacy

The mometasone DPI (Twisthaler)

In many cases, the device used to deliver corticosteroids and other asthma medication can be as important as the medication itself. An 'ideal' inhaler should have a number of critical attributes. These include consistency in dose delivery across a range of inspiratory flow rates and good lung deposition at the site of inflammation to minimise systemic absorption. It should also be easy to teach to use, simple to load, be portable and compact and have a dose counter that indicates the number of doses remaining.[15] Effective use of an inhaler is an important factor in driving patient compliance. DPI devices are now generally preferred over MDIs, as the latter require propellants such as chlorofluorocarbons, which are being phased out due to environmental concerns. In addition, MDIs require effective hand–breath coordination adding complexity to the drug-delivery process.

The mometasone DPI (Twisthaler) has an advanced but simple design that enables precise drug delivery with a simple operating technique, minimising complexity and thereby maximising patient compliance. There are three simple steps in the operation: cap removal, which loads the dose, dose inhalation and cap replacement. The device delivers accurate, uniform and precise dose ranges across a range of inspiratory flow rates, making it acceptable for a variety of patients across a broad age range. Complexity is minimised thus aiding compliance.

In vitro studies show that the mometasone inhaler achieved nearly 100% of dose delivery at uniform inspiratory flow rates of 20–60 L/minute, which is within the range generated by adults with all severities of asthma. Dose-to-dose variability was less than 10% at these inspiratory flow rates.[16] Patients required little instruction on the use of the Twisthaler and, when queried, preferred the device to MDIs, indicating that the ease of administration was the principal reason for this preference.[3]

Anti-inflammatory activity

The effects of budesonide and mometasone on airway eosinophils and neutrophils have been investigated in a double-blind, placebo-controlled, randomised, cross-over study of patients with atopic asthma (n=28).[17] Patients inhaled budesonide, 200 μg twice daily, or mometasone, 400 μg twice daily, or placebo, for 6–8 days, and then underwent an allergen inhalation challenge. Both corticosteroids reduced the early and late asthmatic responses, and the number of allergen-induced sputum eosinophils ($p<0.05$). There was a negative correlation between the number of sputum neutrophils at baseline and the percentage inhibition of allergen-induced sputum eosinophils at 7 hours ($p<0.001$) and 24 hours ($p<0.0001$) after challenge. These results suggest that budesonide and mometasone are less effective in reducing allergen-induced airway inflammation in the presence of high neutrophil levels, and that baseline airway neutrophil levels can be used to predict the effect of inhaled corticosteroids on allergen-induced airway inflammation.

Dose-ranging placebo-controlled studies

Many studies have examined the dose–responses of inhaled corticosteroids on a variety of markers of pulmonary function. These are particularly useful in determining the comparative potency and efficacy of different agents in clinical studies. However, the dose–responses of different corticosteroids are not uniform for all drugs and also vary according to the outcome being assessed.

The dose-dependent effects of inhaled mometasone on airway function and inflammation have been investigated in a number of dose-ranging, placebo-controlled studies. A randomised, double-blind, cross-over study of patients with mild asthma (n=12) detemined whether dose–response relationships existed with inhaled mometasone for a variety of different treatment outcomes after allergen-inhalation challenge. Patients received treatment with mometasone, 50, 100 or 400 μg twice daily, or placebo, via a DPI for 6 days before allergen inhalation challenge.[18] All three doses of mometasone delayed the early asthmatic response to allergen inhalation ($p<0.05$), reduced allergen-induced airway hyper-responsiveness ($p<0.05$) and reduced allergen-induced increases in sputum eosinophils ($p<0.005$ and $p<0.05$ at 7 and 24 hours after challenge, respectively) compared with placebo (Table 3). However, there were no apparent dose–response relationships in these parameters (Table 3), with the exception of the attenuation of the late asthmatic response ($p=0.007$ for the dose–response relationship).

Mometasone delayed the early asthmatic response to allergen inhalation, reduced allergen-induced airway hyper-responsiveness and reduced allergen-induced increases in sputum eosinophils.

In a large, multicentre, randomised, double-blind, placebo-controlled trial, patients with moderate persistent asthma (n=365) received mometasone, 100, 200 or 400 μg twice daily via a DPI, or beclometasone dipropionate, 168 μg twice daily via an MDI,[b] or placebo, for 12 weeks.[19] These patients were already receiving treatment with other inhaled corticosteroids. The mean change in forced expiratory volume in 1 second (FEV_1) from baseline to the last treatment visit (the primary efficacy endpoint) was greater with all four active treatments than with placebo ($p<0.01$), as were secondary measures of pulmonary function (Table 4). There was a consistent trend for greater response with the 200 μg dose of mometasone than with the 100 μg dose, but increasing the dose to 400 μg provided no additional benefit. The results achieved with beclometasone dipropionate were similar to those seen

[b]This dose of beclometasone is considered to be equivalent to a metered dose of 200 μg.

Table 3. Respiratory outcomes in patients with mild asthma receiving treatment with mometasone or placebo via a breath-actuated dry powder inhaler for 6 days before allergen inhalation challenge.[18]

Outcome	Placebo	Mometasone (μg)[a]		
		50	100	400
Early asthmatic response (maximal early per cent fall in FEV_1)	36.8	29.6*	24.2*	26.4*
Late asthmatic response (maximal late per cent fall in FEV_1)	23.5	12.3†	11.0†	5.9†
Airway hyper-responsiveness (doubling concentrations)[b]	1.71	0.62*	0.64*	0.41*
Sputum eosinophil levels 7 hours after challenge ($\times 10^4$ cells/mL)	42.6	11.7†	16.4†	3.7†
Sputum eosinophil levels 24 hours after challenge ($\times 10^4$ cells/mL)	60.2	24.0*	15.3*	6.2*

*$p<0.05$ *vs* placebo; †$p<0.005$ *vs* placebo
[a]Administered twice daily.
[b]Measured as the concentration of methacholine required to produce a decrease in forced expiratory volume in 1 second (FEV_1) of 20%.

Table 4. Change in efficacy endpoints from baseline to last treatment visit after 12 weeks' treatment with mometasone, beclometasone dipropionate or placebo, in patients with moderate persistent asthma.[19]

Efficacy endpoint	Mean change from baseline (%)				
	Mometasone[a]			Beclometasone dipropionate, 168 μg[a]	Placebo
	100 μg	200 μg	400 μg		
FEV_1	4.8	7.1	6.2	3.0	–6.6
FVC	4.7	3.3	3.5	2.0	–4.7
$FEF_{25–75\%}$	6.2	18.8	15.2	7.5	–9.5
Morning PEF	4.6	9.9	9.3	5.7	–7.0
Evening PEF	3.8	9.3	6.4	3.1	–3.9

All measurements $p<0.01$ *vs* placebo.
[a]Administered twice daily.
FEV_1, forced expiratory volume in 1 second; FVC, forced vital capacity; $FEF_{25–75\%}$, forced expiratory flow 25–75%; PEF, peak expiratory flow.

with mometasone, 100 μg twice daily. Symptoms (as assessed subjectively by both patients and study investigators) also improved by a greater extent with all four active treatments than with placebo ($p<0.05$), with similar improvements observed with beclometasone dipropionate and mometasone, 200 and 400 μg. Thus, in conclusion, all three doses of mometasone were clinically superior in efficacy to placebo in patients with moderate persistent asthma over a 12-week treatment period. Mometasone improved all measures of pulmonary function compared with placebo, with the most consistent effect observed with the 200 μg twice-daily dose. Given the lack of additional benefit with the 400 μg twice-daily dose, this study indicated that the optimal dose of mometasone in patients with moderate persistent asthma who were already maintained on other inhaled corticosteroids was 200 μg twice daily. Whether a higher optimal dose is necessary for patients with more severe persistent asthma remains to be confirmed in future clinical studies.

Mometasone improved all measures of pulmonary function compared with placebo, with the most consistent effect observed with the 200 μg twice-daily dose.

In another large multicentre, randomised, double-blind study, adult patients with moderate persistent asthma (n=395) previously treated with inhaled corticosteroids received treatment with mometasone, 56, 200 or 500 μg twice daily, or beclometasone dipropionate, 168 μg twice daily, or placebo, all given via an MDI for 4 weeks.[20] All active treatments significantly improved the FEV_1 by the end of the study compared with placebo ($p<0.01$ for all active treatment groups *vs* placebo). The improvements in FEV_1 seen in the mometasone, 200 and 500 μg, treatment groups (13 and 14%, respectively), were greater than that observed with mometasone, 56 μg (6%; $p<0.01$ for both comparisons). A similar pattern emerged with regard to the secondary efficacy endpoints (i.e. mean change in forced vital capacity [FVC], forced expiratory flow between 25% and 75% of vital capacity [$FEF_{25-75\%}$] and morning and evening peak expiratory flow [PEF] rates). Thus, mometasone, 200 and 500 μg twice daily, were comparable in efficacy, and superior to mometasone, 56 μg twice daily, again indicating that 200 μg twice daily is the optimum dose in patients with moderate persistent asthma.

Finally, in a randomised, double-blind, cross-over study, adult patients with mild asthma (n=15) received mometasone, 50 or 100 μg twice daily, or placebo, via a DPI for 2 weeks.[21] Patients were challenged with adenosine monophosphate (AMP) before and at the end of each treatment period. Both doses of mometasone reduced the bronchoconstrictor response to AMP compared with placebo: the dose–response curve was displaced to the right by 2.81 and 3.11 doubling dilutions for the 50 and 100 μg doses, respectively ($p<0.001$ for both doses *vs* placebo). Furthermore, FEV_1 improved by a greater extent over the 2-week treatment period with mometasone than with placebo, with no significant differences reported between the two mometasone doses (mean changes from baseline in FEV_1: 0.235, 0.34 and 0.09 L for mometasone 50 μg and 100 μg and placebo, respectively; $p\leq0.033$ for both doses *vs* placebo). Increases in FVC and PEF were not significant between the different treatment groups. Thus, both doses of mometasone reduced airway hyper-responsiveness and improved respiratory function compared with placebo.

Meta-analysis of dose–response

Two studies of mometasone in patients with persistent asthma were included in a meta-analysis which evaluated the dose–response

Current recommendations indicate that patients with mild-to-moderate persistent asthma should receive the lowest effective dose of inhaled corticosteroid.

relationships of various inhaled corticosteroids (beclometasone dipropionate, budesonide, fluticasone propionate, flunisolide, mometasone and triamcinolone acetonide).[22–24] The two mometasone studies provided only sufficient information to enable a comparison of the effects of the drug upon FEV_1, and no dose–response relationship was reported with this outcome. The results obtained with other inhaled corticosteroids in this meta-analysis showed that morning and evening PEF rates were sensitive to drug dose (as to a lesser extent was FEV_1), but only at the lower end of the recommended dose ranges. These data suggest that increasing the dose of inhaled corticosteroid does not lead to increased efficacy, and are therefore consistent with the current recommendation that patients with mild-to-moderate persistent asthma should receive the lowest effective dose of inhaled corticosteroid.[24]

Reduction of oral corticosteroid requirement

The use of inhaled mometasone in patients with severe persistent asthma reduces or eliminates the need for oral corticosteroids.[25]
In a multicentre, double-blind, placebo-controlled trial of 132 patients with oral corticosteroid-dependent severe persistent asthma, 12 weeks' treatment with mometasone, 400 or 800 μg twice daily, administered by a DPI, reduced the daily requirement for oral prednisolone by 46.0 and 23.9%, respectively, compared with baseline.[25] By contrast, treatment with placebo led to a 164.4% increase in the need for oral prednisolone ($p<0.05$ for both doses of mometasone *vs* placebo). Furthermore, 40% of patients receiving mometasone, 400 μg twice daily, and 37% of patients receiving mometasone, 800 μg twice daily, did not require oral prednisolone at all, compared with none of the placebo-treated patients (*p*-values not reported). An open-label extension of this study showed that mometasone, 400–800 μg twice daily, continued to reduce the need for oral prednisolone by 54.1% after 9 months of treatment. Overall, 76% of patients who completed both phases of the study were able to eliminate the use of oral prednisolone. Thus, mometasone has a clinically significant oral corticosteroid-sparing effect in patients previously dependent on such medication to manage their severe persistent asthma, and may be a useful alternative to oral corticosteroids in such patients.

Treatment with mometasone reduced the daily requirement for oral prednisolone and was associated with improvements in patients' quality of life.

The study also involved an evaluation of health-related quality of life using various questionnaires (including both a generic and disease-specific measure of quality of life).[26] At baseline, patients showed impaired quality of life compared with the general US population ($p<0.01$). After treatment with inhaled mometasone during the double-blind phase of the aforementioned study, quality of life was shown to improve significantly ($p<0.05$ *vs* placebo), and this improvement was maintained during 3 months of the open-label extension. Thus, the oral steroid-sparing effect of inhaled mometasone was accompanied by a significant improvement in patients' quality of life.

Once-daily vs twice-daily administration

The control of asthma can be hampered by a lack of patient compliance with a prescribed therapy.[3] A number of specific factors can limit a patient's compliance to inhaled corticosteroid therapy. These include fear of side-effects, lack of education regarding the role of 'preventer' medication, failure to observe immediate symptom relief, the complexity of the treatment regimen and the ease of use of the inhaler.[15] Failure to comply to treatment can lead to diminished lung function, increased hospitalisations, exacerbations and impaired quality of life.[3]

Compliance with long-term inhaled corticosteroid therapy also tends to decrease as the daily dosing schedule increases. In a study of inhaled corticosteroids in children, compliance with a twice-daily dosing schedule was 71%, but this decreased to 34% with a three-times daily schedule and 18% with a four-times daily schedule.[27] Thus, less frequent daily dosing schedules may improve overall patient compliance.

The efficacy of once-daily inhaled mometasone was evaluated in a multicentre, randomised, double-blind, placebo-controlled trial.[22] Patients with mild-to-moderate persistent asthma (n=236) who had previously used only short-acting inhaled β_2-agonists were randomised to treatment with mometasone, 200 or 400 µg once daily, in the morning via a DPI, or placebo, for 12 weeks. Both doses of mometasone were more effective than placebo in improving FEV_1 ($p<0.05$ for both doses *vs* placebo), FVC ($p<0.05$ for both doses *vs* placebo) and $FEF_{25-75\%}$ ($p<0.01$ for both doses *vs* placebo) throughout the study and at the study endpoint. Improvements with the higher dose were numerically greater than those with the lower dose, but differences between the two groups were not significant. The higher dose of mometasone was more effective than placebo in improving morning PEF throughout the study and at endpoint ($p<0.01$), whereas differences between the lower dose of mometasone and placebo were not significant. Both doses were also more effective than placebo in improving asthma symptom scores ($p<0.05$), use of rescue medication ($p<0.01$) and the physician-evaluated response to therapy ($p<0.01$). Thus, both doses of mometasone were effective in the treatment of mild-to-moderate persistent asthma when administered once daily, but the higher dose gave a greater improvement in morning PEF.

Two studies have directly compared once- and twice-daily dosing schedules with inhaled mometasone. In a randomised, double-blind, placebo-controlled study, patients with mild-to-moderate persistent asthma (n=306) who had previously used only short-acting inhaled β_2-agonists were randomly assigned to mometasone, 200 or 400 µg once daily in the morning via a DPI, or mometasone, 200 µg twice daily via a DPI, or placebo, for 12 weeks.[23] At the study endpoint (the last evaluable visit), the improvements in FEV_1 were 10.4, 16.0, 16.1 and 5.5%, respectively. The difference in FEV_1 between mometasone, 400 µg once daily or 200 µg twice daily, and placebo was significant ($p<0.02$). However, there was no significant difference between mometasone, 200 µg once daily, and placebo. Secondary efficacy variables (FVC, $FEF_{25-75\%}$, morning and evening PEF, asthma symptom scores, rescue salbutamol use, physician-evaluated response to therapy and time to worsening of asthma) also improved significantly with mometasone, 400 µg once daily or 200 µg twice daily (all $p<0.05$ *vs* placebo), but not with mometasone, 200 µg once daily.

In another study, patients with mild-to-moderate persistent asthma (n=286) who had previously been treated with inhaled corticosteroids were stabilised with mometasone, 200 µg twice daily via a DPI, for 2 weeks.[28] Patients were then randomised to double-blind treatment with one of five treatment regimens for 12 weeks: mometasone, 200 µg twice daily; 200 µg once daily in the morning; 200 µg once daily in the evening; 400 µg once daily in the morning; placebo. Once-daily mometasone, 400 µg in the morning, and twice-daily mometasone, 200 µg, were significantly and equally effective in improving FEV_1 ($p<0.01$), morning PEF ($p<0.01$), FVC ($p<0.01$), $FEF_{25-75\%}$ ($p<0.03$), asthma symptom scores ($p<0.01$), salbutamol use ($p<0.01$), the number of nocturnal awakenings ($p<0.01$) and the physician-evaluated response to treatment ($p<0.01$) compared with placebo. Once-daily mometasone, 200 µg in the evening, was also effective in improving measures of pulmonary function ($p<0.01$ *vs* placebo for improvements in FEV_1, morning PEF, FVC and $FEF_{25-75\%}$) but was not as effective in improving other efficacy measures. Once-daily mometasone, 200 µg given in the morning, was less effective than other dosing schedules in improving pulmonary function ($p<0.01$ *vs* placebo for the improvement in morning PEF, only).

Mometasone administered at a total daily dose of 400 µg is effective in the treatment of mild-to-moderate persistent asthma whether it is taken once or twice daily.

The results of these two studies clearly indicate that mometasone administered as a total daily dose of 400 µg is effective in the treatment of mild-to-moderate persistent asthma whether it is taken once or twice daily. The equivalent efficacy associated with once-daily dosing may aid patient compliance. In addition, once-daily administration with the 200 µg dose appears to be more effective when it is administered in the evening compared with morning administration.

Mometasone vs fluticasone propionate

The relative efficacy of mometasone and fluticasone propionate has been compared in a large, multicentre, randomised, double-blind, parallel-group trial.[29] Patients with moderate persistent asthma (n=733) who were previously maintained on inhaled corticosteroids were randomised to receive mometasone, 100, 200 or 400 µg twice daily via a DPI, or fluticasone propionate, 250 µg twice daily via a breath-actuated delivery system, for at least 12 weeks. All four treatment schedules produced an improvement in FEV_1 by the study endpoint (last evaluable visit) compared with baseline (Table 5). The improvements were similar for the 200 and 400 µg doses of mometasone and fluticasone propionate, and significantly greater with the 400 µg dose of mometasone than with the 100 µg dose ($p=0.02$; Table 5). Improvements in morning PEF were greater with mometasone, 200 and 400 µg, and fluticasone propionate, than with mometasone, 100 µg ($p<0.05$), whilst improvements in $FEF_{25-75\%}$ were greater with mometasone, 400 µg, and fluticasone

Table 5. Changes in respiratory function (expressed as mean change ± SEM) after 12 weeks' treatment with mometasone or fluticasone propionate in patients with moderate persistent asthma.[29]

Respiratory function	Mometasone[a]			Fluticasone propionate[a]
	100 μg	200 μg	400 μg	250 μg
FEV_1 (L)	0.07±0.04	0.16±0.04	0.19±0.04*	0.16±0.04
FVC (L)	0.03±0.05	0.08±0.06	0.11±0.05	0.08±0.05
$FEF_{25–75\%}$ (L/second)	0.04±0.07	0.21±0.07	0.28±0.07*	0.25±0.07*
Morning PEF (L/minute)	15±5	29±6*	30±5*	32±5*

*$p<0.05$ vs mometasone, 100 μg twice daily.
[a]Administered twice daily.
FEV_1, forced expiratory volume in 1 second; FVC, forced vital capacity; $FEF_{25–75\%}$, forced expiratory flow 25–75%; PEF, peak expiratory flow.

propionate ($p<0.05$ *vs* mometasone, 100 μg; Table 5). Changes in FVC were similar in all four treatment groups. Thus, a total daily dose of 400 μg mometasone provided comparable clinical benefit in terms of improvements in measures of pulmonary function as fluticasone propionate, 250 μg given twice daily, in patients with moderate persistent asthma.[29]

The effectiveness of once-daily mometasone was compared with that of twice-daily fluticasone propionate, in an 8-week open-label study in 167 patients with moderate persistent asthma.[30] Mometasone was administered in the evening at a dose of 400 μg via a DPI, whilst fluticasone was given as two 125 μg puffs twice daily via an MDI. At baseline, FEV_1 was 75.5 and 76.2% of the predicted normal value in mometasone and fluticasone treatment groups, respectively, corresponding to actual mean measurements of 2.42 and 2.35 L, respectively (p=0.58). An improvement in FEV_1 was noted as early as 2 weeks into both treatment regimens, with the percentage increases in FEV_1 at 2 weeks measuring 4.70 and 6.67% for mometasone and fluticasone, respectively (p-value not reported). By the study endpoint, the mean improvements in FEV_1 from baseline were 4.58 and 6.98% for mometasone and fluticasone, respectively (p=0.35). The changes from baseline to endpoint in morning PEF were also comparable between treatment groups, measuring 10.9 and 18.4 L/minute for mometasone and fluticasone, respectively (p=0.33). Furthermore, no treatment differences were reported between groups in terms of asthma symptom scores ($p\geq0.06$). The percentage of patients rated by their physician as 'improved' or 'much improved' were 62 and 47% for mometasone and fluticasone, respectively (p=0.007). Mometasone was superior to fluticasone in terms of patient preference, with 46.8% of mometasone-treated patients 'liking the inhaler a lot', compared with 22.4% of fluticasone-treated participants (p=0.01). Both treatments were well tolerated, with adverse events mild-to-moderate in severity. Headache was the most common adverse event in both treatment groups.

Mometasone vs budesonide

Two clinical trials have compared the efficacy of mometasone and budesonide in patients with moderate persistent asthma. These studies have indicated that mometasone is superior to budesonide in terms of measures of respiratory function and asthma control.[31,32]

In a multicentre, randomised, evaluator-blinded trial, patients with moderate persistent asthma (n=730) who had been previously maintained on inhaled corticosteroids were randomised to treatment with either mometasone, 100, 200 or 400 μg twice daily via DPI, or budesonide, 400 μg twice daily via DPI, for 12 weeks.[31] All four treatments led to improvements in FEV_1 compared with baseline, but the improvements with mometasone, 200 and 400 μg twice daily, were greater than that provided by budesonide ($p<0.05$ for both comparisons; Table 6 and Figure 2). Morning PEF also increased with all four treatments compared with baseline; the increases observed with mometasone, 200 and 400 μg twice daily, were greater than that seen with mometasone, 100 μg twice daily, and similar to the increase observed with budesonide. Thus, twice-daily administration of mometasone, 200 μg, had comparable efficacy to mometasone, 400 μg twice daily, and both doses were superior to budesonide in improving the main efficacy outcome of FEV_1.

In another multicentre, double-blind, placebo-controlled trial, patients with moderate persistent asthma (n=262) who had been using inhaled corticosteroids were randomised to receive once-daily morning treatment with either mometasone, 440 μg via DPI, or budesonide, 400 μg via DPI, or placebo, for 8 weeks.[a,32] At the end of this study, the

Table 6. Changes in respiratory function (expressed as mean change ± SEM) after 12 weeks' treatment with mometasone or budesonide in patients with moderate persistent asthma.[31]

Respiratory function	Mometasone[a]			Budesonide[a]
	100 μg	200 μg	400 μg	400 μg
FEV_1 (L)	0.10±0.03	0.16±0.03*	0.16±0.03*	0.06±0.03
FEV_1 (% of predicted value)	79.6±1.1	81.6±1.2*	83.0±1.2*,†	77.9±1.1
FVC (L)	0.07±0.04	0.16±0.04	0.15±0.04	0.06±0.04
Morning PEF (L/minute)	18.2±5.3	37.8±5.4†	37.3±5.2†	24.7±5.3

*$p<0.05$ compared with budesonide; †$p<0.05$ compared with mometasone, 100 μg.
[a]Administered twice daily.
FEV_1, forced expiratory volume in 1 second; FVC, forced vital capacity; PEF, peak expiratory flow.

[a]These are the metered doses delivering 400 μg and 320 μg of mometasone and budesonide, respectively.

Figure 2. Changes from baseline in the forced expiratory volume in 1 second (FEV_1) associated with mometasone and budesonide administration in patents with moderate persistent asthma.[31]

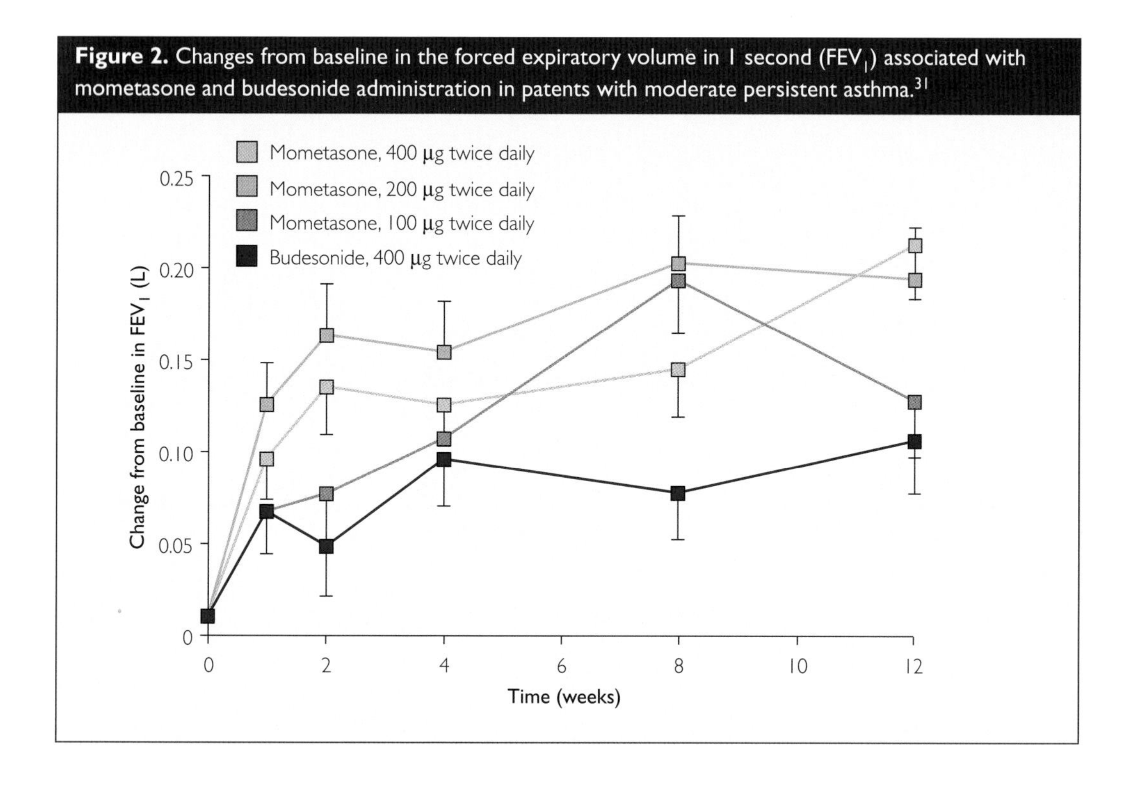

actual and percentage changes in FEV_1 from baseline were greater with mometasone (0.19 L and 8.9%, respectively) than with budesonide (0.03 L and 2.1%, respectively; $p<0.01$ for mometasone *vs* budesonide) and placebo (–0.10 L and –3.9%, respectively; $p<0.01$ for mometasone *vs* placebo). Similarly, secondary efficacy variables ($FEF_{25-75\%}$, morning and evening PEF, rescue salbutamol usage, percentage of symptom-free days and physician-evaluated response to therapy) improved by a significantly greater extent with mometasone than with budesonide or placebo ($p<0.05$). Thus, once-daily morning administration with mometasone was superior to once-daily morning treatment with budesonide in improving pulmonary function and asthma symptoms when given at equivalent microgram dosages.

Once-daily morning treatment with mometasone was superior to once-daily morning treatment with budesonide in improving pulmonary function and asthma symptoms.

Mometasone vs beclometasone dipropionate

Three studies have compared the clinical efficacy of mometasone and beclometasone dipropionate. In two of these studies, the optimum dose of mometasone gave numerically superior results to beclometasone dipropionate though the differences between treatment groups were not statistically significant,[19,33] whilst the third study indicated that mometasone provided significantly greater control of asthma than beclometasone.[20] Thus, mometasone appears to be at least as effective as beclometasone dipropionate in the treatment of asthma.

Two of these studies were essentially dose-ranging studies and have already been reviewed in detail (see Dose-Ranging and Placebo-Controlled Studies and Table 4).[19,20] In one study, beclometasone dipropionate, 168 μg twice daily, was comparable with mometasone, 100 μg twice daily, in improving pulmonary function.[19] This dose of mometasone gave consistently inferior results to mometasone doses of 200 and 400 μg twice daily, although dose-by-dose comparisons were not statistically significant. In addition, beclometasone dipropionate proved comparable with mometasone, 200 and 400 μg twice daily, in improving asthma symptoms.

In a multicentre, randomised, double-blind, placebo-controlled study, patients with moderate persistent asthma (n=227) being maintained with inhaled corticosteroids were allocated to treatment with either mometasone, 100 or 200 μg twice daily via a DPI, or beclometasone dipropionate, 168 μg twice daily via an MDI, or placebo, for 12 weeks.[33] All three treatments significantly improved FEV_1 at endpoint compared with placebo ($p<0.01$ for all comparisons). The improvement in FEV_1 with mometasone, 200 μg twice daily, was almost double that observed with mometasone, 100 μg twice daily, and beclometasone dipropionate, but between group differences were not significant. Similar results were observed with secondary efficacy measures.

Mometasone proved to be superior to beclometasone dipropionate given over 4 weeks in patients with moderate persistent asthma.

In the third study, the improvement in FEV_1 from baseline to the study endpoint was 13 and 14%, respectively, for mometasone, 200 and 500 μg twice daily via a MDI, compared with 4% for beclometasone dipropionate, 168 μg twice daily also administered via an MDI ($p<0.05$ for both doses of mometasone *vs* beclometasone). A similar pattern of superiority emerged for the secondary efficacy measures (i.e. change from baseline in FVC, $FEF_{25-75\%}$, morning PEF, physician's evaluation of asthma symptoms and use of rescue salbutamol use).[20] Thus, in this study, mometasone proved to be superior to beclometasone dipropionate given over 4 weeks in patients with moderate persistent asthma.

In summary, these comparative clinical studies indicate that mometasone appears to be as effective as fluticasone propionate and more effective than budesonide and beclometasone dipropionate in terms of their effects on the principal marker of respiratory function, FEV_1.[10] However, further studies are needed to confirm the dose equivalence of mometasone to these other inhaled corticosteroids, which will enable more accurate comparisons of these agents.

Safety and tolerability

Systemic absorption of inhaled corticosteroids is one of the principal safety concerns associated with the use of these agents. However, data from single-dose pharmacokinetic studies indicate that systemic absorption of mometasone is minimal, although there may be some accumulation with multiple dosing. The use of the Twisthaler device may further minimise the potential for systemic absorption of the drug. In addition, mometasone undergoes a high rate of first-pass metabolism and thus has a low bioavailability.[10] Nevertheless, absorption of mometasone directly from the lungs, may, like other inhaled corticosteroids, have the potential to cause systemic effects.

The currently available evidence indicates that the systemic effects of mometasone are minimal within the licensed dose range, but prescribers should be aware that all inhaled corticosteroids have the potential to cause long-term systemic effects, including growth retardation, decreased bone mineral density, dental erosion and suppression of the HPA axis. These adverse events generally occur in a dose-related fashion and are more frequent with the highest doses of inhaled corticosteroids.[8,34,35] The current recommendation is for inhaled corticosteroids to be used in a step-wise manner to achieve the lowest possible maintenance dose, thus minimising the risk of systemic adverse effects.[8]

Effects on the HPA axis

The effects of inhaled mometasone on the HPA axis have been investigated in three studies performed by the same authors.[6] All three studies were randomised, evaluator-blinded, placebo-controlled, parallel-group trials that lasted for 28 days and involved adults with mild-to-moderate persistent asthma. In the first study, patients (n=60) were randomised to receive inhaled mometasone via a DPI at doses of 200 μg twice daily, or 400, 800 or 1200 μg once daily. At these doses, mometasone had no effect on the AUC for serum cortisol concentrations over 24 hours (AUC_{24}).

In the second study, patients (n=64) were allocated to treatment with either mometasone, 400 or 800 μg twice daily via a DPI, or oral prednisolone, 10 mg once daily.[6] All three treatments reduced the serum cortisol AUC_{24} compared with placebo ($p<0.05$). Oral prednisolone had the greatest effect on cortisol AUC_{24} and the lowest dose of mometasone had the least effect (reductions in cortisol AUC_{24}: mometasone, 400 μg: 19–25% [mean reduction not reported]; mometasone 800 μg: 28.0±8.3%; prednisolone, 10 mg: 67.2±3.6%). The reductions in cortisol AUC_{24} with prednisolone were significantly greater than those observed with either dose of mometasone ($p<0.01$).

In the third study, patients (n=64) received either mometasone, 400 or 800 μg twice daily, or fluticasone propionate, 880 μg twice daily, via an MDI. The lowest dose of mometasone had no effect on serum cortisol AUC_{24} whilst the higher dose elicited a mean decrease of 24.0±3.1% and fluticasone propionate caused a mean decrease of 51.7±3.8%. According to the authors of this study, serum cortisol AUC_{24} levels observed with fluticasone propionate were significantly suppressed compared with those seen with the higher dose of mometasone, although a *p*-value was not reported.

In conclusion, the available evidence indicates that mometasone has only a minimal effect on the HPA axis when administered at high doses. The highest dose used in any of these studies was 1600 μg/day, which is twice the highest recommended clinical dose. This dose appeared to be the lower limit at which consistent suppression of the HPA axis occurred. The authors also suggested that mometasone administered via

Further studies are warranted to fully determine the effects of mometasone on the HPA axis.

an MDI may have less systemic activity (AUC_{24} decreased by 24%) than mometasone delivered via a DPI (AUC_{24} decreased by 28%). However, there has been some criticism of the conclusions drawn from these studies, with some suggestion that significant suppression of the HPA axis does occur with mometasone.[8] Clearly, further studies are warranted to fully determine the effects of mometasone on the HPA axis.

Effects on growth

No data are currently available on the effects of inhaled mometasone on growth or bone mineral density. However, two studies of intranasal mometasone in the treatment of children with allergic rhinitis have indicated that the drug has no significant effect on growth in either the short term (2 weeks) or long term (1 year).[36,37]

Dental health

The acidic pH of inhaled corticosteroids may contribute to a higher incidence of tooth decay and dental erosion in patients with asthma. Powdered formulations appear to be the most problematic as they have the lowest pH values. Thus, tooth decay may be a potential problem with mometasone delivered via a DPI. In view of this, it is recommended that patients should rinse their mouth after using a DPI and should practise good dental hygiene.[35]

Adverse events

In the clinical trial programme of mometasone, the drug has proved to be well tolerated at all the doses investigated. Most adverse events have been mild or moderate in severity and none have been life threatening. The overall incidence of adverse events with mometasone has been similar to that reported with placebo and other comparator inhaled corticosteroids (Table 7). No increase in the incidence of clinically meaningful adverse events has occurred during prolonged (9 months) treatment with mometasone.[25] The most frequently reported adverse events have been headache, oral candidiasis, pharyngitis and dysphonia. No adverse event has occurred more frequently with increasing dose, apart from oral candidiasis, and this condition did not result in treatment discontinuation.[20,29] The incidence of serious adverse events has been low (<2%), as has the incidence of discontinuations due to adverse events. In one study, no evidence of HPA axis suppression was observed,[19] whilst another study found a slight increase (2–5%) in morning plasma cortisol levels after 12 weeks of treatment.[32] In this study, the corresponding figure for budesonide was shown to be 9%.

The most frequently reported adverse events have been headache, oral candidiasis, pharyngitis and dysphonia.

Laboratory parameters

No clinically relevant changes in vital signs, the results of physical examinations or laboratory parameters have been observed with mometasone in clinical trials. In addition, no electrocardiogram abnormalities have been reported.

Table 7. Overall incidence of adverse events (%) in clinical trials of mometasone and comparator drugs.[19,22,23,29,32]

Study	Placebo	Mometasone			Fluticasone propionate, 250 μg twice daily	Beclometasone propionate, 168 μg twice daily	Budesonide, 400 μg once daily
		100 μg twice daily or 200 μg once daily	200 μg twice daily or 400 μg once daily	400 μg twice daily			
Bernstein *et al.*, 1999[19]	22	18	26	28	–	21	–
Kemp *et al.*, 2000[23]	19	23	23	23	–	–	–
Nayak *et al.*, 2000[22]	22	19	25	–	–	–	–
O'Connor *et al.*, 2001[29]	–	20	26	30	29	–	–
Corren *et al.*, 2003[32]	8	–	8	–	–	–	9

Key points

- Mometasone is one of the newer, more potent inhaled corticosteroids for the management of persistent asthma in adults and children over the age of 12 years.
- Single-dose studies suggest that less than 1% of mometasone is absorbed systemically after inhalation. However, multiple-dose studies suggest that absorption may occur after repeated dosing.
- *In vitro* studies have shown that mometasone has a higher affinity for the glucocorticosteroid receptor than other inhaled corticosteroids, and has a variety of anti-inflammatory effects. These effects are comparable with those seen with fluticasone propionate but are more potent than those seen with other inhaled corticosteroids.
- Dose-ranging studies suggest that in patients with mild-to-moderate asthma the optimum daily dose of mometasone is 400 μg. A higher dose of 800 μg does not appear to confer any additional clinical benefit. This lends support to the recommendation that patients with asthma should receive the lowest effective dose of inhaled corticosteroids.
- Use of inhaled mometasone can reduce or eliminate the need for oral corticosteroids. This oral corticosteroid-sparing effect of mometasone is also accompanied by an improvement in patients' quality of life.
- Once-daily dosing with mometasone is as effective as twice-daily dosing, whilst evening dosing appears to be more effective than morning dosing.
- The optimum dose of mometasone (400 μg daily) in patients with mild-to-moderate asthma is comparable in efficacy with fluticasone propionate (500 μg daily) and superior in efficacy to budesonide (800 μg daily).
- Comparisons of mometasone and beclometasone dipropionate are less clear: some studies suggest that the two drugs are comparable in efficacy, whilst others suggest that mometasone is superior.
- Mometasone shows minimal suppression of the HPA axis. However, further studies are warranted to fully clarify the effects of mometasone on the HPA axis.
- Mometasone has proved to be well tolerated in clinical trials, with an incidence of adverse events comparable with that seen with placebo and other inhaled corticosteroids. The most frequently reported adverse events have been headache, oral candidiasis, pharyngitis and dysphonia.

References

A list of the published evidence which has been reviewed in compiling the preceding section of *BESTMEDICINE*.

1. Boulet LP. Once-daily inhaled corticosteroids for the treatment of asthma. *Curr Opin Pulm Med* 2004; **10**: 15–21.
2. Umland SP, Schleimer RP, Johnston SL. Review of the molecular and cellular mechanisms of action of glucocorticoids for use in asthma. *Pulm Pharmacol Ther* 2002; **15**: 35–50.
3. Karpel JP. An easy-to-use dry-powder inhaler. *Adv Ther* 2000; **17**: 282–6.
4. Affrime MB, Cuss F, Padhi D *et al.* Bioavailability and metabolism of mometasone furoate following administration by metered-dose and dry-powder inhalers in healthy human volunteers. *J Clin Pharmacol* 2000; **40**: 1227–36.
5. Pickering H, Pitcairn GR, Hirst PH *et al.* Regional lung deposition of a technetium 99m-labeled formulation of mometasone furoate administered by hydrofluoroalkane 227 metered-dose inhaler. *Clin Ther* 2000; **22**: 1483–93.
6. Affrime MB, Kosoglou T, Thonoor CM, Flannery BE, Herron JM. Mometasone furoate has minimal effects on the hypothalamic-pituitary-adrenal axis when delivered at high doses. *Chest* 2000; **118**: 1538–46.
7. Crim C, Pierre LN, Daley-Yates PT. A review of the pharmacology and pharmacokinetics of inhaled fluticasone propionate and mometasone furoate. *Clin Ther* 2001; **23**: 1339–54.
8. Lipworth BJ, Jackson CM. Safety of inhaled and intranasal corticosteroids: lessons for the new millennium. *Drug Saf* 2000; **23**: 11–33.
9. Derendorf H, Daley-Yates PT, Pierre LN, Efthimiou J. Bioavailability and metabolism of mometasone furoate: pharmacology versus methodology. *J Clin Pharmacol* 2002; **42**: 383–7.
10. Sharpe M, Jarvis B. Inhaled mometasone furoate: a review of its use in adults and adolescents with persistent asthma. *Drugs* 2001; **61**: 1325–50.
11. Smith CL, Kreutner W. *In vitro* glucocorticoid receptor binding and transcriptional activation by topically active glucocorticoids. *Arzneimittelforschung* 1998; **48**: 956–60.
12. Kelly HW. Pharmaceutical characteristics that influence the clinical efficacy of inhaled corticosteroids. *Ann Allergy Asthma Immunol* 2003; **91**: 326–34.
13. Papi A, Papadopoulos NG, Degitz K, Holgate ST, Johnston SL. Corticosteroids inhibit rhinovirus-induced intercellular adhesion molecule-1 up-regulation and promoter activation on respiratory epithelial cells. *J Allergy Clin Immunol* 2000; **105**: 318–26.
14. Zhang X, Moilanen E, Adcock IM, Lindsay MA, Kankaanranta H. Divergent effect of mometasone on human eosinophil and neutrophil apoptosis. *Life Sci* 2002; **71**: 1523–34.
15. O'Connor B. Inhaler devices: compliance with steroid therapy. *Nurs Stand* 2001; **15**: 40–2.
16. Yang TT, Li S, Wyka B, Kenyon D. Drug delivery performance of the mometasone furoate dry powder inhaler. *J Aerosol Med* 2001; **14**: 487–94.
17. Gauvreau GM, Inman MD, Kelly M *et al.* Increased levels of airway neutrophils reduce the inhibitory effects of inhaled glucocorticosteroids on allergen-induced airway eosinophils. *Can Respir J* 2002; **9**: 26–32.
18. Inman MD, Watson RM, Rerecich T *et al.* Dose-dependent effects of inhaled mometasone furoate on airway function and inflammation after allergen inhalation challenge. *Am J Respir Crit Care Med* 2001; **164**: 569–74.
19. Bernstein DI, Berkowitz RB, Chervinsky P *et al.* Dose-ranging study of a new steroid for asthma: mometasone furoate dry powder inhaler. *Respir Med* 1999; **93**: 603–12.
20. Chervinsky P, Nelson HS, Bernstein DI, Berkowitz RA, Siegel SC. Comparison of mometasone furoate administered by metered dose inhaler with beclometasone dipropionate. *Int J Clin Pract* 2002; **56**: 419–25.
21. Holgate ST, Arshad H, Stryszak P, Harrison JE. Mometasone furoate antagonizes AMP-induced bronchoconstriction in patients with mild asthma. *J Allergy Clin Immunol* 2000; **105**: 906–11.
22. Nayak AS, Banov C, Corren J *et al.* Once-daily mometasone furoate dry powder inhaler in the treatment of patients with persistent asthma. *Ann Allergy Asthma Immunol* 2000; **84**: 417–24.
23. Kemp JP, Berkowitz RB, Miller SD *et al.* Mometasone furoate administered once daily is as effective as twice-daily administration for treatment of mild-to-moderate persistent asthma. *J Allergy Clin Immunol* 2000; **106**: 485–92.
24. Bousquet J, Ben-Joseph R, Messonnier M, Alemao E, Gould AL. A meta-analysis of the dose-response relationship of inhaled corticosteroids in adolescents and adults with mild to moderate persistent asthma. *Clin Ther* 2002; **24**: 1–20.
25. Fish JE, Karpel JP, Craig TJ *et al.* Inhaled mometasone furoate reduces oral prednisolone requirements while improving respiratory function and health-related quality of life in patients with severe persistent asthma. *J Allergy Clin Immunol* 2000; **106**: 852–60.
26. Schmier J, Leidy NK, Gower R. Reduction in oral corticosteroid use with mometasone furoate dry powder inhaler improves health-related quality of life in patients with severe persistent asthma. *J Asthma* 2003; **40**: 383–93.
27. Coutts JA, Gibson NA, Paton JY. Measuring compliance with inhaled medication in asthma. *Arch Dis Child* 1992; **67**: 332–3.

28 Noonan M, Karpel JP, Bensch GW *et al.* Comparison of once-daily to twice-daily treatment with mometasone furoate dry powder inhaler. *Ann Allergy Asthma Immunol* 2001; **86**: 36–43.

29 O'Connor B, Bonnaud G, Haahtela T *et al.* Dose-ranging study of mometasone furoate dry powder inhaler in the treatment of moderate persistent asthma using fluticasone propionate as an active comparator. *Ann Allergy Asthma Immunol* 2001; **86**: 397–404.

30 Wardlaw A, Larivee P, Eller J *et al.* Efficacy and safety of mometasone furoate dry powder inhaler vs fluticasone propionate metered-dose inhaler in asthma subjects previously using fluticasone propionate. *Ann Allergy Asthma Immunol.* 2004; **93**: 49–55.

31 Bousquet J, D'Urzo A, Hebert J *et al.* Comparison of the efficacy and safety of mometasone furoate dry powder inhaler to budesonide Turbuhaler. *Eur Respir J* 2000; **16**: 808–16.

32 Corren J, Berkowitz R, Murray JJ, Prenner B. Comparison of once-daily mometasone furoate versus once-daily budesonide in patients with moderate persistent asthma. *Int J Clin Pract* 2003; **57**: 567–72.

33 Nathan RA, Nayak AS, Graft DF *et al.* Mometasone furoate: efficacy and safety in moderate asthma compared with beclometasone dipropionate. *Ann Allergy Asthma Immunol* 2001; **86**: 203–10.

34 Lipworth BJ, Seckl JR. Measures for detecting systemic bioactivity with inhaled and intranasal corticosteroids. *Thorax* 1997; **52**: 476–82.

35 Randell TL, Donaghue KC, Ambler GR *et al.* Safety of the newer inhaled corticosteroids in childhood asthma. *Paediatr Drugs* 2003; **5**: 481–504.

36 Agertoft L, Pedersen S. Short-term lower leg growth rate in children with rhinitis treated with intranasal mometasone furoate and budesonide. *J Allergy Clin Immunol* 1999; **104**: 948–52.

37 Schenkel EJ, Skoner DP, Bronsky EA *et al.* Absence of growth retardation in children with perennial allergic rhinitis after one year of treatment with mometasone furoate aqueous nasal spray. *Pediatrics* 2000; **105**: E22.

Acknowledgement

Figure 2 is adapted from Bousquet *et al.*, 2000.[31]

8. Drug review – Montelukast (Singulair®)

Dr Eleanor Bull
CSF Medical Communications Ltd

Summary

Montelukast is a leukotriene receptor antagonist – a new class of agent recently introduced for the treatment of mild-to-moderate asthma – as an adjunct to an existing corticosteroid treatment regimen. Through the selective blockade of the cysteinyl leukotriene ($cysLT_1$) receptor, montelukast inhibits both the bronchoconstrictive and inflammatory effects of the leukotrienes, which are inflammatory mediators heavily implicated in asthma pathophysiology. In contrast to corticosteroids, which currently represent the first-line treatment option for moderate-to-severe asthma, montelukast has a rapid onset of action, minimal side-effect profile and is administered orally, thus avoiding the complications of an inhaler device. Controlled clinical trials in patients with mild asthma have shown the level of asthma management achieved with montelukast to be comparable to that achieved using inhaled corticosteroids. In the treatment of patients with moderate asthma, there is substantial evidence to suggest that montelukast, as add-on therapy to a corticosteroid regimen, increases asthma control, reduces asthma exacerbations and improves the level of symptomatic relief, and may permit the gradual tapering of the corticosteroid dosage. When compared with the long-acting inhaled β_2-agonist, salmeterol, as add-on therapy, montelukast elicits comparable improvements in asthma control and in clinical parameters of asthma relief. In view of its mechanism of action, favourable side-effect profile and ease of administration, montelukast may be particularly effective in the treatment of asthma in children, in exercise-induced bronchoconstriction (EIB) and in the aspirin-intolerant subgroup of patients. Additionally, montelukast elicits significant symptomatic improvement in patients with allergic rhinitis, a condition that is commonly comorbid with asthma.

Introduction

Currently, inhaled corticosteroids represent the first-line treatment option for the control of chronic asthma, a reflection of their broad spectrum of activity, efficacy across the range of asthma severity and the benefits associated with prolonged use.[1] However, concerns are escalating over the systemic effects of these agents.[2] Consequently, a desire to limit their dosage has driven the development of new asthma therapies with improved tolerability that will provide effective symptomatic relief in a large proportion of patients with asthma.

Ever since asthma was first classified as an inflammatory disease, experimental research has aimed to define the precise contribution of different inflammatory mediators, with a view to tailoring drug therapy to target the specific causes of the disease. One such target is the cysteinyl leukotrienes, a group of inflammatory mediators released from mast cells, eosinophils, macrophages and neutrophils, the actions of which are highly correlated with the pathophysiology of asthma and allergic rhinitis.[3,4] Leukotrienes are derived from the lipoxygenase pathway of arachidonic acid metabolism (Figure 1).[5] Of the three leukotrienes produced in this manner, the LTC_4 and LTD_4 isoforms are the most potent in terms of their inflammatory properties.[6,7] In the airways, leukotrienes mediate allergen-induced airway obstruction, oedema, vascular permeability and the recruitment of inflammatory cells, as well as smooth muscle contraction of both small- and large-calibre airways.[8,9]

Leukotrienes exert their biological actions by binding and activating specific receptors located on the membranes of target cells. Two types of cysLT receptors have been pharmacologically characterised: $cysLT_1$ and $cysLT_2$; of these it is the $cysLT_1$ receptor that is localised to airway smooth muscle, macrophages and other pro-inflammatory cells.[10]

The leukotriene receptor antagonists are the most recently introduced class of anti-asthma agent and act by blocking the effects of leukotrienes at the level of the $cysLT_1$ receptor.[11] By preventing the bronchoconstrictive and inflammatory effects of leukotrienes, these drugs, which include zafirlukast, pranlukast[a] and montelukast, relieve both the acute bronchoconstriction and the chronic inflammation associated with asthma. The leukotriene receptor antagonists have the distinct advantage of being orally active, and thus avoid the treatment adherence issues associated with an inhaler device.[12] Furthermore, their rapid onset of action (within hours of the initial administration)[13] and acceptable side-effect profile, may also promote patient concordance, although they should not be used to relieve an attack of acute severe asthma. Introduced in the UK in 1998, montelukast is currently recommended as an adjunct to inhaled corticosteroids in patients with moderate disease in whom the additive effect of the two drugs is more effective than a standard dose of inhaled corticosteroid alone. This article reviews the properties of montelukast and its efficacy in controlled clinical trials in the context of other available treatments for asthma within the framework of its licensed indications in the UK.

> The leukotriene receptor antagonists have the distinct advantage of being orally active, and thus avoid the treatment adherence issues associated with an inhaler device.

[a]Not licensed in the UK.

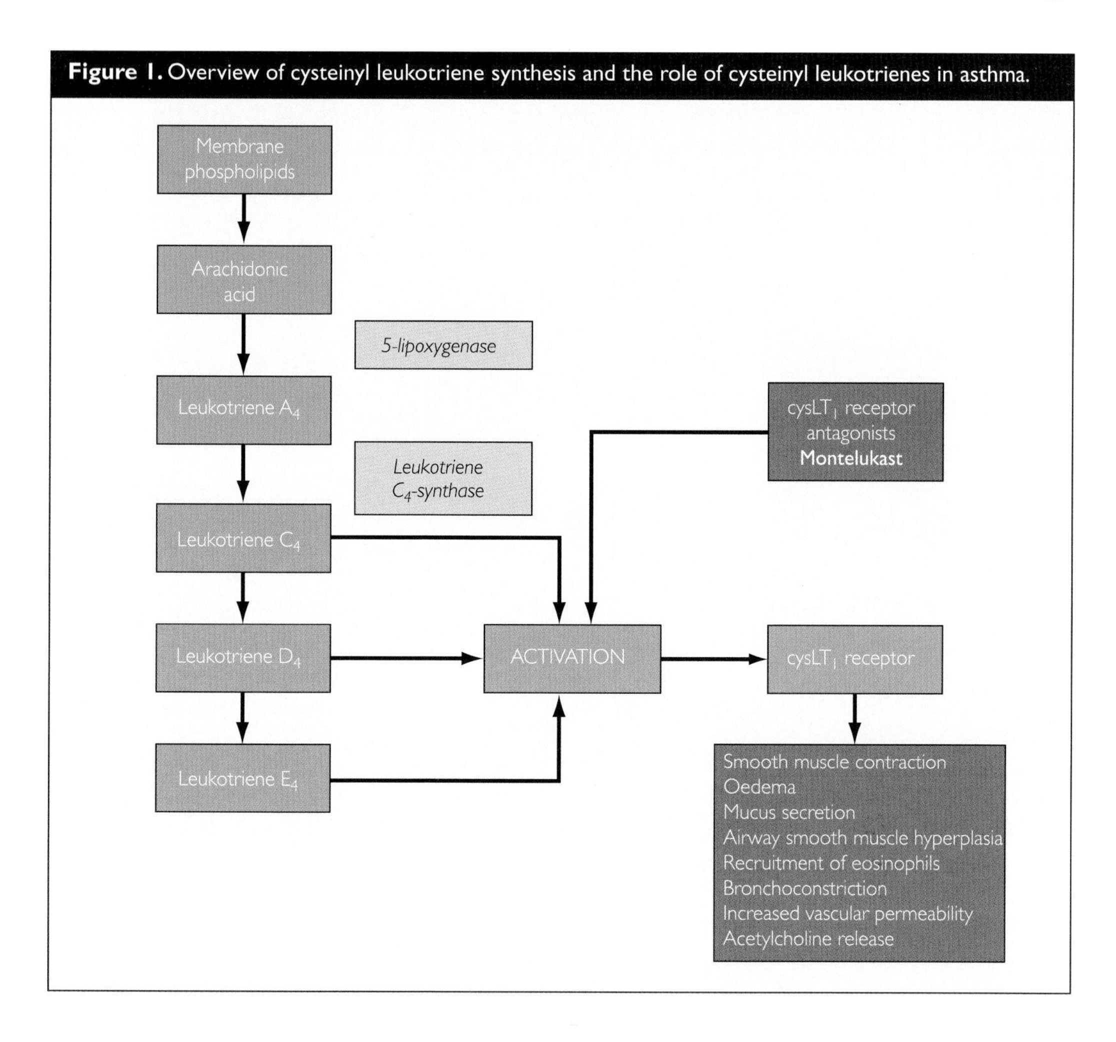

Figure 1. Overview of cysteinyl leukotriene synthesis and the role of cysteinyl leukotrienes in asthma.

Chemistry

The chemical structure of montelukast sodium is illustrated in Figure 2. Montelukast is available as a 10 mg film-coated tablet and as 4 mg and 5 mg chewable tablets. More recently, a granular formulation of montelukast has been introduced, one sachet of which is equivalent to 4 mg montelukast.

☛ *The chemistry of montelukast is of essentially academic interest and most healthcare professionals will, like you, skip this section.*

Figure 2. The chemical structure of montelukast.

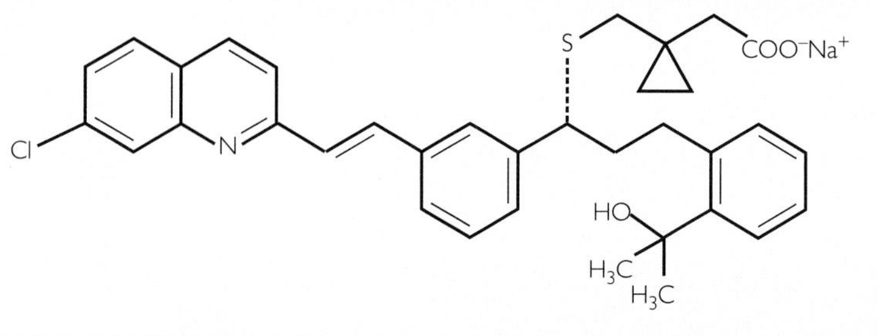

Pharmacology

The leukotriene receptor antagonists exhibit similar *in vitro* and *in vivo* profiles, differing only in terms of relative potency and oral bioavailability.[14] The pharmacological profile of montelukast is reviewed below.

In vitro *activity*

Montelukast is an extremely potent and highly selective LTD_4 receptor antagonist in both guinea pig and human membrane preparations.

Montelukast is an extremely potent and highly selective LTD_4 receptor antagonist in both guinea pig and human membrane preparations.

Receptor binding assays in guinea pig lung cell membranes, measuring the binding of $[^3H]LTD_4$ to the $cysLT_1$ receptor in the presence of montelukast, have revealed an affinity similar to that of zafirlukast (K_i[a] 0.18 nM). These studies also revealed a greater affinity of both drugs for the $cysLT_1$ receptor than that of the endogenous ligand, LTD_4. In differentiated human lung cells, the K_i value was 0.52 nM.[15] Functionally, montelukast antagonises LTD_4-induced contractions of isolated guinea pig trachea (pA_2[b] 9.3; slope 0.8), with a pA_2 value similar to that of zafirlukast.[16] In contrast, montelukast (16 μM) failed to antagonise LTC_4-induced contractions in the presence of serine-borate (an inhibitor of the enzyme responsible for the conversion of LTC_4 to LTD_4), serotonin, acetylcholine, histamine or prostaglandin D_2.[15]

In vivo *activity*

In animal models of pulmonary inflammation, montelukast is active against exogenous and endogenous leukotrienes, antigen-induced bronchoconstriction and various inflammatory markers.

Montelukast is active against exogenous and endogenous leukotrienes, antigen-induced bronchoconstriction and various inflammatory markers.

Intravenous administration of montelukast antagonises LTD_4-induced bronchoconstriction in the anaesthetised guinea pig but does not block the bronchoconstrictive response to arachidonic acid, histamine, serotonin or acetylcholine.[15] When given orally, montelukast blocked LTD_4-induced bronchoconstriction in conscious squirrel monkeys and ovalbumin-induced bronchoconstriction in conscious sensitised rats.[15] A continuous intravenous infusion of montelukast (8 μg/kg/minute) elicited a 70% decrease in the peak early response and a 75% reduction in the late response to ascaris aerosol in allergic conscious sheep.[15] Furthermore, montelukast diminishes the pulmonary response to antigen, tissue eosinophil levels, and the number of cells expressing interleukin-5 mRNA in the Brown Norway rat, suggesting that leukotrienes may also regulate the allergic response through the modulation of cytokine synthesis.[17]

---

[a] K_i, the dissociation constant of an inhibitor.

[b] pA_2, the negative logarithm of the molar concentration of antagonist required to produce an agonist dose ratio equal to 2.

Pharmacokinetics

The pharmacokinetic properties of montelukast, administered as a 10 mg film-coated tablet to fasted adults, are listed in Table 1.[18–21] Montelukast is extensively metabolised by the cytochrome P450 enzymes (CYP) 3A4 and 2C9, and is excreted almost exclusively in the bile.

Generally, the pharmacokinetic properties of montelukast are similar in both elderly and younger adults, and although the plasma half-life is slightly longer in the elderly, no dosage adjustment is necessary.

The pharmacokinetics of a drug are of interest to healthcare professionals because it is important for them to understand the action of a drug on the body over a period of time.

Clinical efficacy

Placebo-controlled trials

The placebo-controlled trials, in which montelukast was administered either alone or in combination with a corticosteroid treatment regimen, are summarised in Table 2. In most of the trials described herein, patients were permitted to use a short-acting β_2-agonist for alleviation of the acute symptoms of an asthma exacerbation. All patients were adults with clinically diagnosed mild persistent asthma.

The administration of montelukast elicited an improvement in at least one aspect of asthma control, compared with placebo.[22–27] A recent survey encapsulating these placebo-controlled trials analysed the effects of montelukast in the treatment of mild persistent asthma.[28] The pooled results demonstrated a treatment effect for montelukast over placebo, both in terms of improvement in the forced expiratory volume in 1 second (FEV_1; 7–8% *vs* 1–4% over baseline, $p \leq 0.02$) free from β_2-agonist medication (22–30% *vs* 8–13% for montelukast and placebo, respectively). In summary, these studies show that in the treatment of mild asthma, montelukast is clearly more effective than placebo and offers a comparable level of asthma control to that achieved using inhaled corticosteroids (Figures 3 and 4).[25,27]

Table 1. The pharmacokinetic properties of montelukast.[18–21]

Pharmacokinetic parameter	
Oral bioavailability (%)	64
t_{max} (hours)	3–4
C_{max} (mg/L)	0.6
C_{min} (mg/L)	0.02
Plasma protein binding (%)	>99
Steady-state volume of distribution (L)	8–11
$t_{1/2}$ (hours)	2.7–5.5
Plasma clearance (mL/minute)	45.5
AUC (mg/L.h)	3.98

AUC, area under the concentration-time curve; t_{max}, time to reach maximum drug plasma concentration; C_{max}, peak plasma concentration; $t_{1/2}$, elimination half life.

Table 2. Summary of placebo-controlled clinical trials of montelukast.[22–27]

Study	Asthma severity	Montelukast dose	Concomitant therapy[a]	Treatment outcomes
Altman *et al.*[22] 6-week Double-blind Multicentre n=343	FEV_1 40–80% of predicted value with a 15% improvement after β_2-agonist therapy	10, 100, 200 mg, once daily *or* 10 or 50 mg, twice daily		Improvement in FEV_1 at all doses, asthma-specific quality of life scores were all significantly improved ($p<0.05$)
Noonan *et al.*[23] 3-week Double-blind Multicentre n=281	FEV_1 40–80% of predicted value with a 15% improvement after β_2-agonist therapy	2, 10, 50 mg, once daily	20% of patients used inhaled corticosteroids	Improvement in FEV_1 (7.1% change from baseline), reduced daily β_2-agonist use, daytime symptoms and nocturnal awakening; 10 and 50 mg doses superior to 2 mg
Reiss *et al.*[24] 12-week Double-blind Multicentre n=681	FEV_1 50–85% of predicted value with a 15% improvement after β_2-agonist therapy	10 mg, once daily	23% of patients used inhaled corticosteroids	Improvement FEV_1, reduced daily β_2-agonist use, daytime symptoms and nocturnal awakenings ($p<0.001$)
Malmstrom *et al.*[25] 12-week Double-blind Parallel-group n=895	FEV_1 50–85% of predicted value	10 mg, once daily	Separate group received inhaled beclometasone (200 µg, twice daily)	Both drugs superior to placebo; change in FEV_1 superior with beclometasone (13.1 *vs* 7.4%; $p<0.01$); overall comparable
Pizzichini *et al.*[26] 4-week Double-blind n=40	>5% sputum eosinophils, FEV_1 >65% of predicted value	10 mg, once daily		Montelukast reduced blood eosinophils ($p=0.009$), asthma symptoms ($p=0.001$), β_2-agonist use ($p<0.001$) and increased morning PEF ($p=0.001$)
Baumgartner *et al.*[27] 6-week Double-blind Parallel-group n=730	FEV_1 50–85% of predicted value with a 15% improvement after β_2-agonist therapy	10 mg, once daily	Separate group received inhaled beclometasone (200 µg, twice daily)	Both drugs superior to placebo; no differences between montelukast and beclometasone in terms of FEV_1 or adverse events

[a]In all studies, patients took short-acting β_2-agonists as needed.

FEV_1, forced expiratory volume in 1 second; PEF, peak expiratory flow.

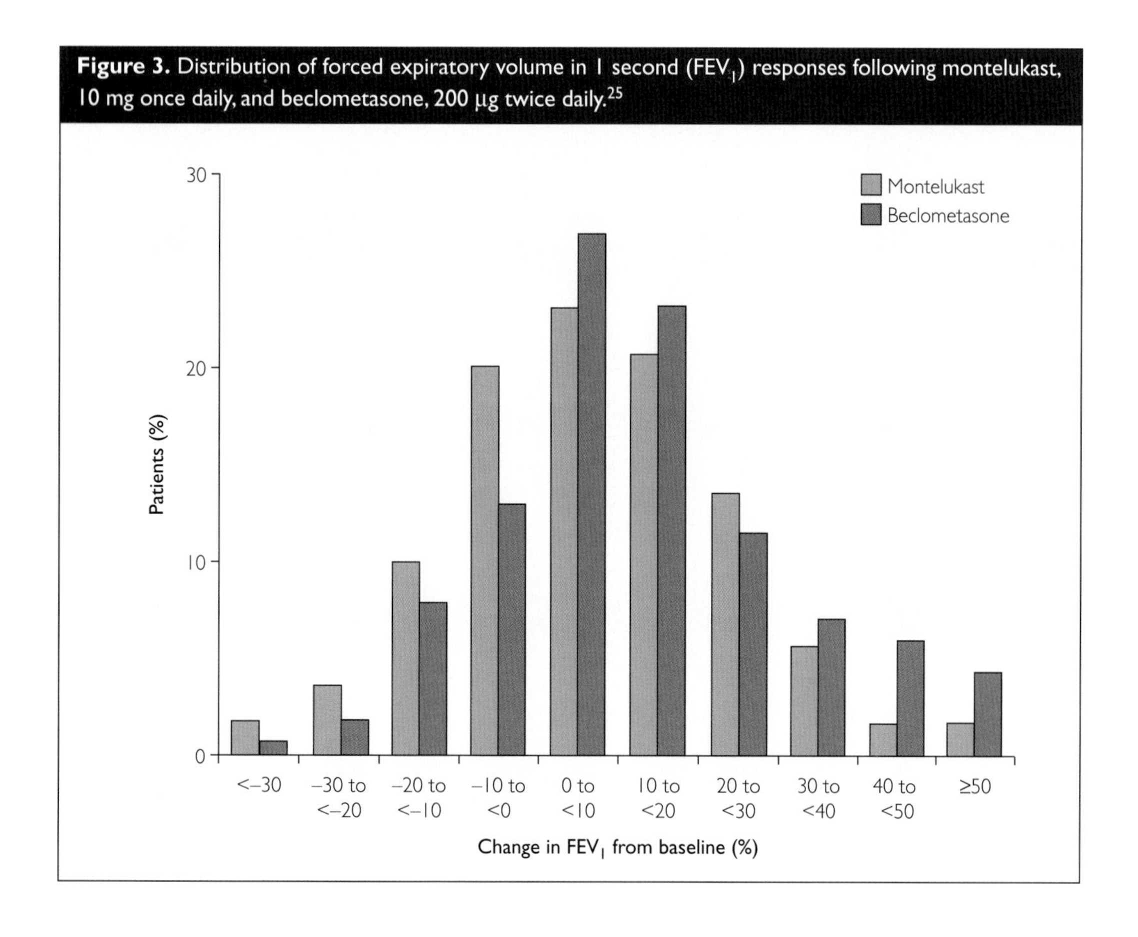

Figure 3. Distribution of forced expiratory volume in 1 second (FEV_1) responses following montelukast, 10 mg once daily, and beclometasone, 200 µg twice daily.[25]

Comparative clinical trials

In a substantial proportion of patients with moderate asthma, low-to-moderate doses of inhaled corticosteroids fail to provide adequate symptom control, possibly because of their inability to prevent the leukotriene-mediated aspects of the inflammatory response. As a leukotriene receptor antagonist, montelukast may prove beneficial by providing additional symptomatic relief whilst avoiding the need to increase the dosage of corticosteroid and the side-effects associated with this.[29,30] Controlled clinical trials that have compared the effects of adding montelukast to an existing corticosteroid treatment regimen are summarised in Table 3. In general, montelukast is inferior to inhaled corticosteroids in the treatment of moderate asthma yet comparable with long-acting β_2-agonists when given in combination with inhaled corticosteroids, in terms of clinical parameters of asthma control.[31,32] In contrast, montelukast appears to be more effective than the long-acting β_2-agonists with respect to anti-inflammatory properties.[33,34]

Montelukast may prove beneficial by providing additional symptomatic relief whilst avoiding the need to increase the dosage of corticosteroid and the side-effects associated with this.

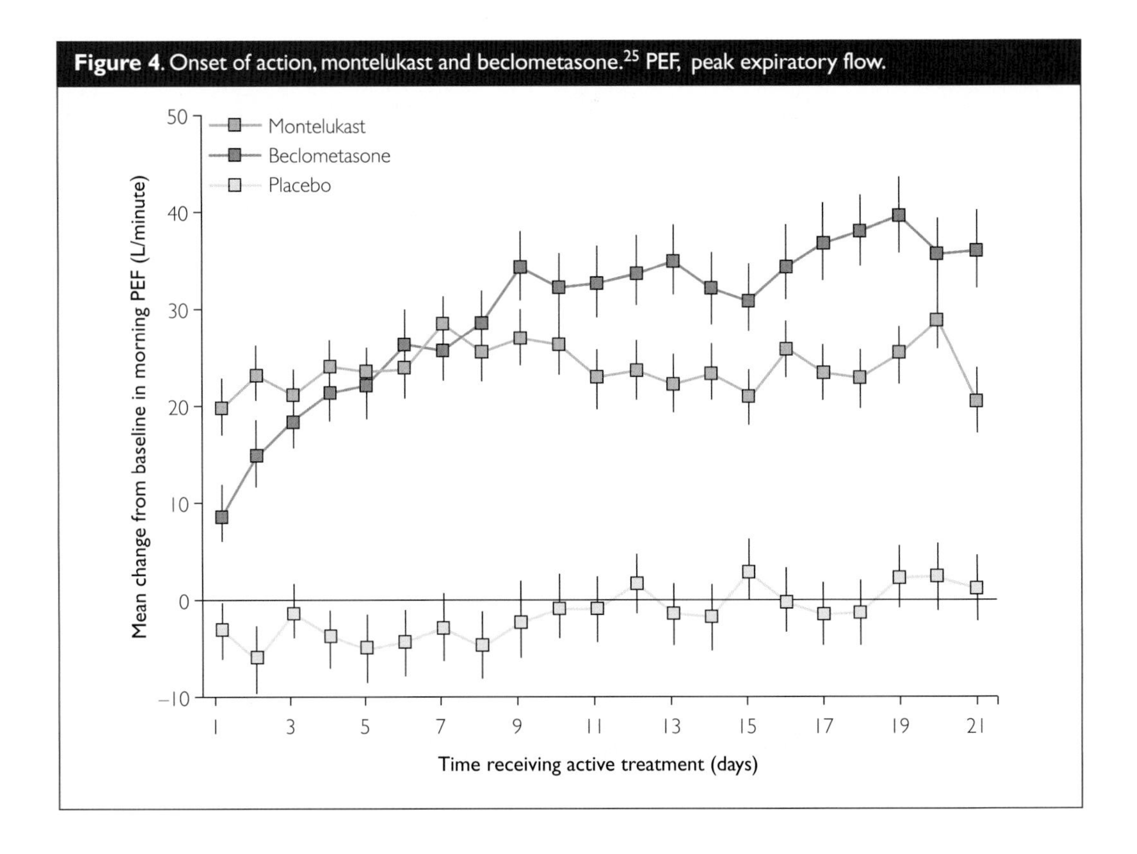

Figure 4. Onset of action, montelukast and beclometasone.[25] PEF, peak expiratory flow.

Montelukast *vs* fluticasone propionate

When montelukast was compared directly with fluticasone propionate, the steroidal treatment provided a superior level of asthma control to that elicited by montelukast alone, as determined by two large-scale trials in patients with persistent asthma with FEV_1 values of 50–80% of the predicted normal value.[31,32] In the first of these trials, 533 patients who remained symptomatic on short-acting β_2-agonists received either montelukast (10 mg once daily) or fluticasone propionate (88 µg, twice daily) for a period of 24 weeks.[31] Fluticasone elicited greater improvements across a range of lung function measurements compared with montelukast. The improvement in morning FEV_1 was 22.9% in the fluticasone group *vs* 14.5% in those patients receiving montelukast ($p<0.001$). Following a similar trend, morning peak expiratory flow (PEF) following fluticasone treatment was 68.5 L/minute compared with 34.1 L/minute following montelukast, decreasing in the evening to 53.9 L/minute and 28.7 L/minute, respectively ($p<0.001$ for both measurements). This superiority was also reflected in the number of night-time awakenings, asthma-free days and asthma symptom scores. The adverse event and asthma exacerbation profiles were similar for the two drugs.[31]

The second study, conducted in 522 patients under an identical treatment regimen, produced a similar pattern of results, with lung

Table 3. A summary of clinical trials comparing montelukast, 10 mg once daily, with corticosteroids and long-acting β-agonists in the treatment of persistent moderate asthma.[30–34]

Study	n	Main outcomes
Montelukast *vs* fluticasone propionate (88 μg, twice daily), 24 weeks[31]	533	• Morning % FEV_1 22.9% following fluticasone *vs* 14.5% following montelukast (p<0.001) • Morning PEF 68.5 L/minute following fluticasone *vs* 34.1 L/minute following montelukast (p<0.001) • Evening PEF 53.9 L/minute following fluticasone *vs* 28.7 L/minute following montelukast (p<0.001) • Symptom-free days 32.0% following fluticasone *vs* 18.4% following montelukast (p<0.001)
Montelukast *vs* fluticasone propionate (88 μg, twice daily), 24 weeks[32]	522	• Morning % FEV_1 22.0% following fluticasone *vs* 14.0% following montelukast (p<0.001) • Morning PEF 63.7 L/minute following fluticasone *vs* 37.6 L/minute following montelukast (p<0.001) • Evening PEF 52.7 L/minute following fluticasone *vs* 27.2 L/minute following montelukast (p<0.001) • Symptom-free days 34.3% following fluticasone *vs* 20.2% following montelukast (p<0.001)
Montelukast plus budesonide (800 μg, once daily) *vs* budesonide (1600 μg, once daily), 16 weeks[30]	889	• Morning PEF days 1–3: 20.1 L/minute following montelukast+budesonide *vs* 9.6 L/minute following budesonide (p<0.001) • Morning PEF last 10 weeks; 33.5 L/minute following montelukast+ budesonide *vs* 30.1 L/minute (NS) • Asthma-free days 86.7% following budesonide *vs* 82.2% following montelukast (NS) • Peripheral blood eosinophil count decrease 0.05×10^9 following budesonide *vs* 0.07×10^9 following montelukast (NS)
Montelukast plus fluticasone propionate (100 μg, twice daily) *vs* salmeterol (50 μg, twice daily) plus fluticasone propionate (100 μg, twice daily), 52 weeks[34]	1490	• % reversibility FEV_1 –11.26 following salmeterol/fluticasone *vs* –7.54 following montelukast/fluticasone (p<0.001) • Morning PEF 34.6 L/minute following salmeterol/fluticasone *vs* 17.7 L/minute following montelukast/fluticasone (p<0.001) • Peripheral blood eosinophil counts reduced from baseline following montelukast/fluticasone but not salmeterol/fluticasone (p<0.001)
Montelukast *vs* salmeterol (50 μg, twice daily) (concomitant corticosteroids in both groups), 12 weeks[33]	948	• Morning PEF 35.0 L/minute following salmeterol *vs* 21.7 L/minute following montelukast (p<0.001) • Symptom-free days 24% following salmeterol *vs* 16% following montelukast (p<0.001) • Rescue-free days 27% following salmeterol *vs* 20% following montelukast (p=0.002)

FEV_1, forced expiratory volume in 1 second; PEF, peak expiratory flow; NS, non-significant.

function, asthma symptom scores, asthma-free days and concomitant β_2-agonist use all significantly improved following fluticasone compared with montelukast (p=0.002 for each comparison). Additionally, patient and physician satisfaction scores were markedly higher in the fluticasone group, with 83% of patients satisfied with their treatment compared with 66% of those patients treated with montelukast (p<0.001). Again, the incidence of asthma exacerbations was similar for each treatment group.[32]

The mean percentage FEV_1 change from baseline following 156 weeks of treatment was comparable between patients receiving montelukast and those receiving beclometasone.

As a more realistic means of assessing the effectiveness of chronic asthma therapy, the long-term use of montelukast, in both adults and children, has been compared with an inhaled corticosteroid in extended controlled settings.[35,36] In a double-blind study of montelukast *vs* beclometasone in adults (n=436), the effects of both drugs were maintained over a 1-year period of continuous therapy.[35] In a second open-label study (n=374) that, for this reason, was perhaps more representative of the real-life clinical situation, the mean percentage FEV_1 change from baseline following 156 weeks of treatment was comparable between patients receiving montelukast and those receiving beclometasone, indicating that long-term treatment adherence issues were not significant with either drug.[35] In children, montelukast has been associated with improved compliance compared with beclometasone over a 6 month period, with 82 *vs* 45% of patients rated highly compliant.[36]

Montelukast *vs* budesonide

Montelukast given as add-on therapy to an inhaled corticosteroid regimen significantly improved asthma control.

The CASIOPEA study group investigated the effect of adding montelukast to a fixed dose of the inhaled corticosteroid, budesonide.[30] Over a 16-week period, patients (n=639) with a baseline FEV_1 of at least 55% of the predicted value and a minimum total daytime asthma score, received either montelukast (10 mg daily) or placebo, in addition to a constant dose of budesonide (400–1600 µg/day). Compared with placebo, montelukast treatment was associated with 35% fewer exacerbations (p=0.03) more asthma-free days (56%; p<0.001), less nocturnal awakening and improved daily β_2-agonist use. Thus, montelukast given as add-on therapy to an inhaled corticosteroid regimen significantly improved asthma control.

In the first study of its kind, the Clinical Outcomes with Montelukast as a Partner Agent to Corticosteroid Therapy (COMPACT) study group compared the effects of adding montelukast to an inhaled corticosteroid regimen that involved doubling the dose of corticosteroid.[29] Patients with asthma that was inadequately controlled on inhaled budesonide received either montelukast (10 mg daily) plus budesonide (800 µg daily) or budesonide (1600 µg daily) for a period of 16 weeks. Overall, the level of asthma control achieved was similar in both treatment groups compared with baseline. Morning PEF was increased to 33.5 L/minute in the montelukast/budesonide group compared with 30.1 L/minute in the double-dose budesonide group. Similar improvements were also observed between treatment groups in terms of β_2-agonist use, daytime symptom scores, nocturnal awakenings, exacerbations and asthma-free days. These data demonstrate that montelukast represents an equally effective alternative to doubling the dose of inhaled corticosteroid.[29]

Montelukast represents an equally effective alternative to doubling the dose of inhaled corticosteroid.

Montelukast *vs* salmeterol

Long-acting β_2-agonists are generally considered to be second-line agents for asthma control and are commonly used as an adjunct to an inhaled corticosteroid regimen. In a large-scale (n=1490) year-long study conducted by the Investigation of Montelukast as a Partner Agent for Complementary Therapy (IMPACT) group, either montelukast (10 mg daily) or salmeterol (50 μg twice daily) was added to an existing inhaled fluticasone propionate regimen (100 μg twice daily) in patients experiencing inadequate asthma control on corticosteroid therapy alone.[34] The montelukast/fluticasone combination was comparable with the salmeterol/fluticasone combination in terms of asthma exacerbations, nocturnal awakenings and asthma-specific quality of life. The salmeterol/fluticasone combination was more effective in terms of FEV_1 and morning PEF (p<0.001) whereas montelukast/fluticasone significantly reduced peripheral blood eosinophil counts (p<0.001).[34]

These findings echo those of an earlier trial in patients with persistent asthma (n=948) who remained symptomatic on inhaled corticosteroids.[33] Montelukast (10 mg once daily) was compared with salmeterol (50 μg twice daily) in patients receiving concomitant inhaled corticosteroid therapy. Again, salmeterol elicited significantly greater improvements in the majority of lung function measurements, including morning PEF (35.0 *vs* 21.7 L/minute; p<0.001), symptom-free days (24 *vs* 16%; p<0.001), therapy-free days (p=0.002) and nocturnal awakenings (p=0.015). Patient opinion also favoured salmeterol over montelukast.[33] In a smaller trial, montelukast, and not salmeterol, produced significant effects on adenosine monophosphate bronchial challenge and blood eosinophil levels, indicative of anti-inflammatory activity.[37]

The efficacies of once-daily montelukast and twice-daily salmeterol were compared in a 1-year, double-blind study of 1473 adult patients with moderate-to-severe persistent asthma that was uncontrolled on low-dose inhaled corticosteroids.[38] Following a 4-week run-in period, during which time all patients received fluticasone propionate, 220 μg/day, participants were randomised to receive either montelukast, 10 mg, or salmeterol, 84 μg, as add-on therapy to the continuing fluticasone regimen, over the remaining 48 weeks of the study. At baseline, FEV_1 was 74.3% of the predicted normal value. The percentages of patients discontinuing treatment prematurely were 17 and 15% for montelukast and salmeterol treatment groups, respectively (p-value not reported). Overall, 80% of montelukast- and 83.3% of salmeterol-treated patients remained free from asthma attacks during 48 weeks of treatment (ratio of montelukast to salmeterol: 1.20), although the study was inconclusive with regard to a difference between treatment groups. Although

Overall, 80% of montelukast- and 83.3% of salmeterol-treated patients remained free from asthma attacks during 48 weeks of treatment.

montelukast significantly reduced blood eosinophil counts compared with salmeterol (difference of –0.04 x $10^3/\mu L$; *p*-value not reported), salmeterol was associated with superior improvements in pre-bronchodilator FEV_1 (difference of –1.98%), asthma-specific quality of life (difference of –0.12), morning PEF (difference of –14.3 L/minute) and nocturnal awakenings (difference of 0.23 nights/week), compared with montelukast.

Paediatric clinical trials

In view of its favourable side-effect profile and oral route of administration, montelukast is particularly useful in children as an alternative to increasing the dosage of corticosteroid.

When treating children, it is particularly important that drug therapy is effective, well tolerated and easily administered. Long-term asthma treatment has prompted parental concern as to the safety of prolonged exposure to any one drug, with particular emphasis on the complications associated with the long-term use of corticosteroids. There is evidence that growth may be impaired in pre-pubertal children receiving steroidal treatment for asthma and so it is prudent to minimise this risk by adding non-steroidal medication to the inhaled corticosteroid regimen where possible, thus allowing the steroid dose to be gradually tapered.[39–41] In view of its favourable side-effect profile and oral route of administration, montelukast is particularly useful in children as an alternative to increasing the dosage of corticosteroid.

Generally, the use of montelukast in children has significant benefits in asthma management compared with placebo. In an 8-week trial conducted in 336 children aged 6–14 years, the daily administration of montelukast, 5 mg, in the form of a chewable tablet, elicited a significant improvement in FEV_1 compared with placebo (8.23 *vs* 3.58% increase from baseline, respectively; $p<0.001$).[42] Approximately 35% of patients were also receiving inhaled corticosteroids and using a β_2-agonist daily.[42] In a similar patient population (n=279; mean age 10 years), the same daily dosage of montelukast was administered as add-on therapy to an existing treatment regimen of the inhaled corticosteroid, budesonide. Montelukast significantly improved asthma control, manifested as an increase in lung function ($p<0.05$) and a decrease in asthma exacerbation days ($p<0.001$), a finding echoed in a smaller study which also examined montelukast as add-on therapy to an existing corticosteroid regimen.[43,44] The number of rescue-free days in which no β_2-agonist or oral corticosteroid intervention was necessary, was markedly reduced in the latter study, and montelukast was associated with a 17% decrease in inhaled corticosteroid dose, compared with a 64% increase in steroid use with placebo. This further demonstrates the steroid-sparing potential of concomitant montelukast administration.[44] One study has directly compared the effects of montelukast (5 mg once daily) with the inhaled corticosteroid, beclometasone.[35] Children aged 6–14 years (n=245) were selected on the basis of an FEV_1 of 50–85% of the predicted value that showed a 15% improvement following administration of a short-acting β_2-agonist. Montelukast was as effective as beclometasone in controlling mild-to-moderate chronic asthma, with both drugs eliciting improvement in multiple parameters of asthma control.[35]

Patient adherence to, and parental preference for, regimens of montelukast and inhaled sodium cromoglicate were compared in a group of 333 children aged between 6 and 11 years in an open-label, cross-over, 12-week study.[45] Children were selected for study entry on the basis of a FEV_1 of 60–85% of the predicted normal value, with reversibility of over 12%. After a 2–3-week run-in period, patients were randomised to receive either 4 weeks of treatment with montelukast (5 mg chewable tablet, once daily) or 4 weeks of inhaled sodium cromoglicate (two puffs, four-times daily from a metered dose inhaler). Following a 2-week wash-out period, treatments were switched. Overall, significantly more patients preferred treatment with montelukast than sodium cromoglicate (82 *vs* 17%, respectively; $p<0.001$), a trend echoed in the parental preference scores (78 *vs* 12%, respectively; $p<0.001$). Seventy-eight per cent of montelukast-treated patients were highly adherent to therapy, compared with 42% of patients receiving sodium cromoglicate ($p<0.001$). The rate of treatment discontinuation was lower amongst patients receiving montelukast compared with sodium cromoglicate (1.0 *vs* 5.0%, respectively; *p*-value not reported). Furthermore, the mean daily use of salbutamol was reduced significantly following montelukast compared with sodium cromoglicate (1.56 *vs* 1.92 puffs/day, respectively; $p=0.003$).[43]

Overall, significantly more patients preferred treatment with montelukast than sodium cromoglicate, a trend echoed in the parental preference scores.

Administration and tolerability issues are particularly pertinent in pre-school children for whom compliance with a drug regimen may prove difficult. In a study examining the effect of montelukast in children aged 2–5 years with persistent asthma (n=689), montelukast (4 mg chewable tablet, once daily) produced significant improvements over placebo in many aspects of asthma control, including asthma symptoms, asthma-free days, nocturnal awakening and concomitant β_2-agonist use.[46] This further emphasises the applicability of montelukast for the treatment of asthma in children.

Exercise-induced bronchoconstriction

EIB is common in patients with chronic asthma, with 80–90% of patients affected.[47] EIB is characterised by post-exercise airways obstruction, resulting in reductions in FEV_1 of greater than 10% compared with pre-exercise values. The cooling and drying of airways as a result of exercise may trigger activation of mast cells and the release of inflammatory mediators such as histamine and leukotrienes, which ultimately lead to bronchoconstriction and airway obstruction. Urinary levels of LTE_4 (the stable metabolite of LTC_4 and LTD_4) are elevated after exercise challenge in patients with asthma.[48] Montelukast has been shown to be protective against EIB.[48–50]

In a study of 110 adults with asthma, selected on the basis of a decrease in FEV_1 of at least 20% following exercise, montelukast (10 mg once daily) provided significant protection against EIB over a 12-week period, compared with placebo.[51] Such protection was dose related and was apparent at doses ranging from 0.4 to 50 mg.[49] In two large studies comparing the bronchoprotective effect of montelukast (10 mg once daily) with that of the long-acting β_2-agonist, salmeterol (50 μg twice daily), montelukast provided superior protection against EIB.[52,53] At Week 8, the percentage inhibition in the maximal percentage decrease in FEV_1 was 57.2% in the montelukast group and 33.0% in the salmeterol group (p=0.002). Whilst the control offered by salmeterol exhibited periodic fluctuations at 4 and 8 weeks, the bronchoprotective effect of montelukast was maintained for 8 weeks with no sign of tolerance (Figure 5).[53]

The prevention and relief of EIB is particularly pertinent in children, for whom physical activity represents an important part of everyday life. The daily use of a 5 mg chewable montelukast tablet was superior to placebo in terms of preventing EIB in children aged 6–14 years.[50] In an exercise challenge study in which children (aged 7–13 years; n=19) completed a treadmill task after a single dose of montelukast, the maximal protective effect was reached 12 hours after dosing, highlighting the prolonged nature of the protection afforded.[54] In a similar patient population, montelukast attenuated the immediate asthma response, and was associated with a lower mean maximum decrease in FEV_1 compared with placebo (17.3 *vs* 35.1%; p<0.05). Furthermore, the late response induced by exercise challenge was completely abolished with montelukast.[55]

Aspirin-induced asthma

The exacerbation of asthma by aspirin and other non-steroidal anti-inflammatory drugs is termed aspirin-induced asthma and affects 3–5% of the patient population.[56] Commonly in these patients, asthma is inadequately controlled by conventional treatments.[57] The cysteinyl leukotrienes appear to be the principal mediators of aspirin-induced asthma, with baseline levels in urine and exhaled air being significantly elevated in patients with the condition.[58,59] Thus, a leukotriene receptor antagonist may be an ideally suited therapy in this setting.

In a placebo-controlled clinical trial, 80 patients with aspirin-induced asthma received montelukast, 10 mg, or placebo for a period of 4 weeks.[60] Ninety per cent of patients were undergoing concomitant corticosteroid treatment at moderate-to-high doses. FEV_1 and PEF measurements showed marked improvement following montelukast treatment compared with placebo, the mean differences between treatment groups being 10.2% for FEV_1 and 28.0 L/minute for morning PEF (p<0.001 for both measurements). Asthma symptoms, nocturnal awakening and patients' quality of life were also improved following montelukast (p<0.05). Such findings merit the use of montelukast as a means of achieving additional control of asthma in this aspirin-intolerant subgroup.

You are strongly urged to consult your doctor before taking, stopping or changing any of the products reviewed or referred to in *BESTMEDICINE* or any other medication that has been prescribed or recommended by your doctor.

Safety and tolerability

Generally, the overwhelming evidence derived from controlled clinical trials indicates that the majority of adverse events observed following treatment with montelukast are mild and self-limiting (Table 4).[61] Headache was one of the most frequently reported complaints, yet the incidence following montelukast was not strikingly different to that

Figure 5. Forced expiratory volume in 1 second (FEV_1) after exercise in patients receiving montelukast (top) and salmeterol (bottom).[53]

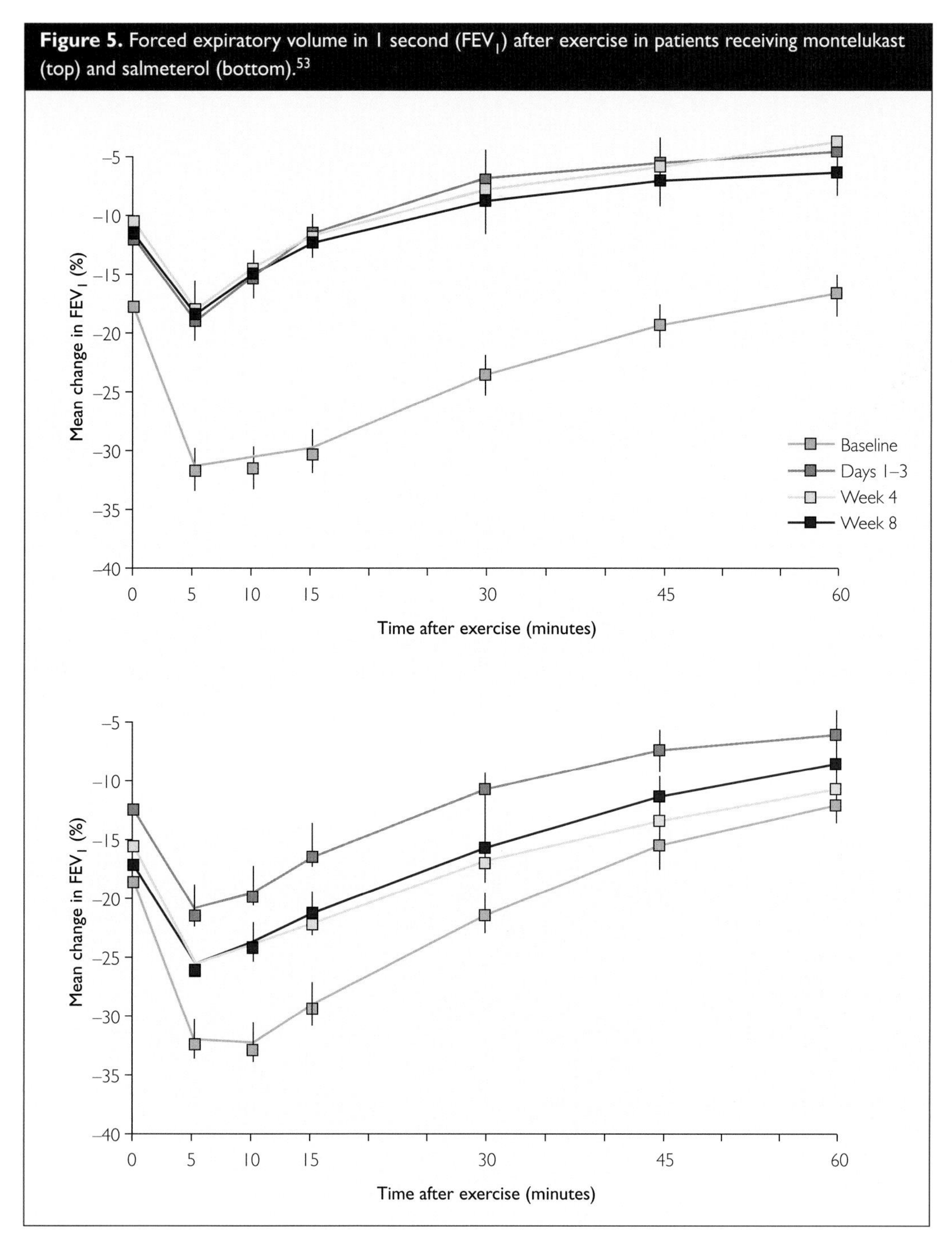

reported in patients receiving placebo.[61] Post-marketing surveillance, conducted across millions of patients worldwide, is consistent with this favourable tolerability profile.[18,19]

Drug interactions associated with montelukast are minimal with no clinically relevant interactions observed with warfarin, digoxin,

Table 4. Most common clinical adverse events, regardless of causality, among adults enrolled in ten phase 2b/3 studies with montelukast.[61] Data are percentage of patients affected.

Adverse event	Placebo (n=1180)	Montelukast (n=1955)	Beclometasone (n=251)
Total patients with >1 adverse event	71.3	66.5	63.7
Upper respiratory infection	24.6	21.5	13.1
Headache	18.1	18.4	18.7
Pharyngitis	7.0	5.4	6.4
Sinusitis	4.3	4.0	2.4
Diarrhoea	3.1	3.1	2.0
Bronchitis	3.6	2.4	2.8
Abdominal pain	2.5	2.9	3.2
Nausea	3.0	2.6	2.0
Rhinitis	1.4	0.8	4.0

terfenadine, fexofenadine, oral contraceptives, theophylline or prednisolone.[18,19] In view of the metabolic pathway of montelukast, clinical monitoring should be employed when co-administering with CYP enzyme inducers such as phenobarbital and rifampin.[18,19]

Churg–Strauss syndrome

The Churg–Strauss syndrome is a rare form of eosinophilic vasculitis that has been, albeit rarely, associated with the use of leukotriene receptor antagonists when used as asthma therapy. Following extensive investigation, it seems likely that Churg–Strauss syndrome can occur after administration of leukotriene receptor antagonists as a result of the emergence of an underlying disease state previously masked by corticosteroid therapy and not as a direct result of the leukotriene antagonist. Symptoms emerge when corticosteroid doses are tapered because of the efficacy of anti-leukotriene therapy.[62–64] Although this pattern is evident in the majority of cases, one case has been reported in the absence of corticosteroid withdrawal and so it is recommended that physicians remain alert to signs of eosinophilia, vasculitic rash, worsening pulmonary symptoms and cardiac complications.[65]

Pharmacoeconomics

Although limited in number, isolated studies have examined the cost-effectiveness of treatment with montelukast as monotherapy compared with the corticosteroid, fluticasone propionate, and/or the long-acting β_2-agonist, salmeterol, as maintenance therapy for mild persistent asthma. The fluticasone/salmeterol combination was found to be a more successful treatment option in terms of the improvement in FEV_1 and symptom-free days achieved. Additionally, the mean daily costs per successfully treated patient were lower in the fluticasone/salmeterol group.[66] This finding has been echoed by similar studies that have analysed the hospitalisation data and pharmacy costs of asthma treatment.[67,68] One study, however, found no significant differences in asthma-related healthcare expenditures between the two therapy options and cited improved patient adherence with montelukast.[69] In a study of a UK primary care database, the chronic use of montelukast was associated with reduced concomitant drug therapy requirements (inhaled corticosteroids, short-acting β_2-agonists and antibiotics) ultimately leading to a reduction in the total cost of asthma therapies ($p<0.05$).[70]

Key points

- Montelukast is a leukotriene receptor antagonist indicated as add-on therapy for the control of moderate-to-severe asthma rather than the immediate relief of asthma symptoms.
- Montelukast acts on the $cysLT_1$ receptor to block the inflammatory and bronchoconstrictive effects of leukotrienes.
- An extremely potent and highly selective LTD_4 receptor antagonist *in vitro*, montelukast is also pharmacologically active in a range of animal models of pulmonary inflammation.
- In clinical trials, montelukast elicited improvement in at least one aspect of asthma management compared with placebo in the treatment of mild asthma. Generally well-tolerated, the beneficial effects of montelukast were maintained for the duration of drug treatment.
- In comparative trials conducted in patients with asthma of moderate severity, montelukast was generally not as effective as inhaled corticosteroids. As add-on therapy to an existing corticosteroid regimen, montelukast exhibited an additive effect that was comparable to interaction with adjunctive long-acting β_2-agonist.
- In children, treatment with montelukast permits the gradual tapering of corticosteroids and thus minimises steroid-associated systemic adverse events.
- Patients with EIB showed greater improvement following montelukast than with the long-acting β_2-agonist, salmeterol.
- Considering the involvement of leukotrienes in aspirin-induced asthma, montelukast may represent an ideal treatment option in these patients, with trials to date indicating a significant improvement following treatment.
- Montelukast encourages patient concordance as a result of its rapid onset of action (with effects observed hours after initial administration), a tolerable side-effect profile and oral route of administration.

References

A list of the published evidence which has been reviewed in compiling the preceding section of *BESTMEDICINE.*

1 Jarvis B, Markham A. Montelukast: a review of its therapeutic potential in persistent asthma. *Drugs* 2000; **59**: 891–928.

2 Lipworth B. Airway and systemic effects of inhaled corticosteroids in asthma: dose response relationship. *Pulm Pharmacol* 1996; **9**: 19–27.

3 Drazen J, Austen K. Leukotrienes and airway responses. *Am Rev Respir Dis* 1987; **136**: 985–98.

4 Henderson WJ. The role of leukotrienes in inflammation. *Ann Intern Med* 1994; **121**: 684–97.

5 Samuelsson B, Dahlen S, Lindgren J, Rouzer C, Serhan C. Leukotrienes and lipoxins: structures, biosynthesis, and biological effects. *Science* 1987; **237**: 1171–6.

6 Barnes N, Kuitert L. Drugs affecting the leukotriene pathway in asthma. *Br J Clin Pract* 1995; **49**: 262–6.

7 Holgate S, Bradding P, Sampson A. Leukotriene antagonists and synthesis inhibitors: new directions in asthma therapy. *J Allergy Clin Immunol* 1996; **98**: 1–13.

8 Holgate S, Sampson A. Antileukotriene therapy. Future directions. *Am J Respir Crit Care Med* 2000; **161**: S147–53.

9 Barnes N, Costello J. Mast-cell-derived mediators in asthma. Arachidonic acid metabolites. *Postgrad Med* 1984; **76**: 148–51.

10 Lynch K, O'Neill G, Liu Q *et al.* Characterization of the human cysteinyl leukotriene CysLT1 receptor. *Nature* 1999; **399**: 789–93.

11 Coleman R, Eglen R, Jones R *et al.* Prostanoid and leukotriene receptors: a progress report from the IUPHAR working parties on classification and nomenclature. *Adv Prostaglandin Thromboxane Leukot Res* 1995; **23**: 283–5.

12 Drazen J. Asthma therapy with agents preventing leukotriene synthesis or action. *Proc Assoc Am Physicians* 1999; **111**: 547–59.

13 Lipworth B. Leukotriene-receptor antagonists. *Lancet* 1999; **353**: 57–62.

14 Aharony D. Pharmacology of leukotriene receptor antagonists. *Am J Respir Crit Care Med* 1998; **157**: S214–19.

15 Jones T, Labelle M, Belley M *et al.* Pharmacology of montelukast sodium (Singulair), a potent and selective leukotriene D4 receptor antagonist. *Can J Physiol Pharmacol* 1995; **73**: 191–201.

16 Krell R, Aharony D, Buckner C *et al.* The preclinical pharmacology of ICI 204,219. A peptide leukotriene antagonist. *Am Rev Respir Dis* 1990; **141**: 978–87.

17 Ihaku D, Cameron L, Suzuki M, Molet S, Martin J, Hamid Q. Montelukast, a leukotriene receptor antagonist, inhibits the late airway response to antigen, airway eosinophilia, and IL-5-expressing cells in Brown Norway rats. *J Allergy Clin Immunol* 1999; **104**: 1147–54.

18 Merck Sharp and Dohme. Singulair® 10 mg tablets/ 4 and 5 mg paediatric tablets. *Summary of product characteristics.* Hoddesdon, Hertfordshire, 2004.

19 Merck Sharp and Dohme Limited. Singulair paediatric 4 mg granules. *Summary of product characteristics.* Hoddesdon, Hertfordshire, 2004.

20 Schoors D, De Smet M, Reiss T et al. Single dose pharmacokinetics, safety and tolerability of MK-0476, a new leukotriene D4-receptor antagonist, in healthy volunteers. *Br J Clin Pharmacol* 1995; **40**: 277–80.

21 Zhao J, Rogers J, Holland S *et al.* Pharmacokinetics and bioavailability of montelukast sodium (MK-0476) in healthy young and elderly volunteers. *Biopharm Drug Dispos* 1997; **18**: 769–77.

22 Altman L, Munk Z, Seltzer J *et al.* A placebo-controlled, dose-ranging study of montelukast, a cysteinyl leukotriene-receptor antagonist. Montelukast Asthma Study Group. *J Allergy Clin Immunol* 1998; **102**: 50–6.

23 Noonan M, Chervinsky P, Brandon M *et al.* Montelukast, a potent leukotriene receptor antagonist, causes dose-related improvements in chronic asthma. Montelukast Asthma Study Group. *Eur Respir J* 1998; **11**: 1232–9.

24 Reiss T, Chervinsky P, Dockhorn R, Shingo S, Seidenberg B, Edwards T. Montelukast, a once-daily leukotriene receptor antagonist, in the treatment of chronic asthma: a multicenter, randomized, double-blind trial. Montelukast Clinical Research Study Group. *Arch Intern Med* 1998; **158**: 1213–20.

25 Malmstrom K, Rodriguez-Gomez G, Guerra J *et al.* Oral montelukast, inhaled beclometasone, and placebo for chronic asthma. A randomized, controlled trial. Montelukast/Beclometasone Study Group. *Ann Intern Med* 1999; **130**: 487–95.

26 Pizzichini E, Leff J, Reiss T *et al.* Montelukast reduces airway eosinophilic inflammation in asthma: a randomized, controlled trial. *Eur Respir J* 1999; **14**: 12–18.

27 Baumgartner R, Martinez G, Edelman J *et al.* Distribution of therapeutic response in asthma control between oral montelukast and inhaled beclometasone. *Eur Respir J* 2003; **21**: 123–8.

28 Barnes N, Wei L, Reiss T *et al.* Analysis of montelukast in mild persistent asthmatic patients with near-normal lung function. *Respir Med* 2001; **95**: 379–86.

29 Price D, Hernandez D, Magyar P *et al.* Randomised controlled trial of montelukast plus inhaled budesonide versus double dose inhaled budesonide in adult patients with asthma. *Thorax* 2003; **58**: 211–16.

30 Vaquerizo M, Casan P, Castillo J *et al.* Effect of montelukast added to inhaled budesonide on control of mild to moderate asthma. *Thorax* 2003; **58**: 204–11.

31 Busse W, Raphael G, Galant S *et al.* Low-dose fluticasone propionate compared with montelukast for first-line treatment of persistent asthma: a randomized clinical trial. *J Allergy Clin Immunol* 2001; **107**: 461–8.

32 Meltzer E, Lockey R, Friedman B *et al.* Efficacy and safety of low-dose fluticasone propionate compared with montelukast for maintenance treatment of persistent asthma. *Mayo Clin Proc* 2002; **77**: 437–45.

33 Fish J, Israel E, Murray J *et al.* Salmeterol powder provides significantly better benefit than montelukast in asthmatic patients receiving concomitant inhaled corticosteroid therapy. *Chest* 2001; **120**: 423–30.

34 Bjermer L, Bisgaard H, Bousquet J *et al.* Montelukast and fluticasone compared with salmeterol and fluticasone in protecting against asthma exacerbation in adults: one year, double blind, randomised, comparative trial. *BMJ* 2003; **327**: 891–7.

35 Williams B, Noonan G, Reiss T *et al.* Long-term asthma control with oral montelukast and inhaled beclometasone for adults and children 6 years and older. *Clin Exp Allergy* 2001; **31**: 845–54.

36 Maspero J, Duenas-Meza E, Volovitz B *et al.* Oral montelukast versus inhaled beclometasone in 6- to 11-year-old children with asthma: results of an open-label extension study evaluating long-term safety, satisfaction, and adherence with therapy. *Curr Med Res Opin* 2001; **17**: 94–104.

37 Wilson A, Dempsey O, Sims E, Lipworth B. Evaluation of salmeterol or montelukast as second-line therapy for asthma not controlled with inhaled corticosteroids. *Chest* 2001; **119**: 1021–6.

38 Ilowite J, Webb R, Friedman B *et al.* Addition of montelukast or salmeterol to fluticasone for protection against asthma attacks: a randomized, double-blind, multicenter study. *Ann Allergy Asthma Immunol* 2004; **92**: 641–8.

39 Crowley S, Trivedi P, Risteli L, Risteli J, Hindmarsh P, Brook C. Collagen metabolism and growth in prepubertal children with asthma treated with inhaled steroids. *J Pediatr* 1998; **132**: 409–13.

40 Russell G. Inhaled corticosteroid therapy in children: an assessment of the potential for side effects. *Thorax* 1994; **49**: 1185–8.

41 Russell G. Childhood asthma and growth – a review of the literature. *Respir Med* 1994; **88**: 31–6.

42 Knorr B, Matz J, Bernstein J *et al.* Montelukast for chronic asthma in 6- to 14-year-old children: a randomized, double-blind trial. Pediatric Montelukast Study Group. *JAMA* 1998; **279**: 1181–6.

43 Simons F, Villa J, Lee B *et al.* Montelukast added to budesonide in children with persistent asthma: a randomized, double-blind, crossover study. *J Pediatr* 2001; **138**: 694–8.

44 Phipatanakul W, Greene C, Downes S *et al.* Montelukast improves asthma control in asthmatic children maintained on inhaled corticosteroids. *Ann Allergy Asthma Immunol* 2003; **91**: 49–54.

45 Bukstein D, Bratton D, Firriolo K *et al.* Evaluation of parental preference for the treatment of asthmatic children aged 6 to 11 years with oral montelukast or inhaled cromolyn: a randomized, open-label, crossover study. *J Asthma* 2003; **40**: 475–85.

46 Knorr B, Franchi L, Bisgaard H *et al.* Montelukast, a leukotriene receptor antagonist, for the treatment of persistent asthma in children aged 2 to 5 years. *Pediatrics* 2001; **108**: E48.

47 Gotshall R. Exercise-induced bronchoconstriction. *Drugs* 2002; **62**: 1725–39.

48 Reiss T, Hill J, Harman E *et al.* Increased urinary excretion of LTE4 after exercise and attenuation of exercise-induced bronchospasm by montelukast, a cysteinyl leukotriene receptor antagonist. *Thorax* 1997; **52**: 1030–5.

49 Bronsky E, Kemp J, Zhang J, Guerreiro D, Reiss T. Dose-related protection of exercise bronchoconstriction by montelukast, a cysteinyl leukotriene-receptor antagonist, at the end of a once-daily dosing interval. *Clin Pharmacol Ther* 1997; **62**: 556–61.

50 Kemp J, Dockhorn R, Shapiro G *et al.* Montelukast once daily inhibits exercise-induced bronchoconstriction in 6- to 14-year-old children with asthma. *J Pediatr* 1998; **133**: 424–8.

51 Leff J, Busse W, Pearlman D *et al.* Montelukast, a leukotriene-receptor antagonist, for the treatment of mild asthma and exercise-induced bronchoconstriction. *N Engl J Med* 1998; **339**: 147–52.

52 Villaran C, O'Neill S, Helbling A *et al.* Montelukast versus salmeterol in patients with asthma and exercise-induced bronchoconstriction. Montelukast/Salmeterol Exercise Study Group. *J Allergy Clin Immunol* 1999; **104**: 547–53.

53 Edelman J, Turpin J, Bronsky E *et al.* Oral montelukast compared with inhaled salmeterol to prevent exercise-induced bronchoconstriction. A randomized, double-blind trial. Exercise Study Group. *Ann Intern Med* 2000; **132**: 97–104.

54 Peroni D, Piacentini G, Pietrobelli A *et al.* The combination of single-dose montelukast and loratadine on exercise-induced bronchospasm in children. *Eur Respir J* 2002; **20**: 104–7.

55 Melo R, Sole D, Naspitz C. Exercise-induced bronchoconstriction in children: montelukast attenuates the immediate-phase and late-phase responses. *J Allergy Clin Immunol* 2003; **111**: 301–7.

56 Szczeklik A, Stevenson D. Aspirin-induced asthma: advances in pathogenesis, diagnosis, and management. *J Allergy Clin Immunol* 2003; **111**: 913–21.

57 Szczeklik A, Stevenson D. Aspirin-induced asthma: advances in pathogenesis and management. *J Allergy Clin Immunol* 1999; **104**: 5–13.

58 Antczak A, Montuschi P, Kharitonov S, Gorski P, Barnes P. Increased exhaled cysteinyl-leukotrienes and 8-isoprostane in aspirin-induced asthma. *Am J Respir Crit Care Med* 2002; **166**: 301–6.

59 Daffern P, Muilenburg D, Hugli T, Stevenson D. Association of urinary leukotriene E4 excretion during aspirin challenges with severity of respiratory responses. *J Allergy Clin Immunol* 1999; **104**: 559–64.

60 Dahlen S, Malmstrom K, Nizankowska E *et al.* Improvement of aspirin-intolerant asthma by montelukast, a leukotriene antagonist: a randomized, double-blind, placebo-controlled trial. *Am J Respir Crit Care Med* 2002; **165**: 9–14.

61 Storms W, Michele T, Knorr B *et al.* Clinical safety and tolerability of montelukast, a leukotriene receptor antagonist, in controlled clinical trials in patients aged ≥ 6 years. *Clin Exp Allergy* 2001; **31**: 77–87.

62 Franco J, Artes M. Pulmonary eosinophilia associated with montelukast. *Thorax* 1999; **54**: 558–60.

63 Wechsler M, Pauwels R, Drazen J. Leukotriene modifiers and Churg–Strauss syndrome: adverse effect or response to corticosteroid withdrawal? *Drug Saf* 1999; **21**: 241–51.

64 Wechsler M, Finn D, Gunawardena D *et al.* Churg–Strauss syndrome in patients receiving montelukast as treatment for asthma. *Chest* 2000; **117**: 708–13.

65 Tuggey J, Hosker H. Churg–Strauss syndrome associated with montelukast therapy. *Thorax* 2000; **55**: 805–6.

66 Sheth K, Borker R, Emmett A, Rickard K, Dorinsky P. Cost-effectiveness comparison of salmeterol/fluticasone propionate versus montelukast in the treatment of adults with persistent asthma. *Pharmacoeconomics* 2002; **20**: 909–18.

67 Armstrong E, Malone D. Fluticasone is associated with lower asthma-related costs than leukotriene modifiers in a real-world analysis. *Pharmacotherapy* 2002; **22**: 1117–23.

68 Pathak D, Davis E, Stanford R. Economic impact of asthma therapy with fluticasone propionate, montelukast, or zafirlukast in a managed care population. *Pharmacotherapy* 2002; **22**: 166–74.

69 Bukstein D, Henk H, Luskin A. A comparison of asthma-related expenditures for patients started on montelukast versus fluticasone propionate as monotherapy. *Clin Ther* 2001; **23**: 1589–1600.

70 Price D, Ben-Joseph R, Zhang Q. Changes in asthma drug therapy costs for patients receiving chronic montelukast therapy in the UK. *Respir Med* 2001; **95**: 83–9.

Acknowledgements

Figures 3 and 4 are adapted from Malmstrom *et al.*, 1999.[25]
Figure 5 is adapted from Edelman *et al.*, 2000.[53]

9. Drug review – Salmeterol (Serevent®)

Dr Anna Palmer
CSF Medical Communications Ltd

You are strongly urged to consult your doctor before taking, stopping or changing any of the products reviewed or referred to in *BESTMEDICINE* or any other medication that has been prescribed or recommended by your doctor.

Summary

Salmeterol is a long-acting β_2-agonist, which relieves symptoms of asthma via its interaction with β_2-adrenoceptors located on bronchial smooth muscle. It shares a similar mechanism of action with the short-acting β_2-agonists, salbutamol or terbutaline, but its bronchodilatory effects are prolonged for up to 12 hours. This extended duration of action permits twice-daily dosing and enables good control of nocturnal asthma. When used to treat mild-to-moderately severe asthma, salmeterol reduces shortness of breath, wheezing and chest tightness and also improves pulmonary function (manifesting as increases in the forced expiratory volume in 1 second [FEV_1] and peak expiratory flow [PEF]). Salmeterol is indicated as add-on therapy in patients already receiving regular inhaled corticosteroid therapy but who still experience asthma symptoms. Salmeterol treatment is also associated with an improvement in patients' quality of life, a reduced requirement for rescue bronchodilator therapy and increases the incidence of symptom-free days and nights. Salmeterol is more effective as a controller therapy than the oral agent theophylline and has equivalent efficacy to other long-term β_2-agonists such as formoterol and bambuterol. In comparison with montelukast, salmeterol mediates greater improvements in lung function (PEF and FEV_1) and provides equivalent improvements in quality of life, incidence of exacerbations and nocturnal awakenings. Salmeterol must always be used in combination with regular inhaled corticosteroid (and not as a monotherapy) and, as such, it provides an effective and well-tolerated therapeutic option for the provision of long-term bronchodilator therapy.

Introduction

Inhaled β_2-adrenoceptor agonists (β_2-agonists) are the most effective and widely used bronchodilators currently available.[1] Historically, the first successful treatment of acute, severe asthma was with subcutaneous injections of adrenaline, though its precise mechanism of action was unknown at that time. It is now known that adrenaline interacts with β_2-adrenoceptors to relieve bronchoconstriction but at the same time also binds to β_1-adrenoceptors resulting in an accelerated heart rate. This observation provided the rationale for the development of more selective β_2-agonists, which provide effective and rapid relief from wheezing and chest tightness associated with asthma. However, the relief provided by the first-generation of these agents is relatively short-lived (4–6 hours) and therefore they must be used fairly frequently according to symptom severity. This led to development of long-acting β_2-agonists, such as salmeterol and formoterol, which have an extended duration of action of up to 12 hours and can be taken twice daily. In addition to reducing the occurrence of nocturnal asthma, salmeterol provides the patient with sustained and effective control of asthma symptoms.[2] Salmeterol is indicated for treatment of reversible airways obstruction (including nocturnal asthma and prevention of exercise-induced bronchospasm) in patients requiring long-term regular bronchodilator therapy.

Salmeterol is indicated for treatment of reversible airways obstruction in patients requiring long-term regular bronchodilator therapy.

Pharmacology

β_2-adrenergic receptors

The adrenergic receptors (or adrenoceptors) are named on the basis of their binding to adrenaline and related catecholamines. The α_1-adrenoceptors are coupled to the phosphoinositide signalling cascade, whilst the β-adrenoceptors are coupled by G-proteins to the adenylate cyclase pathway. The β-adrenergic receptor is a 64 kDa plasma membrane receptor containing seven transmembrane helices. The β_1 and β_2 forms of the adrenergic receptor are classified according to their affinities for adrenaline and noradrenaline, with β_2 receptors interacting primarily with adrenaline. Two other types of β-adrenoceptors also exist: the β_3-adrenoceptor located primarily in adipose tissue where it is involved in lipolysis and thermogenesis, and the β_4-adrenoceptors which – in common with the β_1-adrenoceptors – are found in the heart and act to increase heart rate.

The bronchodilating activity of adrenoceptors was unknown for some time, and adrenoceptor agonists such as adrenaline were thought only to have contractile and constrictor properties as demonstrated in cardiac tissue. In fact, β_2-adrenoceptors have a wide range of physiological actions including vasodilation, bronchodilation, relaxation of the gastrointestinal tract, glycogenolysis in the liver, tremor in skeletal smooth muscle and inhibition of histamine release from mast cells.[1]

β_2 adrenoceptor polymorphism

There is evidence to suggest that polymorphisms of the β_2-adrenoceptor may determine the degree of tolerance and subsensitivity of response that may develop after long-term exposure to β_2-agonists.[3] The homozygous glycine-16 variant occurs in 40% of individuals, the homozygous arginine-16 in around 15% of individuals with the remainder heterozygous for arginine/glycine. The evidence to date suggests that the arginine-16 polymorphism is responsible for subsensitivity and blunted bronchodilator response to the long-acting β_2-agonists with a greater degree of subsensitivity observed with formoterol than with salmeterol.[3] These conclusions were drawn from a retrospective meta-analysis and require confirmation from large-scale controlled prospective studies.

Mechanism of action and chemistry

The function of β_2-agonists in asthma is to mediate dilation of airway smooth muscle, thereby counteracting the bronchoconstriction generated by histamine, acetylcholine, leukotrienes and tachykinins.[1] The relaxant effect of salmeterol on bronchial smooth muscle is reversed by β-adrenoceptor antagonists *in vitro* and restored upon antagonist removal, suggesting that salmeterol interacts competitively with the β-adrenoceptor.[4] Salbutamol and terbutaline are the most widely used short-acting β_2-agonists, whilst salmeterol and formoterol were developed as longer-acting agents.

The chemistry of salmeterol is of essentially academic interest and most healthcare professionals will, like you, skip this section.

Salmeterol and formoterol have a duration of action of at least 12 hours.[1,4,5] Several hypotheses have been proposed to account for the extended duration of action of salmeterol, most of which relate to the long lipophilic N-substituted chain, or spacer arm, linking the two ring components of the molecule (Figure 1). One of the more conceptually appealing, yet presently debated, theories is that the spacer arm allows the drug to bind, not only to the active site of the β_2-adrenoceptor, but also to an additional 'exosite', which serves to anchor the agonist in the correct conformation, resulting in enhanced receptor occupancy.[1,4]

Salmeterol and formoterol have a duration of action of at least 12 hours.

The β_2-agonists are chiral drugs, which are generally formulated as racemic mixtures of an active, (R)-enantiomer, and inactive (L)-stereoisomer. It has been suggested that pure formulations of the

Figure 1. Chemical structure of salmeterol.

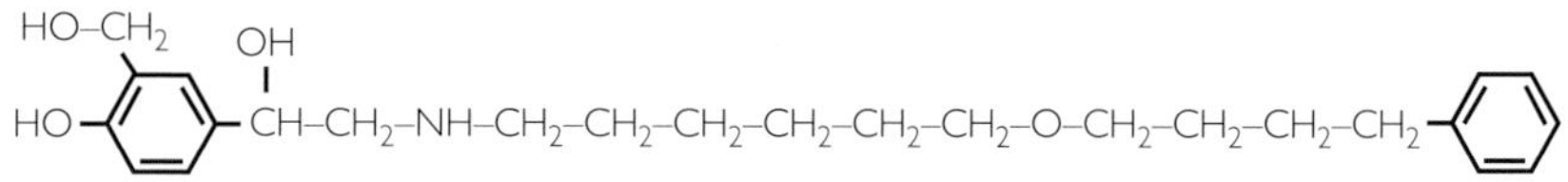

$HO-CH_2$ / OH

$HO-C_6H_3-CH(OH)-CH_2-NH-CH_2-CH_2-CH_2-CH_2-CH_2-CH_2-O-CH_2-CH_2-CH_2-CH_2-C_6H_5$

(R)-stereoisomer may provide equal efficacy to, but greater tolerability than, the current racemic mixtures.[1,6] However, current clinical data provide little support for the replacement of effective racemic formulations of drugs such as salmeterol with pure enantiomeric variants, such as levalbutamol (which is currently licensed in the US, but not in the UK).[1,6]

Dosage and administration

Salmeterol is formulated as the xinafoate (hydroxy-napthoic acid) salt.[4] For prophylactic use in adults and children over 4 years with asthma, salmeterol is administered by inhalation of a 50 μg dose delivered twice daily via either a Diskhaler®or Accuhaler®, which are breath-activated devices that deliver a fixed dose of drug in micronised powder form. Salmeterol stimulates bronchodilation for at least 12 hours following inhalation of a single 50 μg dose.[7] Salmeterol is also available for delivery by a metered-dose inhaler (MDI), which administers fixed doses of salmeterol of 25 μg per inhalation of suspension. This results in an actuated dose of 21 μg. However, for simplicity throughout this review, both aerosol and powder formulations are referred to in terms of the administered dose (i.e. 50 μg rather than 42 μg).

Current guidelines recommend that short-acting β_2-agonists are the first-line treatment for regular control of asthmatic episodes. Salmeterol should not be used for relief of an acute asthma attack due to its relatively slow onset of action and current anxieties about the effects of multiple dosing. The majority of patients also receive inhaled corticosteroids as 'regular inhaled preventer therapy' and if further control is required, long-acting β_2-agonists, such as salmeterol, can then be used as additional controller therapy. As evidence exists to show that salmeterol use may be detrimental in the absence of inhaled corticosteroids, it should only be used alongside existing corticosteroid therapy and must, therefore, not replace it.[2,3,8]

Salmeterol should only be used alongside existing corticosteroid therapy and must not replace it.

It is also important to note that regular use of long-acting β_2-agonists will reduce the requirement for short-acting agents, and therefore salmeterol may mask the overall requirement for reliever therapy. This is important since asthma activity is often quantified – in primary care and in clinical trials – in terms of patient requirement for short-acting β_2-agonist therapy.[3]

The pharmacokinetics of a drug are of interest to healthcare professionals because it is important for them to understand the action of a drug on the body over a period of time.

Pharmacokinetics

Peak plasma concentrations (C_{max}) of 0.15 μg/L are achieved with a twice-daily inhalation of salmeterol, 50 μg.[4] A similar C_{max} (0.16 μg/L) was observed after inhalation of a single dose of salmeterol (100 μg) and the time to peak plasma concentrations (t_{max}) was 5 minutes.[9] A second peak in plasma concentration (0.12 μg/mL) is observed approximately 45 minutes after inhalation and this is believed to result from swallowing a small proportion of the drug.[4] Given the low plasma concentrations of salmeterol delivered by inhalation, the majority of pharmacokinetic parameters are derived by evaluating an orally administered dose of the drug, and are therefore of limited clinical relevance. Impaired liver function may lead to accumulation of salmeterol in plasma since the drug is primarily metabolised hepatically. Peak plasma concentrations have been reported to be lower in patients with impaired renal function than in healthy volunteers.[5]

Salmeterol xinafoate dissociates in solution to salmeterol and 1-hydroxy-2-napthoic acid (xinafoate), each of which are then absorbed, distributed, metabolised and excreted independently, although the xinafoate salt appears to have no pharmacological activity. Salmeterol is approximately 95% bound to human plasma proteins *in vitro*.[5] The terminal elimination half-life ($t_{1/2}$) of salmeterol (100 μg inhaled in combination with fluticasone, 500 μg) was 7.6 hours.[9] Salmeterol is metabolised via the cytochrome P450 (CYP) 3A4 isoenzyme before it is eliminated in the faeces. The majority of orally administered radiolabelled salmeterol (1 mg administered to healthy volunteers) was recovered in the faeces (57.4%) and 23% was recovered in the urine between 24 and 72 hours after administration.[4]

Clinical efficacy

Preliminary evidence

A small clinical trial conducted in eight asthmatic individuals confirmed both the efficacy and the extended bronchodilatory effect of salmeterol compared with salbutamol.[10] Salmeterol (50, 100 and 200 μg) produced mean increases in FEV_1 in the range of 0.5–0.8 L and in PEF of 71–100 L/minute, which were comparable with salbutamol (100 μg). However, the improvements in pulmonary function with salbutamol returned to baseline within 6 hours whereas more than half of the maximum bronchodilatory effect of salmeterol remained 12 hours after dosing.[10]

Improvements in pulmonary function with salbutamol returned to baseline within 6 hours whereas more than half of the maximum bronchodilatory effect of salmeterol remained 12 hours after dosing.

In addition to their bronchodilator properties, β_2-agonists exert other effects via activation of β_2-adrenoceptors expressed on airway cells such as epithelial and mast cells, and on circulating inflammatory cells including eosinophils and neutrophils.[11] In preclinical studies, salmeterol suppresses the release of histamine, leukotrienes and prostaglandin D_2 from mast cells, inhibits tumour necrosis factor (TNF)-α release from monocytes, reduces neutrophil adhesion to bronchial epithelial cells and inhibits the proliferation of Th2 cells.[12] However, in clinical trials the beneficial effects of salmeterol do not appear to be a function of any of these anti-inflammatory properties.[3,13]

Salmeterol and other long-acting β_2-agonists are licensed as additional controller therapy on a background of short-acting β_2-agonists for immediate relief and inhaled corticosteroids as regular preventer therapy. Many patients now receive inhaled corticosteroids and long-acting β_2-agonists in a single combined inhaler and it is therefore interesting to question whether the effects of these two therapies are additive or synergistic.[3,12] It is already well documented that inhaled corticosteroids potentiate β_2-agonist effects via augmentation of β_2-adrenoceptor function. Conversely, the potential for long-acting

β_2-agonist augmentation of the response to inhaled corticosteroids has not been well examined.[3] However, it has been shown that interleukin (IL)-6 synthesis from human lung fibroblasts was unaffected by salmeterol, but the combination of salmeterol and budesonide enhanced the inhibition associated with budesonide alone ten-fold.[12] There are also *in vitro* data, which suggest that both salbutamol and salmeterol increase nuclear translocation of glucocorticoid receptors, which may explain any synergistic effect of the β_2-agonists on corticosteroid function.[3] However, data from several clinical trials provides evidence of additive rather than true synergistic effects of the two treatments used in combination (as would be expected of two drugs with distinct physiological targets).

Dose-ranging studies are particularly important to ensure that the optimum dose of a drug can be determined in order that benefit can be realised with the least risk of side-effects.

Dose-ranging studies

Three studies have compared 25 and 50 μg doses of salmeterol, given twice daily in children with mild-to-moderate asthma, and have reported a trend towards a dose-related improvement in pulmonary function. The effects of treatment were not different whether given by dry powder or aerosol formulations.[4,14] For example, in one study of 847 children (aged 4–16 years), salmeterol, 50 μg twice daily, led to greater improvements in mean morning PEF than the 25 μg twice-daily dose measured at 3 months from baseline (28 *vs* 22 L/minute; $p<0.05$).[15] There was no difference in the incidence of adverse events across treatment groups. A double-blind comparative study of 45 children (aged 5–16 years) did not demonstrate any additional benefit of a 100 μg twice-daily dose compared with a 50 μg twice-daily dose in terms of either morning or evening PEF, symptom control or use of rescue salbutamol.[4] These data suggest that the appropriate dose of salmeterol in childhood mild-to-moderate asthma is 50 μg of inhaled powder or aerosol, taken twice daily.

Dose-ranging studies have also been performed in adults, and the same conclusions were reached. On treatment day 1, maximum improvement was observed with the 50 μg twice-daily dose of salmeterol, with the maximum increase from baseline in FEV_1 (just over 35%), occurring at 3–5 hours and remaining above 25% for the entire 12-hour period.[16] On day 8, all treatment groups (salmeterol, 25, 50 and 100 μg twice daily), except the 12.5 μg twice-daily group, remained significantly improved with regard to per cent change in FEV_1 compared with placebo ($p<0.01$). The degree of improvement in morning PEF was dose related with mean increases ranging from 0.5 to 29.4 L/minute compared with a mean decrease of 15.3 L/minute with placebo ($p<0.001$; Figure 2). Asthma symptom scores and the frequency of undisturbed nights also improved in a dose-dependent manner. An increased incidence of tremor was reported, but this was confined to the 100 μg twice-daily dose of salmeterol. Thus, the 50 μg twice daily dose of salmeterol offers the best balance of efficacy and tolerability in mild-to-moderately severe asthma.

The optimum dose of salmeterol has also been addressed in 283 patients with moderate-to-severe asthma, defined by an FEV_1 less

Figure 2. Comparison of mean percentage change in peak expiratory flow (PEF) measured before and during salmeterol treatment in a dose-ranging study of patients with mild-to-moderate chronic asthma.[16]

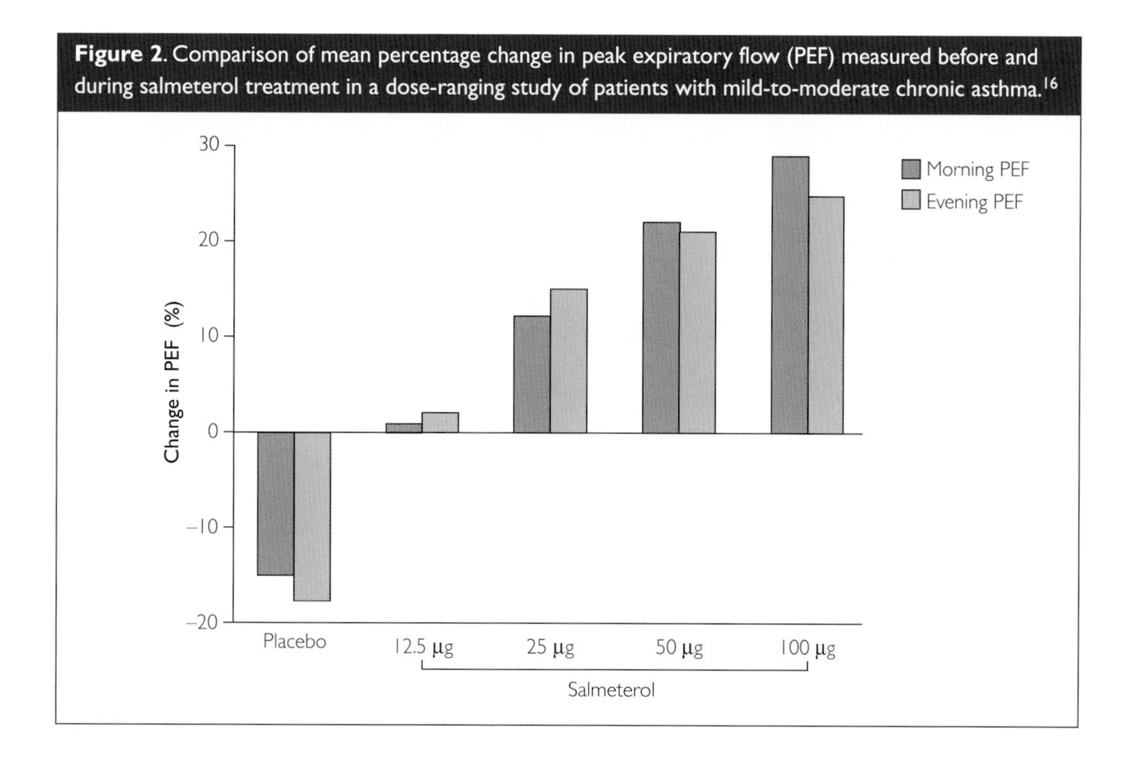

than 50% of the predicted value.[17] Patients were treated with salmeterol, 50 or 100 µg twice daily, via an MDI for 12 weeks and were asked to record symptom scores, their use of rescue medication, and PEF three times each morning and evening using a portable Mini-Wright peak flowmeter. A greater control of peak flow and a reduction in asthma symptoms was observed in the 100 µg salmeterol group compared with those receiving the 50 µg dose, with the greatest improvements observed in more severe asthmatics taking concurrent oral corticosteroids (compared with inhaled corticosteroids or none at all). The mean increases in morning and evening PEF were 55 and 45 L/minute in the salmeterol, 100 µg, group, and 42 and 27 L/minute in the 50 µg group (salmeterol, 50 µg *vs* 100 µg; $p<0.05$). The percentage of days of the 12-week treatment period where no additional salbutamol rescue treatment was required was greater in the salmeterol, 100 µg, group than in the 50 µg group (71 *vs* 32%; $p<0.05$), whilst the percentage of nights with no asthma symptoms was increased in both groups after 4 weeks' treatment (100 and 85.7% with the 100 µg and 50 µg doses, respectively). Improvements in FEV_1 and FVC were observed with both doses of salmeterol and were not different between the two treatment groups. In terms of tolerability, a higher incidence of tremor was recorded in the 100 µg salmeterol group (8 *vs* 0.7%; $p<0.05$). However, the incidence of asthma-related adverse events and of respiratory/chest infection was slightly higher in the salmeterol, 50 µg, group (21.2 and 16.4%, respectively) than in the 100 µg group (17.5 and 9.5%, respectively). Thus, overall, the 100 µg twice-daily dose of salmeterol was more effective in controlling certain aspects of asthma, particularly in those with more severe disease. Therefore, this dose may be more beneficial to patients with severe asthma who do not adequately respond to the 50 μg dose.

Effect of delivery device

The introduction of breath-activated DPI's removes the need to coordinate actuation with inspiration, provide a simpler and more patient-friendly inhaler device.

Appropriate administration of prescribed asthma treatments is a critical factor in eliciting maximal efficacy and until now, metered dose inhalation of aerosolised drugs has been the standard delivery system employed. This provides accurate delivery of the drug to the required site but requires a degree of coordination between breathing and operation of the device, which may be difficult to master, particularly in young children, the elderly or in those with more severe asthma. New technology led to the introduction of breath-activated dry powder inhalers (DPIs), which remove the need to coordinate actuation with inspiration, thereby providing a simpler and more patient-friendly inhaler device.

A randomised, double-blind, placebo-controlled, multicentre study was conducted in 498 sufferers of mild-to-moderate asthma (FEV_1, 50–85% of the predicted value) aged over 12 years in an attempt to determine the comparative efficacy and tolerability of salmeterol administered by these two delivery systems.[18] Peak FEV_1 was increased by 21–24% over baseline by both salmeterol formulations at all time points from 30 minutes to 12 hours post-dosing, and at both week one and week 12 of the study. This contrasted with a 9% increase with placebo (Figure 3). Similarly, mean morning PEF was not different between the salmeterol formulations but was significantly improved in both groups compared with placebo ($p<0.01$). In comparison with placebo, both formulations of salmeterol also decreased the use of rescue salbutamol, decreased the number of nights disturbed by asthma symptoms and increased the percentage of days without asthma symptoms. Again, no differences were observed between the two formulations in these measures. The tolerability, incidence of adverse events and safety measures (i.e. heart rate, blood pressure, electrocardiogram [ECG] readings and haematology) were similar in all three treatment groups, with headache the most common adverse event reported.[18] These and other data, demonstrate that both dry powder and metered dose aerosol inhalation of salmeterol provide comparable improvement in asthma symptoms and pulmonary function.[18,19] Thus, new formulations of β_2-agonists delivered by DPIs are equally well tolerated, acceptable and effective as older MDI systems. As no difference is apparent between these formulations, the remainder of this review will refer only to the dose of salmeterol delivered and will not specify the formulation (aerosol or powder) unless particularly pertinent.

New formulations of β_2-agonists delivered by DPIs are equally well tolerated, acceptable and effective as older MDI systems.

Figure 3. Forced expiratory volume in 1 second (FEV_1) over 12 hours for salmeterol powder, salmeterol aerosol and placebo on treatment day 1 (left) and treatment week 12 (right).[18] Data are mean ±SEM.

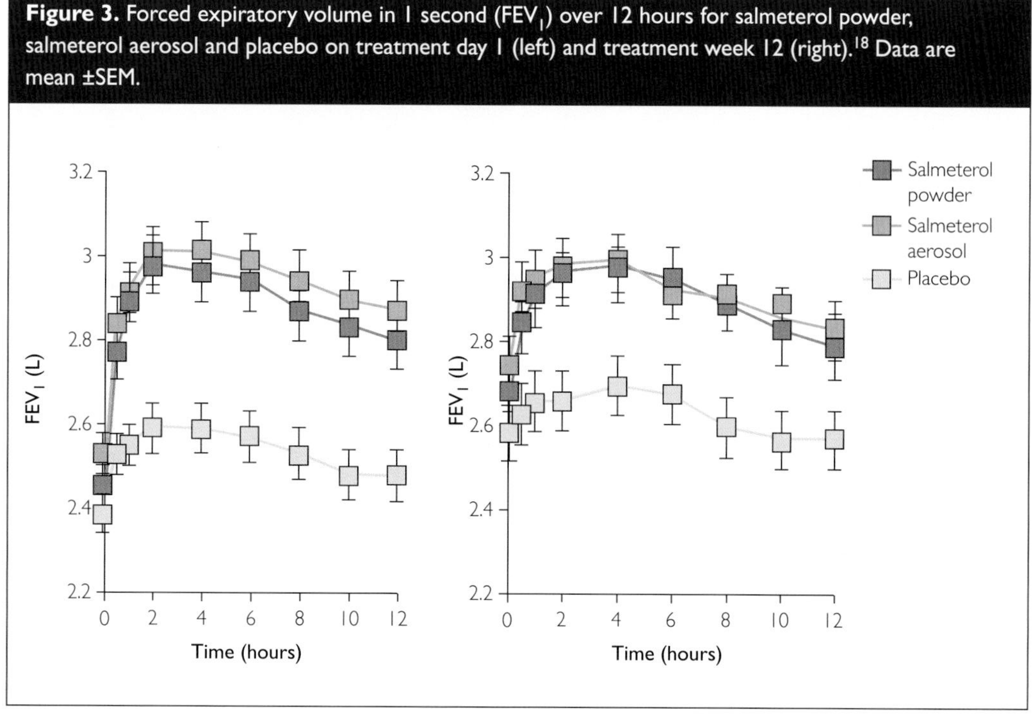

Salmeterol vs inhaled corticosteroid therapy

Initial investigations sought to determine the appropriate role for long-acting β_2-agonists in asthma management. Inhaled corticosteroids are the established long-term controller therapy of choice and the question was whether long-acting β_2-agonists could represent an alternative or an additional therapy.

As inhaled corticosteroids are such well-established therapy for asthma management, few clinical trials have been conducted in asthmatic patients previously unexposed to inhaled corticosteroids. Two such trials have, however, directly compared long-term use of beclometasone with salmeterol in corticosteroid-naïve patients.[20,21] The largest and most recent of these was conducted in 386 adult and adolescent sufferers of persistent asthma (aged >12 years; mean age 30 years) who had not previously received either oral or inhaled corticosteroids in the preceding 6 months.[20] Patients were randomised to receive either salmeterol, 50 µg twice daily, beclometasone dipropionate, 100 µg four-times daily, or placebo, by aerosol inhalation for 6 months. Improvements were observed in both morning and evening PEF with both beclometasone and salmeterol compared with placebo ($p<0.05$). Both treatments also improved FEV_1 from baseline at all time points from week 6 to 26 (0.28, 0.23 and 0.08 L for salmeterol, beclometasone and placebo, respectively; $p<0.05$ for both active treatments *vs* placebo). In contrast with the other treatments, salmeterol was effective as early as

Salmeterol and beclometasone were similar in their ability to increase the percentage of salbutamol-free nights and symptom-free days compared with placebo.

week 2. Salmeterol and beclometasone were also similar in their ability to increase the percentage of salbutamol-free nights and symptom-free days compared with placebo. The two treatments did not differ in reducing the number of asthma exacerbations (16–17%) or in their ability to reduce bronchial hyper-responsiveness (both $p<0.001$ *vs* placebo). There were no clinically important differences in safety profiles, and no difference in the incidence of adverse events, across the different treatment groups (i.e. placebo, beclometasone or salmeterol).[20] Thus, in conclusion, this study demonstrated an equivalent efficacy of salmeterol and beclometasone dipropionate in corticosteroid-naïve patients with persistent asthma.

These data, and those from a further study which compared salmeterol with placebo in corticosteroid-naïve adults, suggest that salmeterol provides effective and sustained improvement in lung function and in the control of asthma symptoms.[13,22] However, studies of corticosteroid-naïve children, and of adults whose corticosteroid treatment was replaced with salmeterol monotherapy, appear to contradict these findings.[13,21] In the latter study, a total of 164 patients (aged 12–64 years) with persistent asthma – well-controlled during a 6-week run-in phase with inhaled triamcinolone (400 µg twice daily) – were randomised to continue triamcinolone or to switch to salmeterol monotherapy (50 µg twice daily delivered in aerosol form), or placebo.[13] At the end of the 16-week treatment period, all patients were switched to placebo for the final 6-week run-out phase. The primary efficacy outcome was the change in morning PEF from week 6 (end of run-in period) to week 22 (end of treatment). Salmeterol demonstrated equivalent efficacy to triamcinolone in improving morning PEF, and maintaining quality of life, asthma symptom scores and use of rescue salbutamol. However, FEV_1 and methacholine responsiveness decreased with salmeterol therapy, whilst inflammatory markers (sputum eosinophils, tryptase and eosinophil cationic protein) and exhaled nitric oxide (a non-invasive measure of airway inflammation) all increased with salmeterol relative to those persisting with their inhaled corticosteroid (Figure 4; all parameters $p<0.05$). This evidence of a resurgence in airway inflammation and loss of asthma control from baseline were similar in the salmeterol and placebo groups. In contrast, in triamcinolone-treated patients, lung function was improved and asthma control was maintained. Even more tellingly, there was no difference between placebo and salmeterol in terms of treatment failure (36 *vs* 24%, respectively) or asthma exacerbations (29 *vs* 20%, respectively), but both were significantly lower in triamcinolone-treated patients (treatment failure: 6%, $p<0.05$; asthma exacerbation: 7%, $p<0.001$). This study appears to confirm that salmeterol is not clinically effective in reducing airway inflammation.[3] It also suggests that the loss of anti-inflammatory activity is a function of corticosteroid withdrawal rather than a direct effect of salmeterol treatment, since a similar pattern is seen with placebo. In conclusion, whilst the use of salmeterol confers improvements in lung function, it is inferior to continued inhaled corticosteroid therapy and indeed, was no more effective than placebo at

Figure 4. Morning peak expiratory flow (PEF [A]), forced expiratory volume in 1 second (FEV_1 [B]), rescue salbutamol use (C) and levels of sputum eosinophils (D) after 16 weeks' treatment with either salmeterol or triamcinolone monotherapy.[13]

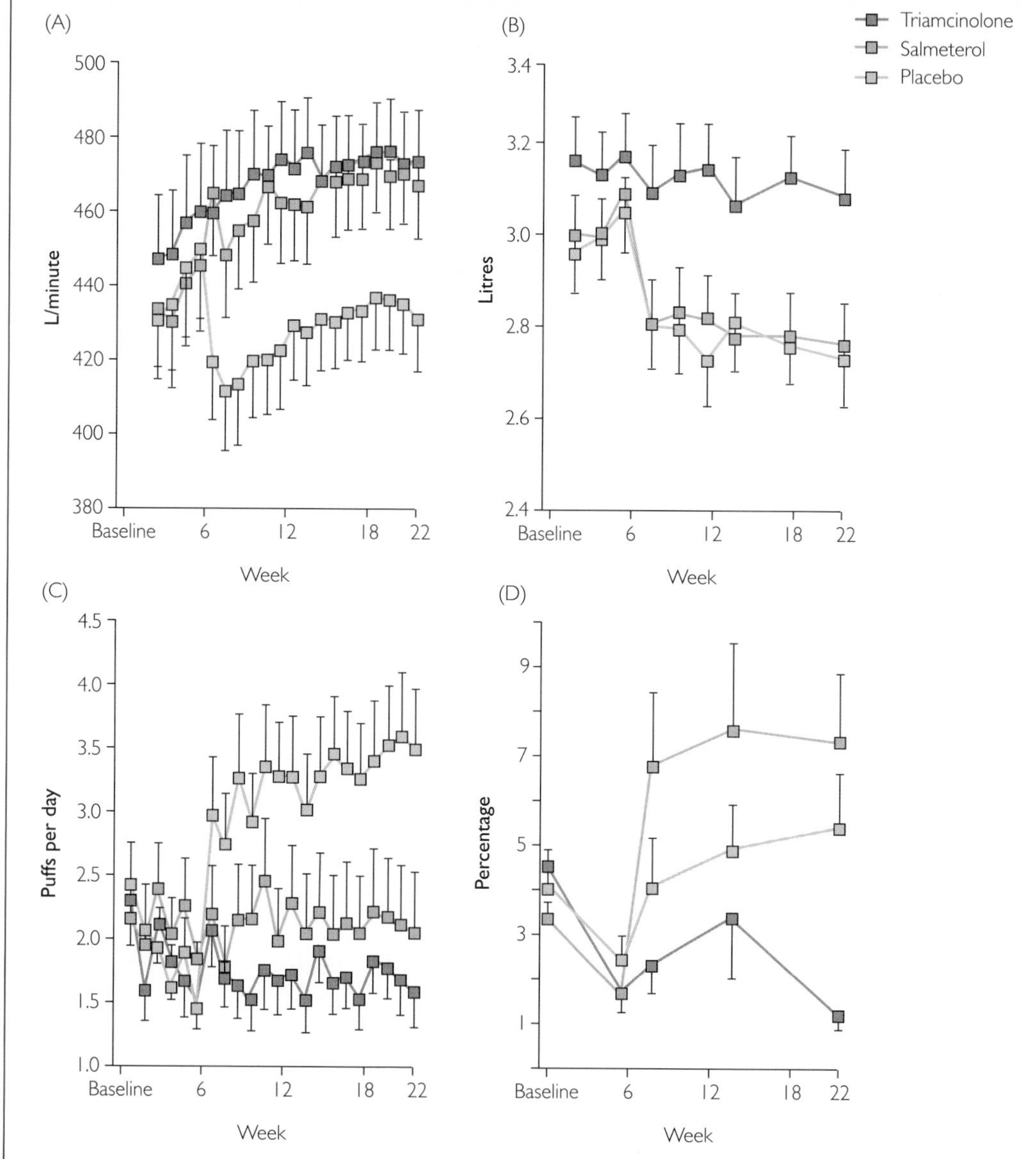

preventing treatment failures and asthma exacerbations.[13] Hence, these data are consistent with current UK guidelines, which advise that salmeterol should be used as an add-on therapy to inhaled corticosteroids and not as a long-term controller monotherapy. This message was reinforced by the abrupt early cessation of the Salmeterol Multicenter Asthma Research Trial.[8] This placebo-controlled trial of approximately 26,000 patients (salmeterol 50 µg twice daily for 28 weeks) was halted early when data from a routine interim analysis revealed a significantly greater occurrence of asthma-related deaths in patients not using inhaled corticosteroids. Among patients using inhaled corticosteroids, however, there was no difference between salmeterol and placebo groups in either primary or secondary outcomes (including respiratory-related deaths and life-threatening events).

Addition of salmeterol was superior to increasing the dose of beclometasone in measures of lung function and the control of symptoms, with no difference in the incidence of asthma exacerbations or adverse events.

Salmeterol in combination with inhaled corticosteroid therapy

The studies described so far provide no evidence to support a policy of replacing inhaled corticosteroids with salmeterol in the long-term control of asthma. Instead, and in accordance with current UK recommendations, salmeterol is generally prescribed as additional therapy to those patients already receiving inhaled corticosteroids but who require further symptom control. Trials have been devised to determine whether such a patient population would benefit more from receiving an increased dose of inhaled corticosteroid or, alternatively, adding salmeterol to their existing corticosteroid treatment regimen. One such study enrolled 429 adults (older than 18 years) who remained symptomatic despite treatment with beclometasone dipropionate, 200 µg twice daily. Patients were randomised to receive either increased beclometasone (500 µg twice daily) or salmeterol, 50 µg twice daily, for 6 months.[23] The results of this study indicate that the addition of salmeterol was superior to increasing the dose of beclometasone in measures of lung function and the control of symptoms, with no difference in the incidence of asthma exacerbations or adverse events.

In brief, the addition of salmeterol mediated greater improvements than higher dose beclometasone in morning PEF at all time points (i.e. PEF at week 13: ≥30 *vs* 15 L/minute; $p<0.001$). Mean evening PEF also increased in the salmeterol group by approximately 19 L/minute at all time points, but did not change from baseline in the higher dose beclometasone group. Salmeterol was also more effective than high-dose beclometasone in reducing night-time awakenings at weeks 1 and 13 ($p<0.05$), and in reducing symptomatic days at weeks 1 and 5 ($p<0.05$). Furthermore, no difference was observed between the two groups in terms of tolerability or safety.[23]

A further study evaluated the effects of using higher doses of both salmeterol and corticosteroid. Thus, patients received either beclometasone, 2000 µg, or beclometasone, 1000 µg, with the addition of salmeterol (50 or 100 µg).[24] Again, the addition of salmeterol to inhaled beclometasone provided greater improvement than a high dose of corticosteroid, in terms of both lung function and symptom control with no alteration in bronchial hyper-responsiveness and no change in exacerbation rates. These data have been supported and extended by a comprehensive meta-analysis.[25] In conclusion, patients remaining symptomatic despite receiving regular inhaled corticosteroids may be prescribed salmeterol as additional asthma management therapy in place of an increased dose of corticosteroid.[26]

Reduction of inhaled corticosteroid dose

Several studies have set out to determine whether the addition of salmeterol to existing corticosteroid therapy may actually permit a reduction in the dose of inhaled corticosteroid used.[27,28]

One study enrolled 101 patients (aged 19–60 years) with mild-to-moderate asthma already receiving inhaled beclometasone dipropionate, and compared the effects of adding salmeterol, 50 μg twice daily, or placebo, given over 6 months.[28] The main outcome measures included reduction in inhaled steroid use, asthma exacerbations and use of oral corticosteroids. Dose reduction of inhaled steroids was controlled by both the patient and their physician according to target PEF and symptom control, and was decreased slowly and in a stepwise manner. Mean inhaled steroid use remained stable over the last 5 months of treatment and was lower with salmeterol than with placebo (daily doses: 561 *vs* 674 μg; $p<0.001$). The use of oral steroids and the incidence of asthma exacerbations did not differ between the salmeterol and placebo groups. In the second study, salmeterol was introduced and triamcinolone was reduced by 50% (for 8 weeks) and then eliminated completely (for a further 8 weeks).[27] Elimination of inhaled steroid from the triamcinolone/salmeterol group resulted in a deterioration in asthma control, again reinforcing current guidelines that salmeterol monotherapy is not appropriate in the absence of an inhaled corticosteroid for effective asthma management. However, the initial introduction of salmeterol resulted in an increased morning PEF and FEV_1, and a decrease in asthma symptom scores and daily use of rescue salbutamol. Moreover, subsequent dose reduction of triamcinolone (to 200 μg) in the salmeterol-treated group led to no significant differences in lung function outcomes compared with those maintained on the higher dose (400 μg) of triamcinolone.[27]

In conclusion, these data indicate that salmeterol can provide effective further control of asthma symptoms when added to existing inhaled corticosteroids, and moreover, can facilitate a careful and controlled reduction in the dose of inhaled corticosteroid required for good asthma management.

Salmeterol can provide effective further control of asthma symptoms when added to existing inhaled corticosteroids, and can facilitate a careful and controlled reduction in the dose of inhaled corticosteroid required for good asthma management.

Placebo-controlled studies

The efficacy of salmeterol has been compared with placebo in patients with mild-to-moderate asthma receiving background therapy with inhaled corticosteroids. Patients receiving placebo in these studies, and indeed in all of the trials discussed hereafter, had access to rescue therapy with inhaled short-acting β_2-agonists (generally salbutamol).

In one 6-month study, lung function and bronchial responsiveness – measured as secondary endpoints – showed improvements for salmeterol over placebo, in terms of FEV_1, FVC, morning and evening PEF, and methacholine hyper-responsiveness (Table 1).[28] Salmeterol treatment also resulted in greater symptom-free days and nights, and a greater percentage of days where bronchodilator rescue therapy was not required. Safety parameters, including serum potassium, heart rate and

Table 1. Lung function and symptom scores in asthmatic patients receiving beclometasone or budesonide with additional placebo or salmeterol, 50 μg twice daily, for 6 months.[28]

Efficacy endpoint	Salmeterol	Placebo	*p*-value
FEV_1 (L)[a]	2.84	2.71	<0.001
FVC (L)[a]	4.01	3.89	<0.001
PEF (L/minute)			
Morning	451	431	<0.001
Evening	456	440	<0.001
PD_{20} methacholine (μmol/L)[b]	2.24	1.46	<0.01
Symptom-free nights (%)	96	86	<0.001
Symptom-free days (%)	82	64	<0.001
Bronchodilator-free days (%)	73	58	<0.001

[a]Mean values are for last 5 months of treatment.
[b]The provocative dose of metacholine causing a 20% fall in FEV_1, determined at 6 months.
FEV_1, forced expiratory volume in 1 second; FVC, forced vital capacity; PEF, peak expiratory flow.

ECG readings, did not differ between the two groups, though salmeterol was associated with more palpitations than placebo.[28]

The long-term efficacy of salmeterol was examined over 1 year in 352 patients (older than 12 years) with mild-to-moderate asthma.[29] At all time points, salmeterol mediated improvements in FEV_1 compared with placebo demonstrating that the bronchodilator effect of salmeterol was sustained over 52 weeks of treatment. Additionally, pre-dose FEV_1 values were increased in the salmeterol group from week 4 of treatment (3.08±0.06 *vs* 2.89±0.05 L with placebo; $p<0.001$), and these were sustained throughout the treatment period. Salmeterol-treated patients also showed greater improvements from baseline in both morning and evening PEF (+35.6 and +25.1 L/minute, respectively) compared with those receiving placebo in whom PEF did not change. Furthermore, the use of rescue salbutamol, the percentage of disturbed nights and asthma symptom scores also declined in salmeterol-treated patients compared with placebo-treated individuals. Finally, salmeterol treatment was associated with a reduction in methacholine-induced bronchial hyper-responsiveness, particularly at weeks 4 and 24 when higher doubling doses of methacholine were required to achieve a required 20% fall in FEV_1 (week 4: 1.02 *vs* 0.4 L for placebo, $p<0.01$; week 24: 1.06 *vs* 0.4 L for placebo, $p<0.05$). Therefore, compared with the use of placebo plus salbutamol rescue therapy, salmeterol was effective in improving lung function over a prolonged period, with no attenuation in its bronchodilatory properties, and with sustained diminution of bronchial hyper-responsiveness to methacholine.

Compared with the use of placebo plus salbutamol rescue therapy, salmeterol was effective in improving lung function over a prolonged period.

Salmeterol has also been compared with placebo in an attempt to determine its impact upon quality of life. Two studies were conducted in over 500 patients (aged over 12 years) who remained symptomatic despite the use of inhaled corticosteroids and both yielded remarkably similar results.[30,31] Changes in asthma-related quality of life scores were determined using the Asthma Quality of Life Questionnaire (AQLQ) and indicate marked improvements in all measured aspects of quality of life with salmeterol compared with placebo (Figure 5).[30] Both studies also confirmed superior improvements relative to placebo in terms of lung function, symptom scores and the use of rescue therapy with salmeterol treatment.[30,31]

Salmeterol vs short-acting β_2-agonists

Other studies have been designed to determine whether the extended duration of action of salmeterol offers better management of asthma than regular administration of a short-acting β_2-agonist, commonly salbutamol (alternatively referred to as albuterol in the US).

Three studies of similar design compared 12 weeks of salmeterol, 50 μg twice daily, with salbutamol, 180 μg four-times daily, in patients with mild-to-moderate asthma.[32–34] A further four studies compared salmeterol (50 μg twice daily) with salbutamol at higher doses of between 200 and 400 μg four-times daily in studies ranging from 12 to 52 weeks in duration.[35–38] Use of inhaled corticosteroids in all studies ranged from 22 to 80% of the study populations.[32–38] In summary, all studies reported that salmeterol was more effective than salbutamol in improving lung function and in minimising the symptoms of asthma.

Salmeterol was more effective than salbutamol in improving lung function and in minimising the symptoms of asthma.

More specifically, FEV_1 was increased by both salbutamol and salmeterol compared with placebo, though salmeterol mediated a

Figure 5. Change in Asthma Quality of Life Questionnaire (AQLQ) from baseline to 12 weeks of salmeterol treatment.[30]

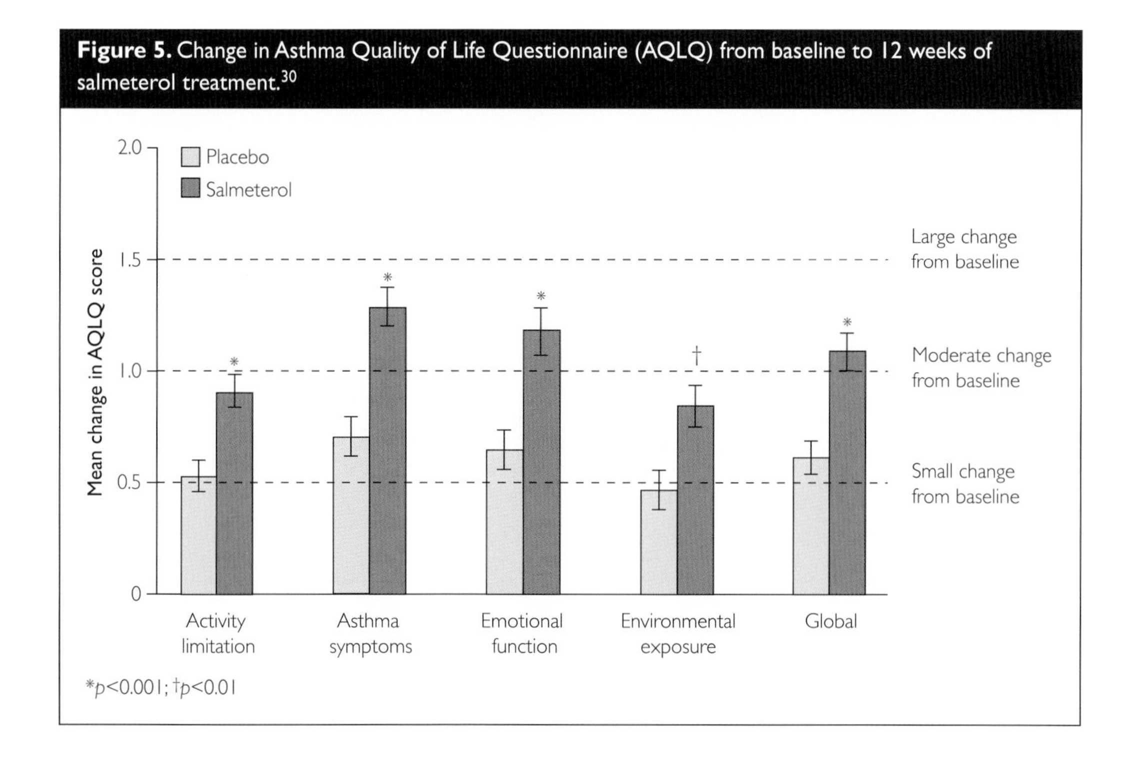

sustained and uniform increase in FEV_1 over a 12-hour period rather than the biphasic improvement that was observed with salbutamol treatment (Figure 6).[33] The mean area under the curve (AUC) for FEV_1 at week 12 was greater in salmeterol- than in salbutamol-treated patients in two of the studies (6.1 *vs* 3.4 L•hours, $p<0.001$; 8.3 *vs* 4.0 L•hours, $p<0.001$).[32,33] Both morning and evening PEF were improved by a significantly greater extent with salmeterol compared with salbutamol in three of the studies which used salbutamol, 180 µg (mean increase in morning PEF 33±6.7 L/minute and evening 21±7.1 L/minute).[32–34] This contrasted with either negligible increases, and in some cases small decreases, in mean PEF with either salbutamol or placebo treatment. The same trends were observed with the higher doses of salbutamol.[35–38] Salmeterol also tended to reduce diurnal variation in PEF, whereas salbutamol and placebo had no effect, and in one case actually increased the degree of diurnal variation.[38] In all cases, salmeterol was more effective than salbutamol in reducing mean symptom scores for asthma, reducing the number of disturbed nights and reducing the use of rescue salbutamol. The most common adverse event reported was headache (followed by either cough or tremor), but the incidence of adverse events was low and was not different between salmeterol, salbutamol and placebo groups. Thus, in conclusion, salmeterol was consistently more effective than regular salbutamol in providing sustained control of the symptoms of asthma.

Salmeterol was consistently more effective than regular salbutamol in providing sustained control of the symptoms of asthma.

Figure 6. Mean change from baseline in forced expiratory volume in 1 second (FEV_1) at week 12 of treatment with either salmeterol, salbutamol or placebo.[33]

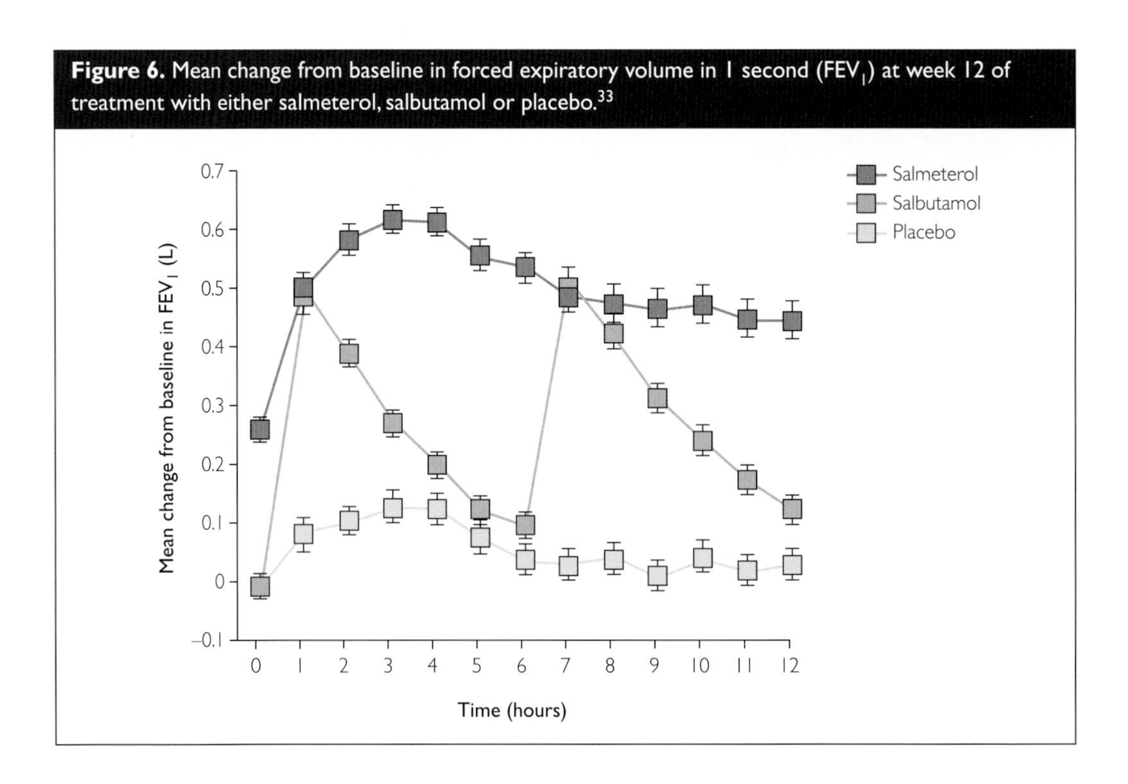

Salmeterol vs oral controller therapies

There are two other drug classes currently recommended for additional control of asthma if symptoms are still apparent after treatment with inhaled corticosteroids. These are modified-release oral theophylline or the leukotriene receptor antagonists including montelukast and zafirlukast (see Disease Overview section).

Salmeterol *vs* theophylline

Theophylline is a bronchodilator belonging to the methylxanthine class of agents. Its use is associated with a number of major clinical disadvantages. At high plasma concentrations the drug causes an unacceptably high incidence of adverse events and thus it must be carefully titrated (10–20 μg/mL) and provides only a narrow window of therapeutic efficacy.[39] A meta-analysis has reviewed data from nine randomised, controlled clinical trials of at least 2 weeks' duration in more than 1330 patients.[39] This indicated that salmeterol was superior in terms of both efficacy and tolerability in the treatment of chronic asthma. Specifically, in comparison with theophylline, salmeterol treatment improved mean morning and evening PEF, increased the percentage of symptom-free days and nights, decreased the use of rescue salbutamol treatment and resulted in a lower incidence of treatment withdrawals.[39] These findings are further substantiated in a more recent study not included in this original meta-analysis.[40]

Salmeterol *vs* leukotriene receptor antagonists

Leukotrienes released by eosinophils and mast cells are important mediators of bronchoconstriction, airway inflammation, oedema and mucus hypersecretion.[41] The leukotriene receptor antagonists (e.g. montelukast and zafirlukast) exert their bronchodilatory effects by targeting the cysteinyl leukotriene 1 ($cysLT_1$) receptor.[41,42] Three randomised, double-blind studies have been reviewed which compared salmeterol (50 μg twice daily) with either montelukast (10 mg once daily) or zafirlukast (20 mg twice daily) in patients already receiving inhaled corticosteroid therapy.[43] Both therapies improved lung function from baseline to the end of each study (4 or 12 weeks), but patients taking salmeterol consistently demonstrated the greatest improvements in mean FEV_1 and morning and evening PEF. Salmeterol also provided greater overall control of asthma with more symptom-free days and nights, reduced asthma exacerbations and reduced use of short-acting bronchodilator rescue therapy compared with either montelukast or zafirlukast. Both treatments were equally well tolerated in these studies.[43]

A recent large-scale (n=1490), randomised study conducted over 1 year specifically compared the effects of salmeterol and montelukast with regard to the frequency of asthma exacerbations and found that the number of patients experiencing exacerbations was similar between the two groups. Thus, 19.1% and 20.1% of salmeterol- and montelukast-treated patients experienced exacerbations. Again, salmeterol exerted greater increases in FEV_1 (0.19 *vs* 0.11 L; $p<0.001$) and morning PEF (34.6 *vs* 17.7 L/minute; $p<0.001$) compared with montelukast. However, there were no differences between the two treatments in the number of nocturnal awakenings or in asthma specific quality of life scores, both of which were improved by both treatments.[42]

Salmeterol appears to mediate greater improvements in lung function than either montelukast or zafirlukast in patients already receiving inhaled corticosteroid therapy.

In summary, salmeterol appears to mediate greater improvements in lung function as shown by PEF and FEV_1 than either montelukast or zafirlukast in patients already receiving inhaled corticosteroid therapy, but has no additional effect in terms of reducing asthma exacerbations.

Both salmeterol and montelukast are also effective in the treatment of exercise-induced bronchoconstriction – a common complication in those with chronic asthma. Several studies have now directly compared the two therapies in this indication.[44,45] A group of 122 asthmatic patients (aged 15–58 years) whose symptoms were uncontrolled by inhaled corticosteroids were given additional salmeterol (50 μg twice daily), montelukast (10 mg once daily) or placebo. Lung function was then assessed after exercise challenge at baseline and again after 1 and 4 weeks of treatment.[44] Although pre-exercise FEV_1 was greatest with salmeterol, patients taking montelukast experienced the greatest protection from exercise-induced bronchoconstriction. In addition, salmeterol treatment was associated with an attenuated response to rescue salbutamol, which was not observed with either placebo or montelukast. Thus, at week 1, salbutamol mediated a rise in FEV_1 from pre-exercise levels of 11.3% in the montelukast group and 12.5% with placebo, which contrasted with a rise of only 2.7% in the salmeterol group. A similar pattern was observed after 4 weeks of treatment where the respective responses were 10.9, 9.3 and 1.7%.[44] Further support for the use of montelukast in the treatment of exercise-induced bronchoconstriction was provided in an 8-week comparator study with salmeterol.[45] Despite equivalent efficacy at day 3 of treatment, the salmeterol-mediated improvement in exercise-induced bronchoconstriction was reduced at weeks 4 and 8, in contrast with montelukast, which showed sustained bronchoprotection over the duration of the study. Thus, there was a greater bronchoprotective effect with montelukast than with salmeterol at weeks 4 and 8 of treatment. Therefore, although neither therapy was universally effective, montelukast may be preferred to salmeterol in the treatment of exercise-induced bronchoconstriction.

Salmeterol vs other long-acting β_2-agonists

Other long-acting β_2-agonists licensed in the UK for asthma include bambuterol and formoterol. Bambuterol is an oral terbutaline prodrug with an extended duration of action of around 24 hours, thus enabling once-daily dosing. Formoterol is an inhaled formulation with a similar duration of action to salmeterol but with a more rapid onset of action (≈1 minute).[19,46]

There appears to be little difference in terms of clinical efficacy of bambuterol and salmeterol. In one 4-week study, both treatments mediated similar improvements in morning PEF compared with baseline, and both were well tolerated.[46] Bambuterol, therefore, provides a useful therapeutic alternative to salmeterol in cases where an oral treatment is preferred over inhaler administration.

Direct comparator studies of formoterol and salmeterol generally indicate equivalent clinical efficacy and tolerability.[19,47] A 6-month study of 482 patients with reversible obstructive airways disease, including asthma, demonstrated similar improvements in morning PEF, the frequency of rescue medication and improved control of respiratory symptoms with formoterol (12 μg twice daily) and salmeterol (50 μg twice daily).[47] A further short-term study of asthmatic patients alone (n=230) also reported equivalent efficacy of both treatments.[19] The only apparent difference was in daytime asthma symptom scores, which were improved by a greater extent with formoterol than with salmeterol ($p<0.05$).[19]

Thus, in summary, the clinical efficacy of salmeterol appears to be equivalent to that of the other long-acting β_2-agonists.

The clinical efficacy of salmeterol appears to be equivalent to that of the other long-acting β_2-agonists.

Role in severe asthma

Most studies that have evaluated the effects of salmeterol are performed in mild-to-moderate asthmatics receiving low doses of inhaled corticosteroids. However, the utility of salmeterol has also been determined in patients with more severe asthma.

A group of 119 adults with chronic asthma (defined in this study as requiring at least 1500 μg of inhaled corticosteroid daily [beclometasone dipropionate or equivalent] and under consideration for maintenance oral corticosteroid therapy) were enrolled into a randomised clinical trial.[48] Salmeterol, 100 μg twice daily, or placebo was administered to these patients over 3 months in order to determine whether salmeterol may provide an acceptable alternative to oral corticosteroid treatment for this severe asthmatic population. The study showed that mean morning PEF (but not evening PEF) was increased by salmeterol over the duration of the study (45±41 *vs* 23±45 L/minute for placebo; $p<0.01$), though no difference was apparent in FEV_1. The incidence of symptom-free nights increased with salmeterol (33±32 *vs* 13±26% with placebo; $p<0.001$) and a reduction was also observed in rescue medication usage (decrease of 5.1±4.7 *vs* 2.5±4.0 puffs with placebo; $p<0.001$). No differences in tolerability, minor or serious adverse events were reported in the salmeterol and placebo groups.[48]

A further study carried out in a group of chronic asthmatics (distinguished by persistent symptoms despite receiving high doses of inhaled corticosteroid [i.e. >1500 μg beclometasone or 1200 μg budesonide daily]) was conducted over 6 weeks, to compare a prescribed regimen of salbutamol, 400 μg four-times a day, with salmeterol, 100 μg twice daily. Additional salbutamol was permitted and its use was recorded as rescue therapy. In contrast with the aforementioned study, salmeterol provided greater improvements in FEV_1 (0.22 L increase from baseline) compared with the salbutamol group (0.05 L; $p<0.05$). In common with the previous study, salmeterol, 100 μg twice daily,

A higher dose of salmeterol provides effective improvement in terms of lung function and symptom scores in patients with chronic asthma.

improved lung function (morning PEF improved by 33 L/minute *vs* salbutamol 4 L/minute, $p<0.001$) and increased the number of symptom-free nights (by 57 *vs* 22% with salbutamol; $p<0.001$), although there was no difference between the groups in the number of symptom-free days.[49]

These data indicate that a higher dose of salmeterol (100 µg, twice daily) provides effective improvement in terms of lung function and symptom scores in patients with chronic asthma who are already receiving high-dose inhaled corticosteroids.

Role in nocturnal asthma

Salmeterol, but not placebo or theophylline, also reduced the incidence of nocturnal awakenings and the use of salbutamol.

Nocturnal asthma occurs in more than 70% of asthma patients and the majority of deaths attributable to asthma are said to occur during the night or early in the morning.[50] Thus, effective treatment for nocturnal symptoms of asthma and night-time lung function is required. Both salmeterol and theophylline have been shown to reduce early morning bronchoconstriction and decrease the incidence of nocturnal asthma symptoms. Two trials have recently compared the efficacy of these two agents and both reported marginal improvements in sleep quality with salmeterol but not theophylline.[50,51] In the second study, the overall mean nocturnal FEV_1 level fell significantly with both placebo and theophylline, but was maintained with salmeterol. Salmeterol, but not placebo or theophylline, also reduced the incidence of nocturnal awakenings and the use of salbutamol.[50] These data support the use of salmeterol in the treatment and control of the symptoms of nocturnal asthma.

Role in exercise-induced asthma

Salmeterol was more effective than salbutamol in the short-term treatment of exercise-induced bronchoconstriction.

Exercise-induced bronchoconstriction is said to affect up to 80% of individuals with clinically diagnosed asthma and in younger sufferers this may be the primary manifestation of their asthmatic symptoms.[52] The value of salmeterol therapy in this type of asthma has been assessed in 161 young adults (aged 12–35 years) who were not receiving any long-term medication (including inhaled corticosteroids or long-acting β_2-agonists). Exercise-induced bronchoconstriction (after an exercise challenge performed 30 minutes after dosing with salmeterol, 50 µg, or salbutamol, 180 µg, or placebo) was completely prevented (<10% decrease in FEV_1 from baseline) by both salbutamol and salmeterol. However, at 5.5 hours post-dose, only salmeterol remained effective in preventing exercise-induced bronchoconstriction (decrease in FEV_1: 8 *vs* 25% with salbutamol; $p<0.001$). Furthermore, at 11.5 hours post-dose, salmeterol continued to provide greater bronchoprotection than either salbutamol or placebo (decrease in FEV_1: 13, 27 and 26% for salmeterol, salbutamol and placebo, respectively; $p<0.001$ in favour of salmeterol). Thus, salmeterol was more effective than salbutamol in the short-term treatment of exercise-induced bronchoconstriction, with a single 50 µg dose offering protection against post-exercise exacerbations for up to 12 hours. However, as described in a previous section of this review, direct comparator studies have found that montelukast is more effective than salmeterol in providing sustained improvements to lung function after exercise, since after 1 week of use, salmeterol attenuated the response to salbutamol.[44,45] Therefore, although salmeterol may provide some relief of the symptoms of exercise-induced asthma in the immediate-term (up to 12 hours) it does not appear to be the therapy of choice for longer-term control of this type of asthma.[53]

Salmeterol in children

A comparison of both salmeterol, 50 μg twice daily, and beclometasone dipropionate, 200 μg twice daily, with placebo has been performed in corticosteroid-naïve children (aged 6–14 years; n=241).[21] Beclometasone was effective in reducing airway hyper-responsiveness whereas salmeterol and placebo had no effect. In terms of lung function, both salmeterol and beclometasone elicited similar improvements in FEV_1 and PEF compared with placebo, but beclometasone mediated better overall control of asthma symptoms. The incidence of adverse events was similar amongst the groups, though beclometasone decreased blood eosinophil counts whilst placebo and salmeterol did not. Also, children treated with beclometasone gained less height over the year-long study (3.96 cm), compared with placebo- (5.04 cm) or salmeterol-treated children (5.40 cm). This study suggests a greater efficacy of inhaled corticosteroid than salmeterol treatment in the control of childhood asthma, though it also raises questions about the influence of inhaled steroid treatment on growth rates in this patient population. Thus, in mild childhood asthma, salmeterol may be preferred since it may have sufficient efficacy to combat the milder symptoms without unwelcome growth-related and systemic effects.[21] However, according to current guidelines, as with adult asthmatic patients, salmeterol is recommended as an add-on therapy to those already receiving inhaled corticosteroids.

Dose-ranging studies performed in a paediatric population (4–11 years) revealed that salmeterol, 50 μg, provided superior control of asthma symptoms than a lower dose (25 μg), although both were more effective in comparison with placebo.[14] An investigation of 207 children with asthma indicated that salmeterol induced significantly greater improvements in both PEF and FEV_1 over the 12-week treatment period compared with placebo.[54] The use of rescue salbutamol was also significantly lower in the salmeterol group (0.8 *vs* 0.3 puffs per day; $p<0.005$), whilst there was also a trend towards an increased percentage of undisturbed nights with salmeterol compared with placebo (9.1 *vs* 4.1%).

A critical review of the role of long acting β_2-agonists in paediatric asthma has confirmed that salmeterol significantly improves lung function but has questioned the role of salmeterol as a clinically useful long-term add-on bronchodilator therapy.[53] Rather, the authors suggest that salmeterol may be more appropriate as an 'as-needed' daily-dose bronchodilator treatment during symptomatic periods. This aside, salmeterol appears to be an effective bronchodilator for children with moderate persistent asthma and is not associated with serious adverse events or cardiovascular changes.

You are strongly urged to consult your doctor before taking, stopping or changing any of the products reviewed or referred to in *BESTMEDICINE* or any other medication that has been prescribed or recommended by your doctor.

Safety and tolerability

The long-acting β_2-agonists are licensed as add-on therapy for asthma in children and adults. However, caution is advised when using all β_2-agonists (both short- and long-acting) in the following conditions:

- hyperthyroidism
- cardiovascular disease
- arrhythmias
- susceptibility to QT-interval prolongation
- hypertension
- pregnancy
- diabetes.

Plasma potassium levels should also be monitored in severe asthma as potentially serious hypokalaemia has been associated with the use of β_2-agonists. Much of this guidance has arisen from theoretical concerns or from preclinical or *in vitro* observations. Hypokalaemia tends to occur on initiation of treatment and to be short-lived, and appears to be more closely linked with β_2-agonists delivered either orally or by a nebuliser.[2] The following section describes studies which have specifically examined the safety of long-acting β_2-agonists in asthmatic patients.

Safety of β_2-agonists

The safety of the short-acting β_2-agonist fenoterol was the subject of much controversy in the 1990s and this led to many questions regarding the mortality effects of the β_2-agonists as a class.[2] The short- and long-term safety of salmeterol, 100 µg/day, has been examined in two large studies conducted in the UK.[55,56] The first study was a double-blind, randomised trial comparing salmeterol with salbutamol in over 25,000 patients, 60% of whom were over 40 years and 28% over 60 years.[56] Upon diagnosis of asthma, patients were prescribed appropriate bronchodilator therapy by their general practitioner and assessed at 4, 8 and 16 weeks. The only observed difference between the two treatment groups was in the incidence of withdrawals from the trial for asthma-related reasons (2.9 *vs* 3.8% for salmeterol and salbutamol, respectively; $p<0.001$). In the salmeterol group (n=16,787) there were 54 deaths (0.32%) from all causes and the majority of these were cardiovascular in nature (0.17%), followed by 12 deaths (0.07%) related to asthma. Death rates were not different in the salbutamol group (n=8393), with 20 deaths recorded from all causes (0.24%), two of which were related to asthma. All deaths due to asthma were in patients with severe asthma and no positive correlation to treatment was drawn.

The second study was a prescription-event monitoring study of 15,407 patients treated with salmeterol for at least 1 year.[55] The patient group was an equal mix of men and women of mean age 54.5 years, and the majority (70.3%) received salmeterol for asthma with the remainder either being treated for chronic obstructive airways disease (12.5%), other respiratory disease (2.0%), or an unrecorded indication (15.2%). Salmeterol was reported to be effective in 70.1% of reports that included an assessment of efficacy. Paradoxical bronchospasm was reported in only three patients from the salmeterol group. The number of deaths recorded in this study was 1022 (6.6%) and 73 of these (0.47%) were attributed to asthma. Only half of these patients were still taking salmeterol in their last month of life and in 90% of these, no association was drawn between salmeterol and cause of death. The death rate in this study was higher than that observed in the previous study described, but the authors attribute this difference to an older and more severely ill study population and to the longer duration of the trial.[55,56]

These data and those from other studies indicate that, despite previous fears of an association between an increased risk of death from asthma and the regular use of inhaled β_2-agonist bronchodilators, salmeterol does not appear to contribute to increased mortality in asthma sufferers.[2,55–60] Rather, any increase in adverse events or death in those using β_2-agonists long-term is thought more likely to be related to the increased severity of disease in such a patient population. However, concerns persist regarding the use of salmeterol therapy in the absence of corticosteroid use, where salmeterol has been positively associated with increased numbers of asthma-related deaths compared with placebo (13 *vs* 4 of ~26,000 study population; *p*-values unavailable).[8] In contrast, no differences in primary events (i.e. the combined number of respiratory related deaths and respiratory related life-threatening experiences, such as intubation or mechanical ventilation) or asthma-related events, including death, were observed in those receiving concomitant corticosteroid therapies. These data, therefore, further reinforce the need to administer inhaled corticosteroids concomitantly and in addition to salmeterol.[3] This requirement also provides much of the rationale for switching patients to combination inhalers containing both corticosteroid and β_2-agonist (i.e. Seretide®, a combination of fluticasone and salmeterol).

Salmeterol does not appear to contribute to increased mortality in asthma sufferers.

Cardiovascular safety of salmeterol

High doses of short-acting β_2-agonists have been associated with adverse cardiovascular events including palpitations, changes in blood pressure and ECG abnormalities.[61] It is thought that any adverse effects on cardiovascular function are caused by cross-stimulation of salmeterol upon the β_1-adrenoceptors in cardiac tissue. Thus, the long-term (1 year) cardiovascular safety of salmeterol powder (50 μg twice daily) was examined in a group of 352 patients aged over 12 years with chronic persistent asthma.[61] No deaths were reported in the study and the incidence of drug-related adverse cardiovascular events (such as raised blood pressure, palpitations or abnormal ECG) was not different between the salmeterol and placebo groups (2% in each). Furthermore, there were no differences in mean pulse rate or mean, maximum or minimum heart rates deduced from 24 hour Holter monitoring. No differences were reported in plasma electrolytes, though two patients from the salmeterol group had low potassium concentrations but levels were in the normal range upon retesting. Greater increases in systolic blood pressure (1–2 mmHg) were observed with salmeterol therapy ($p<0.05$ *vs* placebo), but changes in diastolic blood pressure remained similar in both groups. These small differences were not thought to be of clinical relevance. Similarly, less than 1% of salmeterol-treated patients exhibited abnormal ECGs, which were considered to be clinically significant. In particular, no differences in QTc intervals were observed between salmeterol- and placebo-treated patients at any time-points, with no arrhythmias reported. Despite this, it is still recommended that β_2-agonists are used with caution in those with either arrhythmias, susceptibility to prolonged QT interval, cardiovascular disease or hypertension. However, this and other studies have confirmed that salmeterol is not associated with any adverse cardiovascular events or clinically significant changes in cardiovascular function.[2,3,61,62]

Salmeterol is not associated with any adverse cardiovascular events or clinically significant changes in cardiovascular function.

Use in pregnancy

In the prescription-event monitoring study described above, 93 pregnancies were reported, with 67% taking salmeterol during the first trimester of pregnancy.[55] Of these, two women gave birth to babies who later developed asthma, but given that asthma has a strong heritable component these occurrences are unlikely to be drug-related. It is particularly important that asthma is well controlled during pregnancy, and it is advised that any anti-asthma therapies should be given via inhalation, where possible, to minimise exposure to the foetus.

Drug–drug interactions

The metabolism of salmeterol occurs via the CYP3A4 isoenzyme, thus any inhibitors of this enzyme are likely to increase exposure to fluticasone. Inhibitors of CYP3A4 include grapefruit juice, ketoconazole, itraconazole and ritonavir, and the latter, at 100 mg twice daily, was shown to increase the plasma concentration of fluticasone several hundred fold and markedly reduce serum cortisol levels.[63]

Adverse event profile

There are several minor adverse effects of the β_2-agonists, which one would expect to occur upon absorption into the systemic circulation and subsequent stimulation of non-respiratory β-adrenoceptors.[2] Stimulation of cardiac β_2-adrenoceptors induces increased rate and force of cardiac contractions often manifesting as palpitations, whilst skeletal muscle receptor activation results in tremor and may also contribute to metabolic effects including hypokalaemia and hyperglycaemia. Effects of the β_2-agonists on vascular tissue can cause peripheral vasodilation, which may result in headaches and/or reduced blood pressure.

Stimulation of cardiac β_2-adrenoceptors induces increased rate and force of cardiac contractions often manifesting as palpitations.

In a 12-week, randomised, placebo-controlled, double-blind comparison of salmeterol and salbutamol in 556 subjects (aged

12–73 years) with mild-to-moderate chronic asthma, the most frequent adverse event reported was headache, which occurred at a frequency of 9–10% in all treatment groups. Tremor and dizziness were also reported at a similar frequency in all three groups (1–3%).[62] This low rate of adverse events was corroborated in a further 12-week clinical trial, of similar design, in which all adverse events occurred in less than 1% of patients.[34]

In a dose-ranging trial examining salmeterol (12.5–100 μg twice daily) in sufferers of mild-to-moderate asthma over 1 week, the only adverse event to occur more frequently with active treatment than with placebo was tremor. However, this was observed only in those treated with salmeterol at 100 μg twice daily and occurred in five of the 154 patients enrolled.[16]

Adverse events reported after year-long treatment with salmeterol are summarised in Table 2.[55] The rate ratio is an indicator of whether a specific adverse event is causally associated with drug treatment. Thus, although the incidence of both headache and tremor were reported at a similar frequency during the first month of treatment, only tremor was deemed significantly associated with salmeterol use. Malaise and lassitude, palpitation and tachycardia were also regarded as positively linked to salmeterol treatment.

Although the incidence of both headache and tremor were reported a similar number of times in the first month of treatment, only tremor was deemed significantly associated with salmeterol use.

Table 2. Incidence of adverse events after 1 month of salmeterol therapy.[55]

Event	Number of times reported in month 1 of treatment	Rate ratio[a]
Malaise, lassitude	31	3.4
Malaise	20	4.8
Headache, migraine	54	2.1
Headache	54	2.6
Tremor	47	7.3
Tachycardia	15	5.4
Palpitation	25	4.5
Asthma	221	1.7
Wheezing	38	2.3
Cough	46	2.2
Dyspnoea	45	2.9
Respiratory tract infection	365	1.6
Chest infection	191	1.8
Upper respiratory tract infection	40	1.8
Nausea, vomiting	35	2.5
Non-surgical admissions	100	2.2

[a]Rate ratio, event rate per 1000 patients in month 1 divided by event rate in months 2–6. Event rates exceeding 3 are considered to represent an adverse event related to study drug treatment.

Key points

- Salmeterol is a β_2-adrenoceptor agonist with a prolonged duration of action providing sustained bronchodilation in patients with asthma.
- Salmeterol may be administered via inhalation of either a micronised powder form or aerosol suspension. Both formulations have equivalent clinical efficacy.
- A 50 μg dose of salbutamol, administered twice daily, appears to provide optimal management of asthma in both children and adults, with minimal reported side-effects.
- Salmeterol should always be used in addition to existing inhaled corticosteroid treatment since its use as monotherapy has been linked to an increased risk of asthma-related deaths.
- In comparison with placebo, salmeterol improves patients' quality of life, reduces the need for rescue β_2-agonist therapy and improves the percentage of symptom-free days and nights.
- Salmeterol provides sustained increases in FEV_1 and morning and evening PEF over its 12-hour duration of action.
- Salmeterol is more effective than regular administration of short-term β_2-agonist therapies, such as salbutamol, but provides equivalent clinical efficacy to the other long-acting β_2-agonists, formoterol and bambuterol, in the control of asthma.
- Salmeterol provides effective treatment of nocturnal asthma and chronic asthma but is less effective than montelukast for exercise-induced asthma.
- Salmeterol has an excellent safety and tolerability profile. It is associated with a low incidence of adverse events, with the most common events reported being headache or tremor.

References

A list of the published evidence which has been reviewed in compiling the preceding section of *BESTMEDICINE.*

1 Waldeck B. Beta-adrenoceptor agonists and asthma—100 years of development. *Eur J Pharmacol* 2002; **445**: 1–12.
2 Abramson MJ, Walters J, Walters EH. Adverse effects of beta-agonists: are they clinically relevant? *Am J Respir Med* 2003; **2**: 287–97.
3 Jackson CM, Lipworth B. Benefit-risk assessment of long-acting beta2-agonists in asthma. *Drug Saf* 2004; **27**: 243–70.
4 Adkins JC, McTavish D. Salmeterol. A review of its pharmacological properties and clinical efficacy in the management of children with asthma. *Drugs* 1997; **54**: 331–54.
5 Buchwald A, Hochhaus G. Pharmacokinetic and pharmacodynamic aspects of salmeterol therapy. *Int J Clin Pharmacol Ther* 1998; **36**: 652–60.
6 Boulton DW, Fawcett JP. Beta2-agonist eutomers: a rational option for the treatment of asthma? *Am J Respir Med* 2002; **1**: 305–11.
7 Brogden RN, Faulds D. Salmeterol xinafoate. A review of its pharmacological properties and therapeutic potential in reversible obstructive airways disease. *Drugs* 1991; **42**: 895–912.
8 Wooltorton E. Salmeterol (Serevent) asthma trial halted early. *CMAJ* 2003; **168**: 738.
9 Kirby S, Falcoz C, Daniel MJ *et al.* Salmeterol and fluticasone propionate given as a combination. Lack of systemic pharmacodynamic and pharmacokinetic interactions. *Eur J Clin Pharmacol* 2001; **56**: 781–91.
10 Ullman A, Svedmyr N. Salmeterol, a new long acting inhaled beta 2 adrenoceptor agonist: comparison with salbutamol in adult asthmatic patients. *Thorax* 1988; **43**: 674–8.
11 Hanania NA, Moore RH. Anti-inflammatory activities of beta2-agonists. *Curr Drug Targets Inflamm Allergy* 2004; **3**: 271–7.
12 Johnson M. Effects of beta2-agonists on resident and infiltrating inflammatory cells. *J Allergy Clin Immunol* 2002; 110: S282–90.
13 Lazarus SC, Boushey HA, Fahy JV *et al.* Long-acting beta2-agonist monotherapy *vs* continued therapy with inhaled corticosteroids in patients with persistent asthma: a randomized controlled trial. *JAMA* 2001; **285**: 2583–93.
14 Weinstein S, Chervinsky P, Pollard SJ *et al.* A one-week dose-ranging study of inhaled salmeterol in children with asthma. *J Asthma* 1997; **34**: 43–52.
15 Lenney W, Pedersen S, Boner AL, Ebbutt A, Jenkins MM. Efficacy and safety of salmeterol in childhood asthma. *Eur J Pediatr* 1995; **154**: 983–90.
16 Bronsky EA, Kemp JP, Orgel HA *et al.* A 1-week dose-ranging study of inhaled salmeterol in patients with asthma. *Chest* 1994; **105**: 1032–7.
17 Palmer JB, Stuart AM, Shepherd GL, Viskum K. Inhaled salmeterol in the treatment of patients with moderate to severe reversible obstructive airways disease – a 3-month comparison of the efficacy and safety of twice-daily salmeterol (100 micrograms) with salmeterol (50 micrograms). *Respir Med* 1992; **86**: 409–17.
18 Wolfe J, Kreitzer S, Chervinsky P *et al.* Comparison of powder and aerosol formulations of salmeterol in the treatment of asthma. *Ann Allergy Asthma Immunol* 2000; **84**: 334–40.
19 Campbell LM, Anderson TJ, Parashchak MR *et al.* A comparison of the efficacy of long-acting beta 2-agonists: eformoterol via Turbohaler and salmeterol via pressurized metered dose inhaler or Accuhaler, in mild to moderate asthmatics. Force Research Group. *Respir Med* 1999; **93**: 236–44.
20 Nathan RA, Pinnas JL, Schwartz HJ *et al.* A six-month, placebo-controlled comparison of the safety and efficacy of salmeterol or beclomethasone for persistent asthma. *Ann Allergy Asthma Immunol* 1999; **82**: 521–9.
21 Simons FE. A comparison of beclomethasone, salmeterol, and placebo in children with asthma. Canadian Beclomethasone Dipropionate-Salmeterol Xinafoate Study Group. *N Engl J Med* 1997; **337**: 1659–65.
22 Rosenthal RR, Busse WW, Kemp JP *et al.* Effect of long-term salmeterol therapy compared with as-needed albuterol use on airway hyperresponsiveness. *Chest* 1999; **116**: 595–602.
23 Greening AP, Ind PW, Northfield M, Shaw G. Added salmeterol versus higher-dose corticosteroid in asthma patients with symptoms on existing inhaled corticosteroid. Allen & Hanburys Limited UK Study Group. *Lancet* 1994; **344**: 219–24.
24 Woolcock A, Lundback B, Ringdal N, Jacques LA. Comparison of addition of salmeterol to inhaled steroids with doubling of the dose of inhaled steroids. *Am J Respir Crit Care Med* 1996; **153**: 1481–8.
25 Shrewsbury S, Pyke S, Britton M. Meta-analysis of increased dose of inhaled steroid or addition of salmeterol in symptomatic asthma (MIASMA). *BMJ* 2000; **320**: 1368–73.
26 BTS/SIGN. British guideline on the management of asthma. British Thoracic Society Scottish Intercollegiate Guidelines Network, 2004.
27 Lemanske RF, Sorkness CA, Mauger EA *et al.* Inhaled corticosteroid reduction and elimination in patients with persistent asthma receiving salmeterol: a randomized controlled trial. *JAMA* 2001; **285**: 2594–603.
28 Wilding P, Clark M, Thompson Coon J *et al.* Effect of long-term treatment with salmeterol on asthma control: a double blind, randomised crossover study. *BMJ* 1997; **314**: 1441–6.

29 Kemp JP, DeGraff AC, Jr., Pearlman DS *et al.* A 1-year study of salmeterol powder on pulmonary function and hyperresponsiveness to methacholine. *J Allergy Clin Immunol* 1999; **104**: 1189–97.

30 Kemp JP, Cook DA, Incaudo GA *et al.* Salmeterol improves quality of life in patients with asthma requiring inhaled corticosteroids. Salmeterol Quality of Life Study Group. *J Allergy Clin Immunol* 1998; **101**: 188–95.

31 Busse WW, Casale TB, Murray JJ *et al.* Efficacy, safety, and impact on quality of life of salmeterol in patients with moderate persistent asthma. *Am J Manag Care* 1998; **4**: 1579–87.

32 D'Alonzo GE, Nathan RA, Henochowicz S *et al.* Salmeterol xinafoate as maintenance therapy compared with albuterol in patients with asthma. *JAMA* 1994; **271**: 1412–6.

33 Kemp J, Wolfe J, Grady J *et al.* Salmeterol powder compared with albuterol aerosol as maintenance therapy for asthma in adolescent and adult patients. *Clin Ther* 1998; **20**: 270–82.

34 Wenzel SE, Lumry W, Manning M *et al.* Efficacy, safety, and effects on quality of life of salmeterol versus albuterol in patients with mild to moderate persistent asthma. *Ann Allergy Asthma Immunol* 1998; **80**: 463–70.

35 Boulet LP, Laviolette M, Boucher S *et al.* A twelve-week comparison of salmeterol and salbutamol in the treatment of mild-to-moderate asthma: a Canadian multicenter study. *J Allergy Clin Immunol* 1997; **99**: 13–21.

36 Leblanc P, Knight A, Kreisman H, Borkhoff CM, Johnston PR. A placebo-controlled, crossover comparison of salmeterol and salbutamol in patients with asthma. *Am J Respir Crit Care Med* 1996; **154**: 324–8.

37 Lundback B, Rawlinson DW, Palmer JB. Twelve month comparison of salmeterol and salbutamol as dry powder formulations in asthmatic patients. European Study Group. *Thorax* 1993; **48**: 148–53.

38 Taylor DR, Town GI, Herbison GP *et al.* Asthma control during long-term treatment with regular inhaled salbutamol and salmeterol. *Thorax* 1998; **53**: 744–52.

39 Davies B, Brooks G, Devoy M. The efficacy and safety of salmeterol compared to theophylline: meta-analysis of nine controlled studies. *Respir Med* 1998; **92**: 256–63.

40 Pollard SJ, Spector SL, Yancey SW, Cox FM, Emmett A. Salmeterol versus theophylline in the treatment of asthma. *Ann Allergy Asthma Immunol* 1997; **78**: 457–64.

41 Spahr JE, Krawiec ME. Leukotriene receptor antagonists – risks and benefits for use in paediatric asthma. *Expert Opin Drug Saf* 2004; **3**: 173–85.

42 Bjermer L, Bisgaard H, Bousquet J *et al.* Montelukast and fluticasone compared with salmeterol and fluticasone in protecting against asthma exacerbation in adults: one year, double blind, randomised, comparative trial. *BMJ* 2003; **327**: 891.

43 Ringdal N. Long-acting beta2-agonists or leukotriene receptor antagonists as add-on therapy to inhaled corticosteroids for the treatment of persistent asthma. *Drugs* 2003; **63(Suppl 2)**: 21–33.

44 Edelman JM, Turpin JA, Bronsky EA *et al.* Oral montelukast compared with inhaled salmeterol to prevent exercise-induced bronchoconstriction. A randomized, double-blind trial. Exercise Study Group. *Ann Intern Med* 2000; **132**: 97–104.

45 Storms W, Chervinsky P, Ghannam AF *et al.* A comparison of the effects of oral montelukast and inhaled salmeterol on response to rescue bronchodilation after challenge. *Respir Med* 2004; **98**: 1051–62.

46 Crompton GK, Ayres JG, Basran G *et al.* Comparison of oral bambuterol and inhaled salmeterol in patients with symptomatic asthma and using inhaled corticosteroids. *Am J Respir Crit Care Med* 1999; **159**: 824–8.

47 Vervloet D, Ekstrom T, Pela R *et al.* A 6-month comparison between formoterol and salmeterol in patients with reversible obstructive airways disease. *Respir Med* 1998; **92**: 836–42.

48 Boyd G. Salmeterol xinafoate in asthmatic patients under consideration for maintenance oral corticosteroid therapy. UK Study Group. *Eur Respir J* 1995; **8**: 1494–8.

49 Faurschou P, Steffensen I, Jacques L. Effect of addition of inhaled salmeterol to the treatment of moderate-to-severe asthmatics uncontrolled on high-dose inhaled steroids. European Respiratory Study Group. *Eur Respir J* 1996; **9**: 1885–90.

50 Wiegand L, Mende CN, Zaidel G *et al.* Salmeterol *vs* theophylline: sleep and efficacy outcomes in patients with nocturnal asthma. *Chest* 1999; **115**: 1525–32.

51 Selby C, Engleman HM, Fitzpatrick MF *et al.* Inhaled salmeterol or oral theophylline in nocturnal asthma? *Am J Respir Crit Care Med* 1997; **155**: 104–8.

52 Kemp JP, Dockhorn RJ, Busse WW, Bleecker ER, Van As A. Prolonged effect of inhaled salmeterol against exercise-induced bronchospasm. *Am J Respir Crit Care Med* 1994; **150**: 1612–15.

53 Bisgaard H. Long-acting beta(2)-agonists in management of childhood asthma: A critical review of the literature. *Pediatr Pulmonol* 2000; 29: 221–34.

54 Weinstein SF, Pearlman DS, Bronsky EA *et al.* Efficacy of salmeterol xinafoate powder in children with chronic persistent asthma. *Ann Allergy Asthma Immunol* 1998; **81**: 51–8.

55 Mann RD, Kubota K, Pearce G, Wilton L. Salmeterol: a study by prescription-event monitoring in a UK cohort of 15,407 patients. *J Clin Epidemiol* 1996; **49**: 247–50.

56 Castle W, Fuller R, Hall J, Palmer J. Serevent nationwide surveillance study: comparison of salmeterol with salbutamol in asthmatic patients who require regular bronchodilator treatment. *BMJ* 1993; **306**: 1034–7.

57 Spitzer WO, Suissa S, Ernst P *et al.* The use of beta-agonists and the risk of death and near death from asthma. *N Engl J Med* 1992; **326**: 501–6.
58 Suissa S, Hemmelgarn B, Blais L, Ernst P. Bronchodilators and acute cardiac death. *Am J Respir Crit Care Med* 1996; **154**: 1598–602.
59 Williams C, Crossland L, Finnerty J *et al.* Case-control study of salmeterol and near-fatal attacks of asthma. *Thorax* 1998; **53**: 7–13.
60 Shrewsbury S, Hallett C. Salmeterol 100 microg: an analysis of its tolerability in single- and chronic-dose studies. *Ann Allergy Asthma Immunol* 2001; **87**: 465–73.
61 Chervinsky P, Goldberg P, Galant S *et al.* Long-term cardiovascular safety of salmeterol powder pharmacotherapy in adolescent and adult patients with chronic persistent asthma: a randomized clinical trial. *Chest* 1999; **115**: 642–8.
62 Nathan RA, Seltzer JM, Kemp JP *et al.* Safety of salmeterol in the maintenance treatment of asthma. *Ann Allergy Asthma Immunol* 1995; **75**: 243–8.
63 Allen and Hanburys Ltd. Serevent® (salmeterol). *Summary of product characteristics.* Uxbridge, Middlesex, 2004.

Acknowledgements

Figure 2 is adapted from Bronsky *et al.*, 1994.[16]
Figure 3 is adapted from Wolfe *et al.*, 2000.[18]
Figure 4 is adapted from Lazarus *et al.*, 2001.[13]
Figure 5 is adapted from Kemp *et al.*, 1998.[30]
Figure 6 is adapted from Kemp *et al.*, 1998.[33]

10. Drug review – Seretide®

Dr Rebecca Fox-Spencer
CSF Medical Communications Ltd

You are strongly urged to consult your doctor before taking, stopping or changing any of the products reviewed or referred to in *BESTMEDICINE* or any other medication that has been prescribed or recommended by your doctor.

Summary

Seretide® is a combination therapy comprising an inhaled corticosteroid, fluticasone propionate, and a long-acting β_2-agonist, salmeterol xinafoate. It is licensed for the prophylactic management of asthma, in adults and children whose asthma is inadequately controlled by inhaled corticosteroids and as-needed short-acting β_2-agonists, or already adequately controlled by inhaled corticosteroids and long-acting β_2-agonists. In addition to a clear superiority over placebo and its constituent monotherapies, Seretide improves pulmonary function and symptom control by a greater extent than a doubling of fluticasone dosage. It is also at least as effective as a combination of fluticasone and the oral leukotriene receptor antagonist, montelukast, further reinforcing the recommendation that long-acting β_2-agonists are the first-line option for add-on therapy in poorly-controlled asthma. The only other combination product available in the UK, Symbicort® – a combination of budesonide and formoterol fumarate – has been shown to offer comparable benefit to Seretide. The combination of salmeterol and fluticasone is equally well tolerated as fluticasone monotherapy, whilst the safety concerns regarding the risk of respiratory related life-threatening events with salmeterol monotherapy do not appear to apply when it is used in combination with inhaled corticosteroids.

Introduction

Inhaled corticosteroids are recommended by national and international guidelines as the maintenance therapy of choice for persistent asthma. This class of drugs effectively combats the underlying inflammatory processes associated with asthma, which if poorly controlled, can lead to permanent airway remodelling. Although inhaled corticosteroids remain unrivalled as the first-line treatment option for persistent asthma in all but the mildest of cases, a considerable proportion of patients remain symptomatic on low-to-moderate doses. Dose escalation is an option available to physicians, but concern persists over the systemic adverse event profile of high doses of inhaled corticosteroids. This is particularly pertinent in the case of paediatric patients with asthma, who form a considerable proportion of the total asthmatic population, and in whom reduced growth velocity has been demonstrated following treatment with certain inhaled corticosteroids.[1] Aside from the safety concerns associated with dose escalation, it is also recognised that inhaled corticosteroids have a relatively flat dose–response curve.[2] Given these considerations, it is recommended that the preferable strategy in these patients is to supplement steroid treatment with a second 'add-on' drug with a complementary mechanism of action.[3]

Long-acting β_2-agonists are currently recommended as the first-line add-on therapy for concurrent use with inhaled corticosteroids, in patients whose asthma is inadequately controlled by corticosteroids alone.

Alongside airway inflammation, bronchoconstriction has a major role in the pathogenesis of asthma. Thus, long-acting β_2-agonists are currently recommended as the first-line add-on therapy for concurrent use with inhaled corticosteroids, in patients whose asthma is inadequately controlled by corticosteroids alone.[3,4] Pioneering studies in the 1990s reported greater average effects on asthma control as a result of adding salmeterol to beclometasone dipropionate therapy compared with doubling the dose of the corticosteroid, though there was considerable variation in the response.[5,6] Since then, robust clinical benefits have been further demonstrated for concurrent use of these two drug classes. Nonetheless, the efficacy of inhaled therapy for asthma remains subject to limitations determined by patient compliance. In the light of these considerations, combination therapies have now been introduced that are delivered from a single inhalation device. Seretide, which consists of the inhaled corticosteroid fluticasone propionate (hereafter referred to as fluticasone) and the long-acting β_2-agonist salmeterol xinafoate (hereafter referred to as salmeterol) combined in a single inhalation device, is the subject of this review.

Although the dose of salmeterol in Seretide is fixed at 50 μg, the dosage of the fluticasone component is variable at 100, 250 or 500 μg. Thus, the doses of Seretide referred to in this review are identified as 50/100, 50/250 or 50/500 μg. Where fluticasone and salmeterol are not administered in a single inhalation device, but concurrently in individual inhalers, the combination is referred to as the two component drugs rather than as Seretide *per se*, though the doses are expressed in the same way.

The most common means by which Seretide is administered is via a dry powder inhaler (DPI). Drug delivery from a DPI is breath actuated, thus it is particularly suitable for those with poor hand–breath coordination, such as young children. The DPI device used for administration of Seretide in the UK is branded the Accuhaler®, whist in the US (and much of the rest of the world) the equivalent device is called the Diskus®, and the drug marketed as Advair®. Alternatively, Seretide may be delivered via a metered dose inhaler (MDI). This device delivers a fixed dose of drug per actuation, such that lung deposition, unlike with the DPI, is independent of inspiratory flow rate. As a result, some MDI doses referred to in this review do not conform to the standard three doses of Seretide described previously. Although the dose of drug administered ('ex-valve') may be 50/100 μg, for example, the actual doses delivered may be given as 42 and 88 μg, respectively.[7] Correct use of the MDI requires some hand–breath coordination, the need for which can, however, be reduced by use of a spacer device. When delivered by MDI, Seretide must be formulated with a propellant. Traditionally, chlorofluorocarbons (CFCs) have been used for this purpose. Due to environmental concerns, however, international guidelines have called for the phasing out of CFC-dependent inhalation devices.[8] A non-CFC formulation of Seretide is now available in the UK, utilising hydrofluoroalkane (HFA) 134a as the propellant molecule. This formulation of Seretide is delivered by an MDI device with the trade name Evohaler®.

Pharmacology

Chemistry

The chemical structures of fluticasone propionate and salmeterol xinafoate are shown in Figure 1. It has been suggested that the two drugs form particle agglomerations within the inhaler, and that these persist following delivery from the device.[9] This interaction may have the potential to alter the deposition patterns of the two drugs administered concurrently via separate inhalers. Further investigation is required, however, into the nature of the physical interaction between the two drugs.

The chemistry of Seretide® is of essentially academic interest and most healthcare professionals will, like you, skip this section.

Figure 1. The chemical structures of fluticasone (bottom) and salmeterol (top).

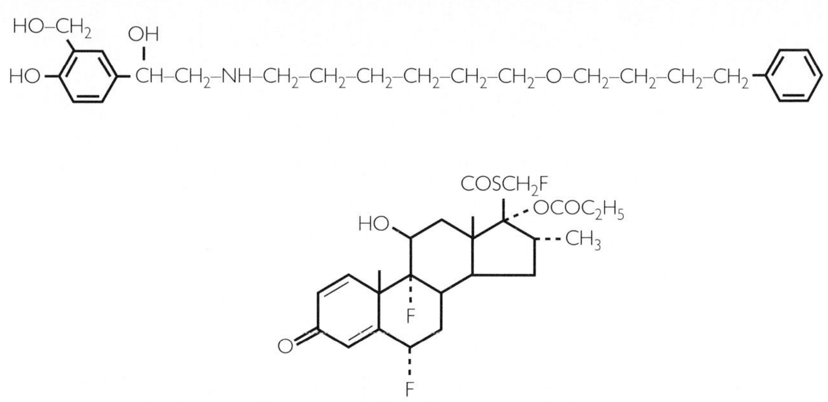

Mechanism of action

Fluticasone

Inhaled corticosteroids act to reduce levels of inflammation in the airways. Following inhalation, fluticasone is taken up into the cytoplasm of the cells lining the airways, where it binds to glucocorticoid receptors. Following translocation of the corticosteroid–receptor complex to the cell nucleus, it down-regulates the transcription of a range of inflammatory mediators (e.g. histamine, leukotrienes, cytokines and eicosanoids). Corticosteroids also reduce mucosal oedema and mucus secretion, whilst persistent, long-term use is associated with a reduction in the number of mast cells in the airways. Importantly in the context of concurrent use of fluticasone with a long-acting β_2-agonist, inhaled corticosteroids also appear to potentiate β-adrenergic responsiveness and increase the rate of synthesis of β_2-adrenoceptors.[10]

Salmeterol

β_2-agonists are derivatives of adrenaline, the natural agonist of β_2-adrenoceptors. Adrenaline acts rapidly to dilate the airways, by inducing relaxation of bronchial smooth muscle. Although adrenaline has historically been used in a clinical setting, and is still used in certain emergency situations for the treatment of asthma, β_2-agonists are associated with fewer side-effects. Salmeterol is a long-acting β_2-agonist, inducing bronchodilation which persists for at least 12 hours. As a result, it is protective against bronchoconstriction induced by histamine, methacholine, cold air and against exercise-induced asthma.

Fluticasone and salmeterol in combination

Fluticasone increases the responsiveness and number of β_2-adrenergic receptors, though it has not yet been consistently demonstrated that salmeterol exerts any meaningful anti-inflammatory activity *in vivo*.

By virtue of their complementary modes of action, the combination of fluticasone and salmeterol forms a more complete defence against asthma exacerbations than either drug in isolation. Furthermore, there is some evidence to suggest that two components of Seretide may interact synergistically rather than merely having additive clinical effects.[11] Fluticasone, for example, increases the responsiveness and number of β_2-adrenoceptors, and therefore has the potential to augment the efficacy of salmeterol (Figure 2).[12] However, the mechanism by which salmeterol impacts upon the anti-inflammatory properties of fluticasone is less clear. In support of a potentiating effect upon the anti-inflammatory response of fluticasone, it has been reported that salmeterol enhances the ability of fluticasone to induce apoptosis in eosinophils by between three- and five-fold.[10] Furthermore, *in vitro* data have suggested that long-acting β_2-agonists may prime the corticosteroid receptor for ligand binding and, subsequent to this, enhances the translocation of the corticosteroid–receptor complex to the nucleus (Figure 2).[13] In patients with mild persistent asthma receiving inhaled fluticasone, supplementary treatment with salmeterol was reported to improve airway hyper-responsiveness to methacholine (a surrogate marker of airway inflammation) compared with fluticasone treatment alone.[14] Aside from

Figure 2. Schematic diagram to demonstrate priming of inactive corticosteroid receptors by β_2-agonists (top) and up-regulation of the number of β_2-adrenoceptors and their sensitivity to β_2-agonists by corticosteroids (bottom).[12]

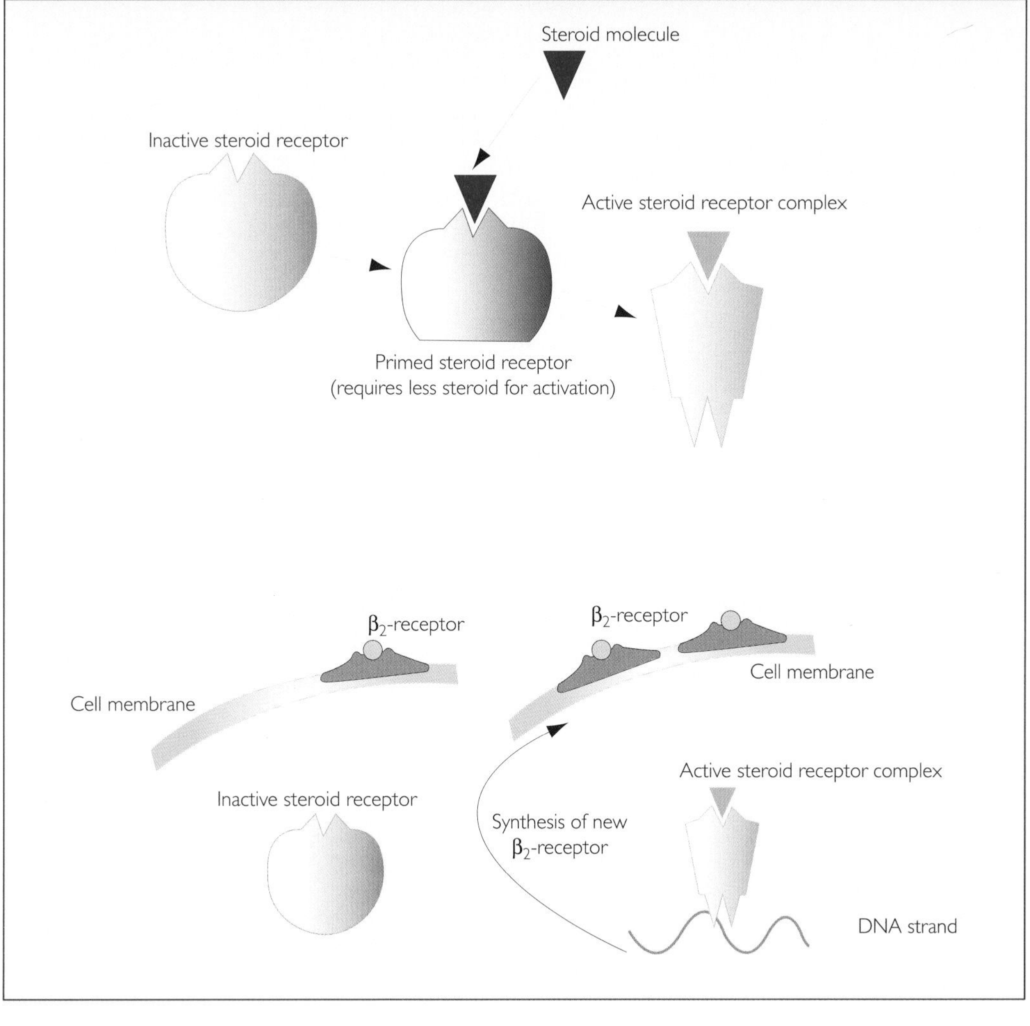

this report and the *in vitro* data, however, it has not yet been consistently demonstrated that salmeterol exerts any meaningful anti-inflammatory activity *in vivo*. Indeed, it has been reported that in patients with moderate persistent asthma, long-acting β_2-agonists afford no additional anti-inflammatory action when co-administered with an inhaled corticosteroid (as determined by measuring levels of exhaled nitric oxide and eosinophilic cationic protein).[13]

The pharmacokinetics of a drug are of interest to healthcare professionals because it is important for them to understand the action of a drug on the body over a period of time.

Pharmacokinetics

Both salmeterol and fluticasone are highly lipophilic, and therefore absorption into the bronchial mucosa is slow, increasing the time both agents spend in contact with the lung surface.[15] As a result, pharmacokinetic data for inhaled salmeterol and fluticasone are limited, since both drugs act locally in the lung, and plasma concentrations following inhaled doses are practically undetectable.[15] For example, the maximum detectable plasma concentration of inhaled salmeterol is only 200 pg/mL.[16] The absolute systemic bioavailability of fluticasone is approximately 12–26% of the inhaled dose, with systemic absorption occurring mainly through the lungs.[17] Plasma protein binding of fluticasone is high, at approximately 91%.[18] Fluticasone is subject to extensive first-pass metabolism, but corresponding data is not available for salmeterol due to its low plasma concentrations.[17,19]

There appears to be no pharmacokinetic or pharmacodynamic interaction between the two drugs when they are administered in combination.

There appears to be no pharmacokinetic or pharmacodynamic interaction between the two drugs when they are administered in combination. A study of healthy volunteers has compared Seretide (100/500 μg) with the two monotherapies and a placebo group, each administered by a DPI.[20] In the 28 subjects, aged between 21 and 48 years, the pharmacokinetics and systemic exposure of each drug was found to be unaffected by co-administration with the other. It has been reported that patients treated with repeated doses of β_2-agonists often develop tachyphylaxis in response. However, in this study, the development of salmeterol-induced tachyphylaxis to cumulative doses of salbutamol was unaffected by the co-administration of fluticasone, and the combined therapy was not associated with any resensitisation of systemic β_2-adrenoceptors.[20]

Both salmeterol and fluticasone are metabolised in the liver by the cytochrome P450 (CYP) 3A4 isozyme.[20] Following an oral dose of fluticasone, 87–100% is excreted in the faeces, with renal clearance accounting for less than 0.02% of the total clearance.[15,17] At least 75% of the excreted drug is in the form of the parent compound, but an inactive metabolite (a 17β-carboxylic acid derivative) is also detectable.[15,17] Salmeterol is also excreted predominantly in the faeces (57.4% [*vs* 23% in the urine]), primarily in the form of the metabolite α-hydroxy-salmeterol.[15]

Clinical efficacy

Seretide vs fluticasone and salmeterol as monotherapy

A number of clinical trials have evaluated the relative benefits of Seretide (fluticasone and salmeterol combination delivered from a single DPI device), in comparison with equivalent doses of the individual drugs that make up the combination. Two such studies took the form of randomised, placebo-controlled trials, and are summarised in Table 1.[21,22] Aside from the fact that one was double- and the other single-blinded, these trials were virtually identical in design, and, for the most part, concurred in their findings. Following 12 weeks' treatment, Seretide was shown to be significantly superior to placebo in all efficacy parameters measured (forced expiratory volume in 1 second [FEV_1], area under the 12-hour serial FEV_1 curve relative to baseline, morning and evening peak expiratory flow [PEF], asthma symptom score, percentage days with no asthma symptoms, percentage days with no awakenings

Table 1. Summary of placebo-controlled trials examining the efficacy and safety of Seretide, salmeterol and fluticasone.[21,22]

Study design and dosage regimen	Asthma severity at baseline	Main outcomes
Kavuru *et al.*, 2000[21] Double-blind 12 weeks Patients aged ≥12 years (n=356) Seretide (50/100 μg), salmeterol (50 μg), fluticasone (100 μg), or placebo Each administered twice daily via a DPI	Asthma requiring pharmacotherapy for at least 6 months Mean FEV_1 40–85% of predicted value Increase in FEV_1 of ≥15% 30 minutes after inhaled salbutamol (180 μg)	• The mean change from baseline in FEV_1 (L) at 12 weeks was significantly greater ($p \leq 0.027$) than placebo (+0.01) following treatment with Seretide (+0.51) or fluticasone (+0.28), but not after salmeterol treatment (+0.11). Seretide was also significantly superior to fluticasone ($p<0.001$) and salmeterol ($p \leq 0.013$). • The mean AUC relative to baseline at 12 weeks was significantly greater than placebo in all treatment groups (Seretide, 8.94; salmeterol, 6.3; fluticasone, 5.41; placebo, 3.01; $p \leq 0.027$). • The mean change from baseline in morning PEF (L/minute) at 12 weeks was significantly greater ($p \leq 0.013$) than placebo (–23.7) following treatment with Seretide (+52.5), fluticasone (+17.3) or salmeterol (–1.7). Seretide was also significantly superior to fluticasone ($p \leq 0.025$) and salmeterol ($p \leq 0.023$). • The mean change from baseline in evening PEF (L/minute) at 12 weeks was significantly greater ($p \leq 0.013$) than placebo (–13.3) following treatment with Seretide (+35.0) or fluticasone (+18.0), but not with salmeterol (–7.4). Seretide was also significantly superior to fluticasone ($p \leq 0.025$) and salmeterol ($p \leq 0.023$). • The mean change from baseline in asthma symptom score at 12 weeks was significantly greater ($p \leq 0.013$) than placebo (+0.4) following treatment with Seretide (–0.7), fluticasone (–0.2) or salmeterol (–0.1). Seretide was also significantly superior to fluticasone ($p \leq 0.025$) and salmeterol ($p \leq 0.023$). • The mean change from baseline in percentage of days with no asthma symptoms at 12 weeks was significantly greater ($p \leq 0.013$) than placebo (–3.8) following treatment with Seretide (+22.6) or salmeterol (+8.0), but not with fluticasone (+7.2). Seretide was also significantly superior to fluticasone ($p \leq 0.025$) and salmeterol ($p \leq 0.023$). • The mean change from baseline in percentage of nights with no awakenings at 12 weeks was significantly greater ($p \leq 0.013$) than placebo (–16.5) following treatment with Seretide (+4.6), fluticasone (+2.4) or salmeterol (–5.3). Seretide was also significantly superior to salmeterol ($p \leq 0.023$) but not fluticasone.

AUC, area under the 12-hour serial FEV_1 curve; DPI, dry powder inhaler; FEV_1, forced expiratory volume in 1 second; PEF, peak expiratory flow.

Table 1. Continued

Study design and dosage regimen	Asthma severity at baseline	Main outcomes
Kavuru *et al.*, 2000[21] *(continued)*		• The mean change from baseline in salbutamol use (puffs/day) at 12 weeks was significantly greater ($p \leq 0.013$) than placebo (+1.7) following treatment with Seretide (–1.9), fluticasone (–0.4) or salmeterol (–0.3). Seretide was also significantly superior to fluticasone ($p \leq 0.025$) and salmeterol ($p \leq 0.023$). • The percentage of patients who withdrew before 12 weeks due to worsening asthma was 49% with placebo, 3% with Seretide, 35% with salmeterol and 11% with fluticasone. The probability of remaining in the study without being withdrawn because of worsening asthma was significantly greater in the Seretide group than in any other group ($p \leq 0.02$), and in the salmeterol and fluticasone groups than placebo ($p \leq 0.007$). • There were no serious drug-related adverse events in any treatment group. Adverse events occurring with a frequency of ≥2% that were considered possibly, probably or almost certainly related to drug treatment were headache, throat irritation, hoarseness/dysphonia and oropharyngeal/unspecified candidiasis. There were no significant cardiovascular changes.
Shapiro *et al.*, 2000[22] Single-blind 12 weeks Patients aged ≥12 years (n=349)	Asthma requiring pharmacotherapy for at least 6 months Mean FEV_1 40–85% of predicted value	• The mean change from baseline in FEV_1 (L) at 12 weeks was significantly greater ($p \leq 0.028$) than placebo (–0.11) following treatment with Seretide (+0.48), fluticasone (+0.25) or salmeterol (+0.05). Seretide was also significantly superior to both fluticasone ($p=0.003$) and salmeterol ($p \leq 0.025$). • The mean AUC relative to baseline at 12 weeks was significantly greater ($p \leq 0.028$) than placebo (3.29) following treatment with Seretide (7.25), but not with fluticasone (4.53) or salmeterol (4.36). Seretide was also significantly superior to both fluticasone ($p=0.003$) and salmeterol ($p \leq 0.025$). • The mean change from baseline in morning PEF (L/minute) at 12 weeks was significantly greater ($p \leq 0.036$) than placebo (–14.1) following treatment with Seretide (+53.5) or fluticasone (+15.2), but not with salmeterol (–11.6). Seretide was also significantly superior to fluticasone ($p \leq 0.015$) and salmeterol ($p \leq 0.003$).

AUC, area under the 12-hour serial FEV_1 curve; DPI, dry powder inhaler; FEV_1, forced expiratory volume in 1 second; PEF, peak expiratory flow.

Table 1. Continued

Study design and dosage regimen	Asthma severity at baseline	Main outcomes
Shapiro *et al.*, 2000[22] *(continued)* Seretide (50/250 μg), salmeterol (50 μg), fluticasone (250 μg), or placebo Each administered twice daily via a DPI	Increase in FEV_1 of ≥15% 30 minutes after inhaled salbutamol (180 μg)	• The mean change from baseline in morning PEF per cent predicted at 12 weeks was significantly greater ($p \leq 0.036$) than placebo (–3.1) following treatment with Seretide (+11.8) or fluticasone (+3.3), but not with salmeterol (–2.2). Seretide was also significantly superior to salmeterol ($p \leq 0.003$) but not fluticasone. • The mean change from baseline in evening PEF (L/minute) at 12 weeks was significantly greater ($p \leq 0.036$) than placebo (–15.8) following treatment with Seretide (+45.4) or fluticasone (+7.9), but not with salmeterol (–13.7). Seretide was also significantly superior to fluticasone ($p \leq 0.015$) and salmeterol ($p \leq 0.003$). • The mean change from baseline in asthma symptom score at 12 weeks was significantly greater ($p \leq 0.036$) than placebo (+0.4) following treatment with Seretide (–0.8), fluticasone (–0.4) or salmeterol (+0.1). Seretide was also significantly superior to fluticasone ($p \leq 0.015$) and salmeterol ($p \leq 0.003$). • The mean change from baseline in percentage of days with no asthma symptoms at 12 weeks was significantly greater ($p \leq 0.036$) than placebo (–7.9) following treatment with Seretide (+33.8) or fluticasone (+15.4), but not with salmeterol (+2.1). Seretide was also significantly superior to fluticasone ($p \leq 0.015$) and salmeterol ($p \leq 0.003$). • The mean change from baseline in percentage of nights with no awakenings at 12 weeks was significantly greater ($p \leq 0.036$) than placebo (–12.0) following treatment with Seretide (+7.2) or fluticasone (+2.8), but not with salmeterol (–8.0). Seretide was also significantly superior to fluticasone ($p \leq 0.015$) and salmeterol ($p \leq 0.003$).

AUC, area under the 12-hour serial FEV_1 curve; DPI, dry powder inhaler; FEV_1, forced expiratory volume in 1 second; PEF, peak expiratory flow.

Table 1. Continued

Study design and dosage regimen	Asthma severity at baseline	Main outcomes
Shapiro *et al.*, 2000[22] *(continued)*		• The mean change from baseline in salbutamol use (puffs/day) at 12 weeks was significantly greater ($p \leq 0.036$) than placebo (+0.9) following treatment with Seretide (–2.3), fluticasone (–0.9) or salmeterol (0). Seretide was also significantly superior to fluticasone ($p \leq 0.015$) and salmeterol ($p \leq 0.003$). • The percentage of patients who withdrew before 12 weeks due to worsening asthma was 62% with placebo, 4% with Seretide, 38% with salmeterol and 22% with fluticasone. The probability of remaining in the study without being withdrawn because of worsening asthma was significantly greater in the Seretide group than in any other group ($p \leq 0.002$), and in the salmeterol and fluticasone groups than placebo ($p < 0.001$). • There were no serious drug-related adverse events in any treatment group. Adverse events occurring with a frequency of ≥2% considered to be related to drug treatment were cough and oropharyngeal/unspecified candidiasis. There were no significant cardiovascular changes. • At 12 weeks, the percentage of patients with morning plasma cortisol concentrations <5 mg/dL was similar between groups (placebo, 6%; Seretide, 3%; fluticasone, 6%; salmeterol, 0%). • At 12 weeks, the percentage of patients with post-stimulation (with synthetic corticotrophin) plasma cortisol concentrations <18 mg/dL was similar between groups (placebo, 6%; Seretide, 3%; fluticasone, 6%; salmeterol, 0%).

AUC, area under the 12-hour serial FEV_1 curve; DPI, dry powder inhaler; FEV_1, forced expiratory volume in 1 second; PEF, peak expiratory flow.

and rescue salbutamol use). Seretide was also significantly superior to either fluticasone or salmeterol administered individually, with the exception of percentage of nights with no awakenings in one study, and morning PEF of the per cent predicted in the other, in which Seretide treatment was considered to be statistically equivalent to fluticasone.[21,22] In terms of superiority over placebo, fluticasone provided the more profound effects of the two monotherapies in both studies. All three active treatments were well tolerated, with no serious adverse events reported in any group which were considered by the investigator to be related to the study treatment. The most commonly occurring drug-related adverse events were headache, throat irritation, cough, hoarseness/dysphonia and candidiasis (oropharyngeal or of unspecified site). Withdrawals due to worsening asthma favoured Seretide over each of the monotherapies or in comparison with placebo (Figure 3). Electrocardiography (ECG) data did not reveal any cardiovascular safety issues with any of the active treatments. One of the studies also assessed the effect of treatment on the hypothalamic–pituitary–adrenal (HPA) axis, and reported that there was no evidence of adrenal suppression in any of the treatment groups compared with placebo-treated patients.

> Seretide was significantly superior to placebo on all efficacy parameters measured and was also significantly superior to either fluticasone or salmeterol administered individually.

Seretide has also been compared with fluticasone and salmeterol as monotherapies in another study that did not include a placebo arm.[7] In contrast with the previous studies, treatment was administered via an MDI and, to reflect the imminent phasing out of CFCs as propellants for inhalation devices,[8] the HFA-based formulation of Seretide was used. HFA–Seretide (fluticasone 88 µg [100 µg ex-valve]; salmeterol 42 µg

Figure 3. Probability of remaining in a 12-week comparative trial. Withdrawals were due to worsening asthma.[22]

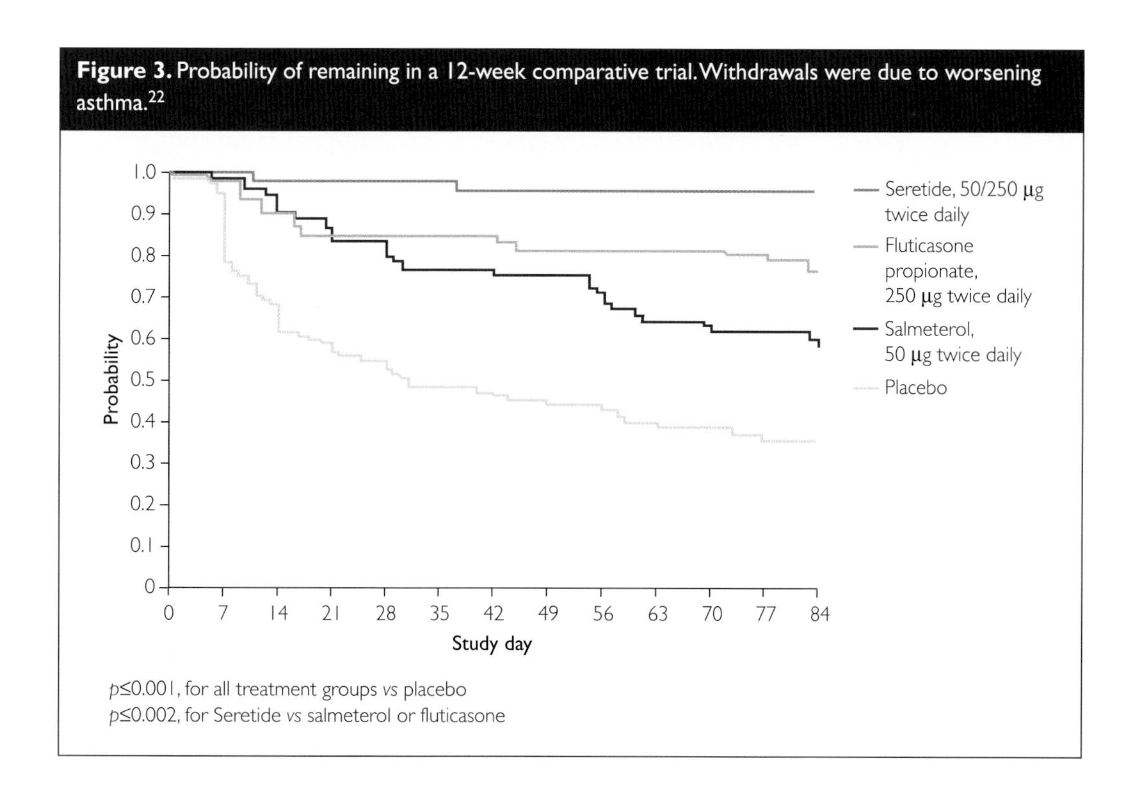

$p \leq 0.001$, for all treatment groups *vs* placebo
$p \leq 0.002$, for Seretide *vs* salmeterol or fluticasone

[50 μg ex-valve]) was evaluated against the equivalent doses of the individual components, both administered as CFC-based formulations. The patients recruited to this study were over the age of 12 years with a medical history of asthma requiring pharmacotherapy for at least 6 months. In the month prior to study entry patients were treated with a short-acting β_2-agonist only. At baseline, patients had a mean FEV_1 of 40–85% of the predicted normal value, and an increase of at least 15% in FEV_1 30 minutes after inhaled salbutamol (180 μg).

Following a 2-week single-blind screening period, during which time patients received HFA–placebo, 283 individuals were randomised to 12 weeks of active treatment. The combined therapy was reported to be statistically more effective than fluticasone ($p \leq 0.028$) and salmeterol ($p<0.001$) in terms of mean area under the 12-hour serial FEV_1 curve relative to baseline and also for the mean change from baseline at 12 weeks in FEV_1, morning PEF, morning PEF as a percentage of the predicted value and evening PEF. Seretide was statistically superior to fluticasone ($p \leq 0.028$) but not to salmeterol in terms of the percentage of days without any requirement for rescue medication. However, the combination therapy did not afford significant benefits over either monotherapy in terms of daily asthma symptom scores, the percentage of days with no asthma symptoms, the percentage of nights with no awakenings or percentage of nights without need for salbutamol use.

When these data are compared with data from the previous studies, in which all treatments were delivered by a DPI, it is evident that there is a less robust response with the HFA formulation of Seretide delivered by an MDI.[21,22] This could indicate that the reformulation Seretide with HFA impacts negatively on its clinical efficacy, but a direct comparative trial of the two formulations used in the same study population is yet to be reported. There do not appear to be any safety implications from reformulating Seretide with HFA. Drug-related adverse events occurred in 17, 16 and 15% of those treated with Seretide, fluticasone and salmeterol, respectively, and none were considered to be serious. Consistent with the placebo-controlled studies described above, the most frequent adverse events were throat irritation, hoarseness/dysphonia, headaches, cough and candidiasis of the mouth or throat.

There are clear benefits of treatment with Seretide in terms of pulmonary function and symptom amelioration compared with the two monotherapies or placebo.

In summary, therefore, there are clear benefits of treatment with Seretide in terms of pulmonary function and symptom amelioration compared with the two monotherapies or placebo. Of the two monotherapies, salmeterol appears to be less effective individually. This highlights that complete replacement of inhaled corticosteroid therapy with a long-acting β_2-agonist is not an appropriate strategy in terms of efficacy, which is consistent with current treatment guidelines.[3,23]

Combination therapy vs increased dose of fluticasone

The use of a long-acting β_2-agonist as add-on therapy is recommended for the treatment of patients who remain symptomatic whilst receiving low-to-moderate doses of inhaled corticosteroids.[3,18] Therefore, a more clinically relevant assessment of the efficacy of Seretide is its performance compared with an increased dose of an inhaled corticosteroid. As such, a number of studies have compared Seretide with a dose of fluticasone higher than that used within the combination treatment arm.

A 24-week randomised, double-blind, double-dummy,[a] parallel group trial enrolled 437 patients with asthma of at least 6 months duration prior to study entry and an FEV_1 at baseline of 40–80% of the predicted normal, with at least 15% reversibility in response to salbutamol (180 µg).[24] A 2–4-week screening period was used to identify those patients who remained symptomatic on open-label fluticasone (88 µg twice daily, administered via an MDI). These patients were then randomised to active treatment with concurrent fluticasone (88 µg twice daily) and salmeterol (42 µg twice daily) or fluticasone alone (220 µg twice daily), all administered via MDIs. Over the course of the study, the improvements in morning and evening PEF were significantly greater following concurrent therapy (mean change from baseline +46.5 and +38.2 L/minute) than treatment with fluticasone alone (+23.8 and +21.2 L/minute; $p \leq 0.001$ for both comparisons). Concurrent therapy was also superior in terms of improvements in combined symptom score (–0.43 *vs* –0.26; $p \leq 0.015$). Moreover, there was also a significantly greater increase in the percentage of symptom-free days associated with concurrent therapy than with fluticasone monotherapy ($p \leq 0.014$). Concurrent therapy was also superior to fluticasone monotherapy in increasing the percentage of nights with no awakenings due to asthma (14.9 *vs* 10.1%; $p<0.001$). The use of rescue salbutamol therapy was reduced by 51% with concurrent therapy and by 29% in the fluticasone group ($p<0.001$). Concurrent therapy was also superior to fluticasone alone in its effect on treatment satisfaction scores, which increased by 1.30 and 1.05, respectively ($p=0.001$).

There was a significantly greater increase in the percentage of symptom-free days associated with concurrent therapy than with fluticasone monotherapy.

Treatment-related adverse events were reported by 10 and 14% of patients in the concurrent therapy and fluticasone groups, respectively. One patient from each group reported a serious adverse event, but neither was considered to be treatment-related. Five patients, all in the fluticasone monotherapy group, withdrew as a consequence of adverse events. There was no significant difference between the number of patients in each group reporting one or more than one asthma exacerbations.

A similarly designed double-blind study compared Seretide (50/100 µg) in a single DPI inhaler with fluticasone (250 µg), also via a DPI, each administered twice daily.[25] The patients recruited into this study were at least 12 years of age, had experienced asthma for at least 6 months prior to entry into the study, and received inhaled corticosteroids for at least 30 days before screening. At screening, patients were selected for randomisation if they demonstrated an FEV_1 of 65–95% of the predicted normal value, and an increase in FEV_1 of at least 12%, 30 minutes after between two and four puffs of salbutamol. A three-part run-in period was used, first to identify those patients whose asthma was controlled on fluticasone, 250 µg twice daily, secondly to

[a]A double-dummy design ensures blinding of patients and investigators in a situation where two treatments are required and cannot be made to look the same.

further narrow the population to those whose asthma was unstable on fluticasone 100 μg twice daily, and finally to select those patients in whom asthma control was regained on reverting to treatment with fluticasone, 250 μg twice daily. This process identified 558 patients for randomisation, of whom 308 were selected for an extended 24 weeks of treatment. In the Seretide and fluticasone groups, 12 and 15% of patients, respectively, discontinued the study during weeks 1–12, and 4% in each group withdrew during weeks 13–24.

The mean changes from baseline were significantly greater in the Seretide group than in the fluticasone group in terms of FEV_1 (12 weeks, $p \leq 0.001$; 24 weeks, $p \leq 0.007$), morning PEF (12 weeks, $p \leq 0.001$), evening PEF (12 weeks, $p=0.001$; 24 weeks, $p=0.039$), percentage of symptom-free days (12 weeks, $p=0.028$), salbutamol use (12 weeks, $p=0.045$; 24 weeks, $p=0.022$) and percentage of days free of rescue medication (12 weeks, $p=0.008$; 24 weeks, $p=0.032$). There was no significant difference between the treatment groups at either time point in daily asthma symptom score or the number of night-time awakenings. Both treatments were well tolerated. Drug-related adverse events occurred in 4 and 5% or patients in the Seretide and fluticasone groups, respectively, in weeks 1–12, and this frequency was reduced to less than 1 and 3%, respectively, during weeks 13–24. Asthma exacerbations occurred in 3% of the Seretide-treated group and 2% of the fluticasone-treated patients during weeks 1–12 and in 2% of Seretide-treated patients during weeks 13–24 (rate not reported for fluticasone), neither of which translated to a statistically significant difference.

This superiority of administering salmeterol concurrently with fluticasone compared with a doubling in the dose of fluticasone has been reported to extend to even higher doses of fluticasone. A double-blind trial of 347 patients evaluated two treatment groups – Seretide (50/250 μg) and fluticasone (500 μg), each administered twice daily via a DPI.[26] Patients were aged between 18 and 70 years, and were diagnosed with asthma at least 6 months prior to enrolment into the study. Their asthma was described, in terms of both symptoms and FEV_1, as moderately severe, with at least 15% reversibility in response to salbutamol (200 μg). All patients had been treated with inhaled corticosteroids (beclometasone dipropionate, budesonide or fluticasone) for at least 3 months. Following 12 weeks of treatment, Seretide was superior compared with double-dose fluticasone in increasing morning PEF (52 *vs* 36 L/minute; $p=0.0356$). The same was true in terms of increases in evening PEF (46 *vs* 29 L/minute; $p=0.0178$), reduction in asthma symptom score (1.5 *vs* 1.0; $p=0.0005$), increase in the percentage of symptom-free days (49 *vs* 38%; $p=0.038$) and reduction in salbutamol use (1.6 *vs* 1.0 puffs/day; $p=0.0001$). However, there was no significant difference between treatment groups in terms of the per cent predicted FVC, FEV_1 or PEF. Both treatments were associated with increases in asthma-related quality of life, with a trend towards superiority for Seretide. The percentage of physicians rating treatment as excellent or good was 82.4% for Seretide and 72.3% for fluticasone. The corresponding values for patient ratings were similar, at 81 and 74%.

Both Seretide and fluticasone were associated with increases in asthma-related quality of life, with a trend towards superiority for Seretide.

During the 12-week duration of the study, asthma exacerbations occurred in one patient receiving Seretide, and four of those receiving fluticasone monotherapy. Adverse drug reactions were reported in 13 Seretide-treated and 17 fluticasone-treated patients, whilst adverse events possibly or probably related to study treatment were reported in 15 and 13 patients, respectively. Only one serious adverse event which was possibly related to the study drug, an asthma exacerbation, occurred during the 12 weeks, and this was in a patient receiving fluticasone alone. Cardiovascular parameters remained stable in both groups throughout.

A double-blind, double-dummy study comparing fluticasone and salmeterol with fluticasone alone highlighted the value of including an additional group who continued on the initial run-in dose of fluticasone.[27] It was argued by these investigators that such a design would allow for an assessment of the real effect of adding a second drug over and above any trial-related effect, thus acting as a form of internal control. The treatment groups in this trial consisted of fluticasone (250 μg) and salmeterol (50 μg) (unspecified whether administered concurrently or via a single inhaler), double dose fluticasone (500 μg) and normal dose fluticasone (250 μg), each administered twice daily by MDI. The patients included in this trial were aged between 16 and 75 years, and were symptomatic despite treatment with inhaled corticosteroids (beclometasone dipropionate at 500–800 μg twice daily, or equivalent). All patients had a PEF under 85% of that determined 15 minutes after inhalation of salbutamol (400 μg). A total of 502 patients were randomised to 6 months of treatment with the active drugs.

The mean improvement in morning PEF with concurrent fluticasone and salmeterol therapy was significantly greater ($p<0.001$) than that with either dose of fluticasone alone, which were statistically equivalent. Patients included in this study had a diurnal variation in PEF of at least 15% prior to study entry, and the 4.9% reduction in this parameter afforded by concurrent therapy was statistically greater than the 3.0 and 2.2% reductions resulting from high- and low-dose fluticasone, respectively ($p<0.001$ *vs* both doses of fluticasone). Surprisingly, FEV_1 and FVC showed almost no change from baseline in any of the three treatment groups. Concurrent therapy was superior to either fluticasone group, which were equivalent to each other, in terms of the mean percentage of symptom-free days and nights throughout the study (Figure 4). The superiority of concurrent therapy extended to the mean percentage of days and nights during which rescue medication was not required ($p\leq0.001$).

Although all patients in this study had experienced more than two asthma exacerbations in the previous year, the majority of patients completing the study experienced no further exacerbations during the 6-month period (66% of the concurrent therapy group, and 59% and 65% of those receiving low- and high-dose fluticasone, respectively). The rate of severe asthma exacerbations was less than 0.25 patients per year in all treatment groups. Seven patients withdrew from the concurrent

Figure 4. Median change from baseline in percentage of patients experiencing no day- or night-time symptoms during treatment with salmeterol/fluticasone (50/250 µg twice daily), fluticasone (500 µg twice daily) or fluticasone (250 µg twice daily).[27]
NS, non-significant.

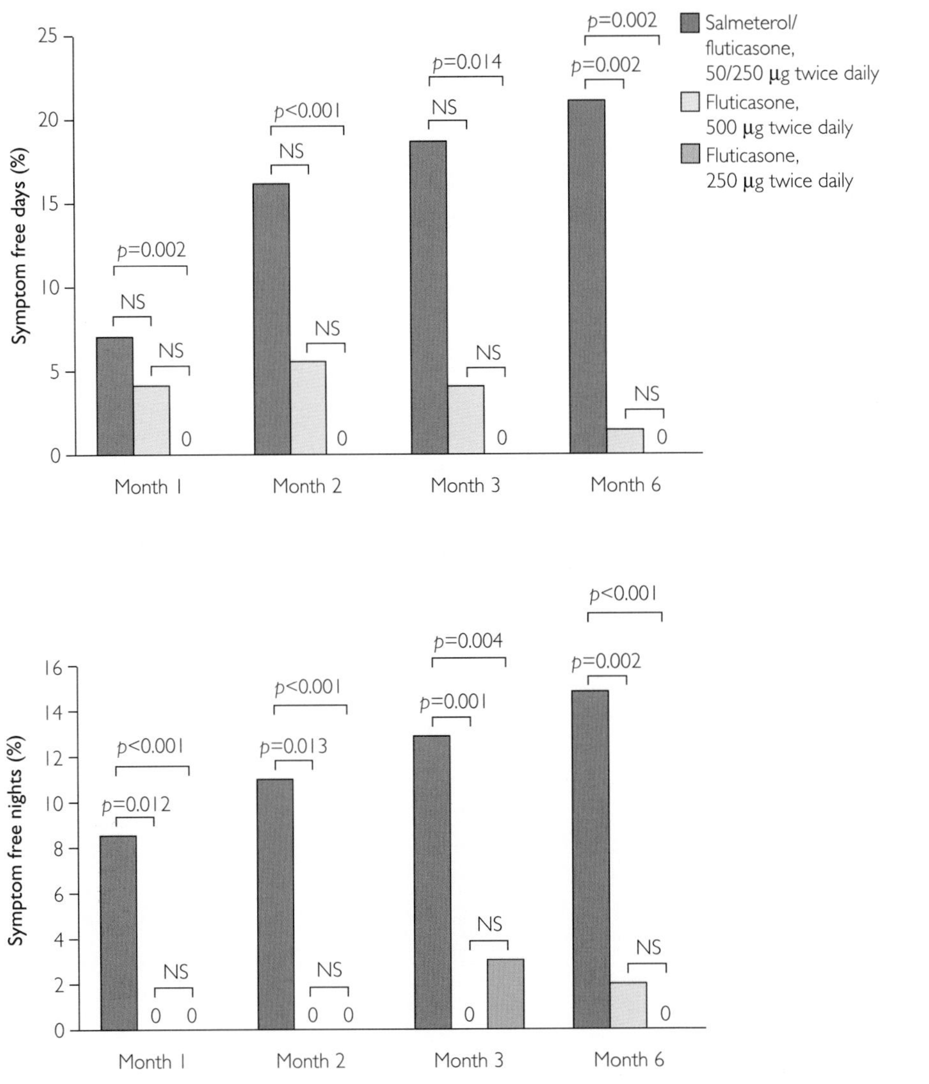

therapy group as a result of adverse events, compared with two and six patients in the low- and high-dose fluticasone groups, respectively.

A year-long study has demonstrated that Seretide offers greater benefits over fluticasone alone in terms of achieving comprehensive, sustained asthma control.[28] Evidence has shown that over 95% of patients fail to achieve the level of optimal control defined by treatment guidelines.[29] The Gaining Optimal Asthma Control (GOAL) study was a randomised, double-blind, parallel group, three-phase study comparing the effectiveness of Seretide with fluticasone treatment in achieving this control. During the first phase, the dose of either drug was 'stepped up' every 12 weeks until either totally controlled asthma was achieved or the maximum study dose was reached (Seretide 50/500 μg twice daily, fluticasone 500 μg twice daily). Following 12 weeks of treatment with the maximum dose, or at the point where total asthma control was reached, patients entered phase II. They then remained on their final phase I dose until the end of the 1-year period. Those patients whose asthma was not totally controlled by the end of phase II were entered into a third, open-label phase, during which they were treated with oral prednisolone (up to 60 mg/day for 10 days) and Seretide (50/500 μg twice a day for 4 weeks).

Patients included in the GOAL study were aged between 12 and 80 years and had at least a 6-month history of asthma, with a documented FEV_1 reversibility of at least 15% in response to inhalation of a short-acting β_2-agonist. In order to be included, patients were required to have uncontrolled asthma, demonstrated by a failure to demonstrate at least two well-controlled asthma weeks during the 4-week run-in period, during which they received their usual dose of inhaled corticosteroid treatment. Of the 3416 patients who were randomised, 3039 completed phase I and 2890 completed phase II. Within each treatment group, patients were divided into three strata: patients in stratum 1 had received no inhaled corticosteroids in the previous 6 months, patients in stratum 2 had received beclometasone dipropionate (500 μg daily or equivalent) and patients in stratum 3 had received beclometasone dipropionate (between 500 and 1000 μg daily or equivalent). The outcomes of this study included the proportion of patients who achieved well- and totally controlled asthma – composite measures incorporating PEF, rescue medication use, symptoms, night-time awakenings, exacerbations, emergency visits and adverse events.

During phase I, more patients treated with Seretide than fluticasone achieved well-controlled asthma (stratum 1, 71 *vs* 65%, p=0.039; stratum 2, 69 *vs* 52%, p<0.001; stratum 3, 51 *vs* 33%, p<0.001). The same pattern was reported for patients achieving totally controlled asthma (stratum 1, 42 *vs* 31%; stratum 2, 32 *vs* 20%; stratum 3, 19 *vs* 8%; all p<0.001). Furthermore, during the first 12 weeks, asthma control was achieved significantly faster with Seretide than with fluticasone ($p \leq 0.002$). The superiority of Seretide persisted through phase II in terms of the proportion of patients achieving well-controlled asthma (stratum 1, 78 *vs* 70%, p=0.003; stratum 2, 75 *vs* 60%, p<0.001; stratum 3, 62 *vs* 47%, p<0.001) and totally-controlled asthma (stratum 1, 50 *vs* 40%; stratum 2, 44 *vs* 28%; stratum 3, 29 *vs* 16%; all p<0.001). Of those achieving well- or totally controlled asthma during phase I, 62–83% maintained this status throughout phase II.

More patients treated with Seretide than fluticasone achieved well-controlled asthma.

The final week of the second phase was characterised by well-controlled asthma in 77% of those receiving Seretide and 68% of those receiving fluticasone alone. Of the remainder, who were entered into the 4-week open-label phase, relatively few showed any additional benefit from prednisolone/Seretide treatment, though more of those who did had received fluticasone during the double-blind phase. During the study, the mean annual rate of exacerbations requiring oral corticosteroids and/or hospitalisation or emergency visits were significantly lower in the Seretide group in all strata ($p \leq 0.009$). Asthma Quality of Life Questionnaire (AQLQ) scores were also significantly better in the Seretide group in strata 2 ($p=0.008$) and 3 ($p=0.006$) by the end of phase II. Improvements to mean morning pre-bronchodilator FEV_1 were significantly larger in the Seretide group at the end of phase II ($p<0.001$ for all strata). The overall incidence of drug-related adverse events was 10% in both groups. At the end of phase II, no significant differences were observed between treatments in the geometric mean of the cortisol/creatinine ratio. This study demonstrated that 'total asthma control' is, in fact, achievable in a considerable proportion of patients (41% in this case). Seretide offered sustained control in more patients, more rapidly and at a lower corticosteroid dose than fluticasone alone.

Seretide is superior to fluticasone alone, even when it is administered at more than double the dose used in the combination drug.

Thus, taken together, all of these data indicate that Seretide is superior to fluticasone alone, even when it is administered at more than double the dose used in the combination drug, in terms of pulmonary function, symptoms and patient/physician satisfaction with treatment. Tolerability appears similar whether increasing the dose of fluticasone or adding salmeterol treatment.

Seretide vs fluticasone and salmeterol given concurrently

A number of the studies comparing the relative efficacy of the fluticasone/salmeterol combination with an increased dose of fluticasone did not use Seretide itself, but rather concurrent fluticasone and salmeterol administered via separate inhaler devices. Use of the single combination inhaler does not affect the delivered dose or the pharmacokinetics of the component drugs.[20] Accordingly, a number of trials have investigated whether the combination product affords at least equivalent benefits in terms of pulmonary function and symptom control as fluticasone and salmeterol administered concurrently via separate inhalers.[30–32]

Three trials employing double-blind, double-dummy designs reported on the comparable efficacy and safety of concurrent fluticasone and salmeterol therapy with Seretide at its three licensed dosages, all administered twice-daily via DPI. All three studies recruited patients with a PEF of 50–85% of the maximum PEF recorded 15 minutes after administration of inhaled salbutamol (400 μg). Included patients also demonstrated a symptom score of at least 2 on at least 3 (in one study) or 4 (in the other two) of the last 7 consecutive days prior to the study.[30–32]

The study using the lowest dose combination (50/100 μg) recruited 244 patients over the age of 12 years.[30] Compliance to treatment was reported to be good in both treatment groups: 91% in those treated with Seretide and 89% in those receiving concurrent therapy with the two component drugs at equivalent doses. The adjusted mean change in morning PEF during the course of the 12-week study was 42 and

33 L/minute in the Seretide and concurrent treatment groups, respectively, whilst the corresponding values for evening PEF were 36 and 30 L/minute, respectively. In neither parameter was there a statistically significant difference between the two groups. The adjusted mean change from baseline at week 12 in FEV_1 was 6% in both treatment groups. Seretide and concurrent treatment also generated significant and statistically equivalent benefits in day and night-time symptom scores, the percentage of symptom-free days and nights, and the percentage of days and nights when rescue salbutamol treatment was not required. Both treatment regimens were equally well tolerated and neither generated any clinically significant changes in laboratory values, physical examinations or vital signs. Adverse events considered by the investigator to be drug related occurred in 15% of patients treated with Seretide and 14% of those receiving concurrent therapy. A total of 9% of patients in the Seretide group and 7% in the concurrent therapy group withdrew from the study due to adverse events.

A further study comparing Seretide (50/250 µg) with the corresponding doses of salmeterol and fluticasone administered concurrently evaluated 371 patients over the age of 12 years.[31] The inclusion criteria for this study required that patients should still be symptomatic after receiving beclometasone dipropionate, budesonide (800–1200 µg/day for both) or fluticasone (400–600 µg/day) prior to study entry. Mean compliance to treatment during weeks 1–12 was 96% in Seretide-treated patients and 95% in the concurrent treatment group. The mean adjusted changes from baseline in morning PEF were 43 and 36 L/minute for Seretide and concurrent therapy, respectively. Over the course of 12 weeks, this difference was not significant, though at weeks 3 and 4, there was a significant difference that favoured Seretide (p=0.037 and p=0.043, for each time point, respectively). Seretide and concurrent therapy were associated with increases in evening PEF of 35 and 25 L/minute, respectively. Statistically significant differences in evening PEF favoured Seretide at all time points, as well as over the whole 12-week treatment duration (p=0.008). No significant difference between treatment groups was reported for asthma symptom scores, the percentage of patients with symptom-free days and nights, or the percentage of days and nights without the need for rescue salbutamol therapy. Safety evaluations continued for an extended period of 28 weeks. A total of 12 patients in the Seretide group and nine patients in the concurrent therapy group withdrew from the study due to adverse events, which were asthma-related in five patients in each group. No clinically significant changes were reported in laboratory values, physical examinations or vital signs. Mean serum cortisol concentrations were also reported to be equivalent in the two groups.

The third of these studies compared Seretide (50/500 µg) with the corresponding doses of the component drugs administered concurrently.[32] It also included an additional treatment group, who received fluticasone monotherapy (500 µg). Included patients (n=503) were aged 12 years and over and had received inhaled corticosteroid treatment continuously for 12 weeks prior to run-in. Baseline FEV_1 in these patients was at least 50% of the predicted normal value. As in the previous study, efficacy data were recorded for 12 weeks, with an extended safety assessment continuing up to 28 weeks. Mean compliance over the entire 28-week period was reported at 93–94% in all three treatment groups. The adjusted mean changes from baseline in morning PEF were 35, 33 and 15 L/minute in the Seretide, concurrent therapy and fluticasone monotherapy groups, respectively. The corresponding values for evening PEF were 29, 23 and 9 L/minute. In both cases, Seretide and concurrent therapy were statistically equivalent, but each was superior to treatment with fluticasone alone (all comparisons $p<0.001$). The same relationship was reported in terms of the percentage of symptom-free days and nights and the percentage of days and nights without any need for rescue medication, though no statistical data was reported with regard to the superiority of Seretide and concurrent therapy over fluticasone alone. The incidence of drug-related adverse events over 28 weeks was 17% with Seretide, 14% with concurrent therapy and 19% with fluticasone alone. The proportions of patients withdrawing due to adverse events in the three groups were 10, 9 and 13%, respectively.

These studies provide consistent evidence that fluticasone and salmeterol administered in a single DPI inhaler are at least as effective and as well tolerated as the two drugs when administered alone. It has been suggested that the use of a single product containing both individual drugs may increase patient compliance for combination therapy.[33] It should be borne in mind that the trials discussed above are of a double-blind, double-dummy design, and effects upon efficacy as a result of difference in compliance are unlikely to emerge from such studies. Indeed, the levels of compliance reported in all three of these studies were comparable, and greater than 90% for both Seretide and concurrent therapy. It is well-established that compliance in clinical practice is directly related to the complexity of the treatment regimen, though the number of drugs required to impact negatively upon compliance is not known.[34] Longer-term open-label trials, which are more reflective of actual clinical practice, are more likely to highlight discrepancies in compliance, and the resulting impact on efficacy, between Seretide and concurrent therapy.

Fluticasone and salmeterol administered in a single DPI inhaler are at least as effective and well tolerated and safe as the two drugs when administered alone.

In support of potential compliance benefits of Seretide, a 12-month retrospective, observational cohort study has demonstrated that Seretide treatment is associated with greater refill persistence than that reported for the fluticasone component of concurrently administered fluticasone with salmeterol or fluticasone with montelukast.[34] Refill rates were defined as number of monthly prescription claims for the cohort regimens over the 12-month follow-up period. Thus the level of refill persistence indicates patients' adherence to their allocated treatment. Seretide treatment was also associated with less supplemental use of short-acting β_2-agonists than either of the two concurrent treatment regimens. On both parameters, Seretide treatment was equivalent to orally administered montelukast alone. Oral treatment with montelukast is generally associated with greater patient compliance than inhaled corticosteroid therapy.[35] The equivalence of Seretide therapy in terms of compliance is presumably a result of the improved perceived efficacy and convenience conferred by salmeterol – a conclusion which is supported by the fact that refill persistence during Seretide treatment was significantly greater than that reported for fluticasone alone. A further benefit of Seretide in this respect is that it does not allow selective non-compliance between the corticosteroid and the β_2-agonist.

Seretide vs alternative controller therapies

Seretide *vs* budesonide

The value of switching patients who remain symptomatic on budesonide (800–1200 μg/day, or an equivalent inhaled corticosteroid dose[b]) to treatment with Seretide has been evaluated in a randomised, double-blind, double-dummy trial.[36] Patients in this study (n=353) had an FEV_1 or PEF of 50–85% of the predicted normal value, and also demonstrated an increase of at least 15% in FEV_1 or no more than 85% in morning PEF in response to inhalation of a short-acting β_2-agonist. The symptom score was at least 2 on at least 4 of the last 7 consecutive days before the run-in phase. Patients were then randomised to active treatment with Seretide (50/250 μg) or budesonide (800 μg), each administered twice daily by a DPI.

Over the course of the 24-week study, Seretide was associated with a greater adjusted mean morning PEF (406 *vs* 380 L/minute; $p<0.001$), mean evening PEF (416 *vs* 398 L/minute; $p<0.001$) and a lower adjusted mean diurnal variation in PEF (6 *vs* 8%; $p<0.001$) compared with budesonide. There was a trend towards superiority for Seretide in terms of FEV_1 (absolute value and per cent of predicted normal), though it did not reach statistical significance at week 24. The percentage of symptom-free days ($p<0.001$), salbutamol-free days ($p\leq0.001$) and salbutamol-free nights ($p=0.029$) was significantly greater in the Seretide group over the course of 24 weeks. There was no superiority of Seretide in terms of symptom-free nights. The number and severity of asthma exacerbations in the two groups were also similar, with one Seretide-treated patient and two budesonide-treated patients experiencing at least one severe exacerbation. Adverse events considered by the investigator to be related to study treatment occurred in 25 and 31 patients, respectively. None of the serious adverse events reported were considered to be treatment-related.

Seretide was associated with a greater adjusted mean morning PEF, mean evening PEF and a lower adjusted mean diurnal variation in PEF compared with budesonide.

A second comparative study of Seretide and budesonide focused specifically on the relative benefits of treatment upon asthma-related quality of life.[37] This randomised, double-blind, double-dummy trial recruited patients (n=113) aged at least 12 years, who had received budesonide (800–1200 μg/day, or an equivalent dose of an inhaled corticosteroid[b]) for at least 4 weeks prior to the trial. Asthma-related quality of life was assessed using the AQLQ at baseline and after

[b]Beclometasone, 800–1200 μg/day, or fluticasone, 400–600 μg/day.

12 weeks of treatment, or at study withdrawal. The study included two treatment groups: Seretide (50/250 μg) or budesonide (800 μg), both of which were administered twice daily via DPI. Both treatments afforded significant benefits on all domains of the AQLQ in terms of mean change from baseline at 12 weeks or at early withdrawal. However, Seretide was shown to be superior to budesonide within each domain (i.e. activity limitation, $p=0.032$; asthma symptoms, $p=0.002$; emotional functioning, $p=0.004$; environmental exposure, $p=0.014$) and also in terms of overall AQLQ score ($p=0.002$).

Seretide *vs* montelukast or fluticasone/montelukast combination

The relative efficacy and safety of Seretide (50/100 μg twice daily, given via DPI) and the leukotriene receptor antagonist montelukast (10 mg once daily, in orally administered capsules) have been evaluated in a double-blind, double-dummy trial.[38] Patients included in the study population (n=432) were aged at least 15 years, had experienced asthma for at least 6 months and had at least a 6-week history of treatment with short-acting β_2-agonists, during which time their symptoms were inadequately controlled. The study population had an FEV_1 of 50–80% of the predicted normal value at baseline, which increased by at least 12% within 30 minutes of an inhaled dose of salbutamol (180 μg). Prior to treatment randomisation, patients were entered into an 8–14-week run-in period, during which time all short-acting β_2-agonists were replaced with inhaled salbutamol.

Over the course of this 12-week study, Seretide was consistently superior to montelukast ($p\leq0.001$) in terms of mean change from baseline on numerous efficacy variables (FEV_1, morning PEF, evening PEF, combined symptom score, percentage of symptom-free days, salbutamol use, percentage of days without need for rescue medication and percentage of nights with no awakenings). Both treatment regimens generated significant improvements in asthma-related quality of life, according to the AQLQ, but the effect on quality of life was greater with Seretide ($p\leq0.001$). Significantly more Seretide- than montelukast-treated patients reported being satisfied with their study medication, along with how rapidly it worked and the duration of its effects ($p<0.001$). Asthma exacerbations were reported in 3% of the Seretide group and 6% of the montelukast group. Adverse events which were considered by the investigator to be related to the study drug occurred in 8 and 11% of patients, respectively. One patient in the Seretide group withdrew due to adverse events which were potentially related to study treatment, compared with four patients in the montelukast group. There were no reports in either group of any serious drug-related adverse events leading to withdrawal from the study.

Seretide was consistently superior to montelukast in terms of mean change from baseline on numerous efficacy variables.

Given that low-dose fluticasone in isolation provides better control of lung function and asthma symptoms than oral montelukast, and that Seretide offers greater improvements to asthma control than a doubling in the dose of fluticasone, it is perhaps not surprising that Seretide appears so robustly superior to montelukast when given in isolation.[39,40]

However, as oral leukotriene receptor antagonists are licensed in the UK as add-on therapy for patients inadequately controlled on low-to-moderate doses of inhaled corticosteroids alone[c], it is more clinically relevant to compare Seretide with montelukast administered in combination with an inhaled corticosteroid.

A number of randomised double-blind, double-dummy trials have evaluated the relative benefits of adding salmeterol and montelukast to fluticasone therapy.[41–43] Two of these studies included the lowest available Seretide dose (50/100 µg, administered twice daily via a DPI), and compared it with a combination of fluticasone (100 µg, twice daily via a DPI) and oral montelukast (10 mg once daily).[41,42] The first of these trials recruited patients aged at least 15 years who had asthma for at least 6 months and who had been receiving low-to-moderate doses of an inhaled corticosteroid for at least 30 days prior to screening. In these patients, FEV_1 was between 50 and 80% of the predicted normal value, and increased by at least 12% within 30 minutes of receiving an inhaled dose of salbutamol (180 µg). Patients included in the study (n=447) remained symptomatic following a 3-week run-in period, during which time they were treated with fluticasone monotherapy (100 µg twice daily, administered by a DPI).

Both treatment regimens provided significant benefits on all efficacy measures over the course of the 12-week study ($p<0.001$). However, Seretide was significantly superior to the fluticasone/montelukast combination in terms of the mean change from baseline in morning PEF ($p<0.001$), evening PEF ($p<0.001$), FEV_1 ($p<0.001$), percentage of days with no salbutamol use ($p=0.032$), total salbutamol use ($p=0.014$) and shortness of breath score ($p=0.017$). The two treatment strategies were equivalent in terms of chest tightness score, wheeze score and overall daytime symptom scores. However, asthma exacerbations occurred less frequently in Seretide- than fluticasone/montelukast-treated patients (2 *vs* 6%; $p=0.031$). Visits to the physician were required in 50% of those treated with Seretide and 69% of those receiving fluticasone/montelukast. One patient in the fluticasone/montelukast treatment group required treatment in an emergency department. Four patients in the Seretide group and two in the fluticasone/montelukast group withdrew from the study due to adverse events considered by the investigator to be related to study treatment.

Asthma exacerbations occurred less frequently in Seretide- than fluticasone/montelukast-treated patients.

The second study comparing Seretide (50/100 µg twice daily, administered via a DPI) with fluticasone (100 µg twice daily, administered via a DPI) plus oral montelukast (10 mg once daily) recruited asthmatic patients aged at least 15 years with FEV_1 at least 50% of the predicted normal value, with at least 15% reversibility in response to salbutamol (up to 800 µg; n=806).[42] These patients had received inhaled corticosteroids for at least 4 weeks prior to entry into the study. During this period, patients had not changed their asthma medication, had a respiratory tract infection or required hospitalisation

[c]Oral leukotriene agents are, however, used in isolation for the treatment of exercise-induced asthma.

for an acute asthma exacerbation. Despite this stability, patients' asthma was shown to be inadequately controlled by fluticasone (100 μg twice daily, via a DPI) during a subsequent 4-week run-in period.

Over the course of the 12-week treatment period, Seretide was significantly superior to fluticasone/montelukast in terms of mean change from baseline in morning PEF (p=0.0001), evening PEF (p=0.0001), FEV_1 (p=0.0001), percentage of symptom-free days (p=0.017), percentage of symptom-free nights (p=0.033) and percentage of days free of rescue medication use (p=0.03). There was no difference between the two treatments in terms of the percentage of nights free of rescue medication use. However, there was a significant difference in favour of Seretide treatment in terms of the percentage of patients who experienced at least one asthma exacerbation (9.6 *vs* 14.6%; $p<0.05$), though this advantage was not reported when the percentage of patients experiencing asthma exacerbations of moderate or severe intensity was considered (4.8 *vs* 8.4%; p=0.07). The time until first asthma exacerbation was also significantly longer in the Seretide group ($p<0.05$; Figure 5). Seretide was superior in terms of the percentage of patients satisfied or very satisfied with their treatment (92.9 *vs* 83.5%; $p<0.05$) and for physician ratings of satisfaction (79.6 *vs* 72.6%; $p<0.05$).

The incidence of adverse events was similar in Seretide- and fluticasone/montelukast-treated patients (44 *vs* 42%), and there were no serious drug-related adverse events in either group. The rate of treatment

Figure 5. Number of patients remaining free from asthma exacerbations over 12 weeks, as a percentage of the number who started treatment. Patients received salmeterol/fluticasone (50/100 μg twice daily) or montelukast (10 mg once daily) plus fluticasone (100 μg twice daily).[42]

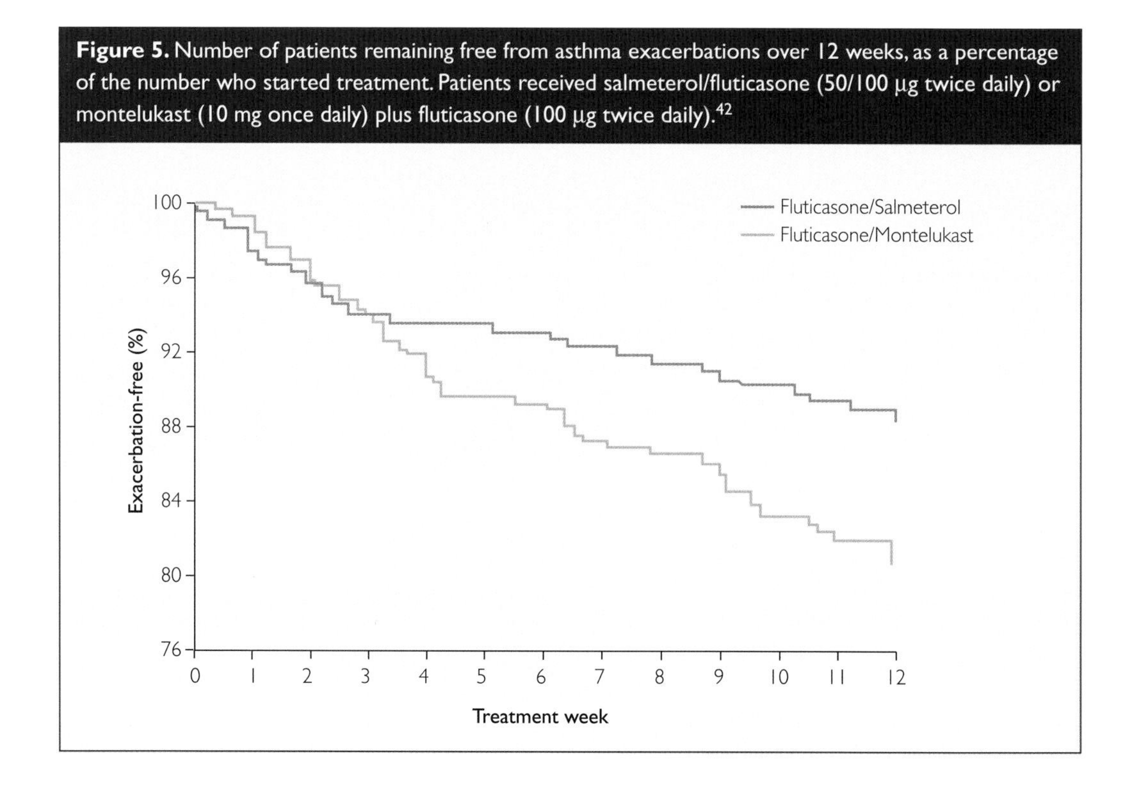

withdrawals was significantly lower in the Seretide group (5 *vs* 10%; $p<0.05$).

A third trial has compared salmeterol/fluticasone (50/100 µg twice daily, via MDI and DPI, respectively) with oral montelukast (10 mg once daily) and fluticasone (100 µg twice daily, via DPI).[44] In this trial, patients (n=1490) were aged between 15 and 72 years, and demonstrated a baseline FEV_1 between 50 and 90% of the predicted normal, with at least 12% reversibility in FEV_1 or morning PEF following β_2-agonist inhalation. Of the patients in the salmeterol/fluticasone group, 19.1% experienced at least one asthma exacerbation during the course of the 52-week study, compared with 20.1% in the montelukast/fluticasone group – a 1% difference which was not statistically significant. Indeed, there was no significant difference in the distribution of patients according to the number of asthma exacerbations between the two groups, and the characteristics of these exacerbations were identical. The two treatment strategies were also statistically equivalent in terms of reducing nocturnal awakenings and improving asthma-specific quality of life.

The salmeterol/fluticasone combination, however, was significantly more effective than montelukast/fluticasone at increasing pre-bronchodilator FEV_1 over baseline (0.19 *vs* 0.11 L; $p\leq0.001$), though there was no significant difference in terms of post-bronchodilator FEV_1. The salmeterol/fluticasone group showed a significantly greater decrease from baseline in percentage reversibility of FEV_1 compared with the montelukast/fluticasone group (11.26 *vs* 7.54%; $p\leq0.001$). Morning PEF was increased by a greater extent in the salmeterol/fluticasone group than in the montelukast/fluticasone group (34.59 *vs* 17.73 L/minute; $p\leq0.001$). Montelukast/fluticasone significantly reduced eosinophil counts in peripheral blood and sputum, whereas salmeterol/fluticasone did not.

Patients receiving salmeterol/fluticasone reported a significantly higher incidence of drug-related adverse events than those receiving montelukast/fluticasone (10.0 *vs* 6.3%; $p=0.01$) and of serious adverse events (7.4 *vs* 4.6%; $p=0.022$). One patient in the salmeterol/fluticasone group died due to a severe asthma attack, 15 days after the initiation of treatment. This was reported by the investigator to be possibly related to study treatment. One patient in the salmeterol/fluticasone group and none in the montelukast/fluticasone group reported serious laboratory adverse experiences.

In summary, the addition of montelukast to inhaled corticosteroid therapy appears to be as effective as adding salmeterol in terms of preventing asthma exacerbations. Despite this comparable clinical effectiveness, however, salmeterol induced greater improvements in pulmonary function than montelukast. However, the anti-leukotriene agent could be argued to be a preferable add-on option in terms of drug-related adverse events.

Finally, a year-long double-blind, double-dummy study has compared concurrent fluticasone/salmeterol treatment (110/42 µg twice daily, each administered via a separate MDI) with the fluticasone (110 µg twice daily, via MDI)/montelukast (10 mg once daily) combination.[43] This large-scale study included patients (n=1473) with chronic asthma (experienced for at least 1 year), which was not optimally controlled using inhaled corticosteroids alone. Patients were between the ages of 14 and 73 years and had an FEV_1 of 50–90% of the predicted normal value, which increased by at least 12% in response to inhaled salbutamol.

No significant difference between the fluticasone/salmeterol and the fluticasone/montelukast groups was reported for the percentage of patients remaining free of asthma exacerbations (80.0 *vs* 83.3%, respectively). Add-on therapy with montelukast was favoured in terms of visits to emergency departments and hospitalisations, whereas salmeterol was favoured in terms of doctor's visits and frequency of oral corticosteroid use. Only the discrepancy in the number of doctor's visits was significant. There was a slight but non-significant difference in favour of add-on salmeterol treatment in terms of daytime symptom scores, asthma-related quality of life scores and a composite score of asthma activity. Salmeterol was superior to montelukast at increasing pre-salbutamol but not post-salbutamol FEV_1 values. Supplemental salbutamol use in both groups indicated that asthma control remained sub-optimal. The authors suggested that persisting need for rescue medication may have been due to inadequate control of underlying inflammation.

Thus, in conclusion, Seretide is clearly superior to montelukast administered as monotherapy in providing control of asthma symptoms. Furthermore, the use of Seretide is consistent with current recommendations, which advise that long-acting β_2-agonists are the first-line option for add-on therapy to inhaled corticosteroids in persistent asthma, with leukotriene receptor antagonists as an alternative option.[3,4]

Seretide *vs* budesonide/formoterol fumarate combination

As reported in this review, Seretide has consistently been demonstrated to offer superior efficacy compared with placebo, fluticasone (including a double dose), salmeterol or montelukast. There are also some indications of superiority for Seretide over treatment with fluticasone and montelukast given concurrently. Given the clear benefits of an inhaled corticosteroid/long-acting β_2-agonist combination therapy, it is of interest to conduct a head-to-head comparison with the only other combination of these two drug classes that is currently available as a single inhaled product. Symbicort® is a combined formulation of budesonide and formoterol fumarate (hereafter referred to as formoterol), which has been shown to provide superior benefits in terms of pulmonary function and symptom control over placebo and the component drugs administered individually.[45–48]

Seretide has been compared with the budesonide/formoterol combination in a double-blind, double-dummy trial of 428 patients who remained symptomatic after budesonide treatment (1000–1600 µg/day or the equivalent inhaled corticosteroid dose[d]).[49] Patients were aged between 16 and 75 years, and had an FEV_1 of 50–85% of the predicted normal value which increased by at least 15% within 15 minutes of an inhaled dose of salbutamol (400 μg). In order to confirm that patients remained symptomatic on inhaled corticosteroids alone, they were only selected if they had a symptom score of at least 2, or had used salbutamol for symptom relief on at least two occasions, on at least 4 of the last 7 evaluable days of the run-in period. In this study, budesonide (800 μg twice daily) and formoterol (12 μg twice daily) were administered concurrently in separate DPI inhalers. This combination was compared with Seretide (50/250 μg twice daily, administered via a single DPI).

The difference in the mean morning PEF following 12 weeks of treatment was 3.2 L/minute in favour of Seretide, but this was not significantly different (p=0.593). Both drug combinations were also equivalent in reducing percentage diurnal variation in PEF and absolute FEV_1. Seretide was, however, significantly more effective than the budesonide/formoterol combination at reducing the asthma exacerbation rate (129 *vs* 206 exacerbations experienced; p<0.001). Seretide was also associated with a higher percentage of nights without awakening (p=0.02), nights without symptoms (p=0.04) and with a symptom score of under 2 (p=0.03). Seretide-treated patients made more primary care visits, whereas there were more than twice as many unscheduled specialist visits and in-patient hospital days in the budesonide/formoterol group.

Adverse events considered to be related to study drug occurred in 8.5% of Seretide- and 10.6% of budesonide/formoterol-treated patients. The most common of these events were oral candidiasis (1 *vs* 9 patients, respectively), hoarseness/dysphonia (6 *vs* 2), throat irritation (4 *vs* 1), worsening asthma control (0 *vs* 4), tremors (0 *vs* 3), tachycardia (3 *vs* 0) and muscle cramp/spasm (0 *vs* 3). There was one serious adverse event (polymyalgia), which was considered to be possibly related to study treatment, and this occurred in the Seretide group. It is not mentioned on what basis the polymyalgia was diagnosed, and its occurrence is somewhat surprising given that steroid treatment would be expected to reduce inflammation.

The two combinations of drugs have also been compared in a study which used the single inhalation device for each.[50] This direct comparison of Seretide and Symbicort adopted a double-blind, double-dummy design for 1 month, and also included a 6-month open-label extension period. Patients (n=658) were at least 12 years of age, had experienced asthma for at least 6 months and had been using inhaled corticosteroids for at least 3 months prior to study entry. At baseline, the mean FEV_1 was at least 50% of the predicted normal value. During the double-blind period, patients received either Symbicort (formoterol, 4.5 μg; budesonide, 160 μg) or Seretide (50/250 μg), each administered

---

[d]Beclometasone or flunisolide, 1000–1600 μg/day, or fluticasone, 500–800 μg/day.

twice daily via a DPI. During the 6-month open-label extension period, an additional treatment arm was included, in which patients were able to adjust their dose of Symbicort according to pre-defined dose-adjustment criteria. Patients in this 'adjustable maintenance dosing' group were allowed between one and four inhalations of Symbicort twice daily. However, there was no corresponding adjustable dosing permitted with Seretide, and so for the purpose of this review, the most important comparison is between the two fixed-dosing groups.

The odds of achieving a well-controlled asthma week were statistically equivalent between the fixed-dose Symbicort and Seretide groups.

Asthma control in this study was measured in terms of 'well-controlled asthma weeks', which were defined in terms of the number of night-time awakenings due to asthma, the frequency of asthma exacerbations and changes in asthma treatment due to adverse events, as well as criteria for symptom scores, use of rescue medication and PEF. The odds of achieving a well-controlled asthma week were equivalent between the fixed-dose Symbicort and Seretide groups. During the open-label extension phase, however, the adjustable maintenance dosing Symbicort group reported significantly more well-controlled asthma weeks than the group receiving a fixed-dose of the same drug, but not significantly more than the group receiving a fixed-dose of Seretide (Figure 6). The total number of asthma exacerbations was equivalent in the adjustable- and fixed-dose Symbicort groups, but the adjustable-dose Symbicort group reported fewer exacerbations than the fixed-dose

Figure 6. Mean percentage of patients with a well-controlled asthma week (WCAW). Patients in the fixed-dose (FD) groups received Symbicort (4.5/160 μg, two inhalations twice daily) or Seretide (50/250 μg, one inhalation twice daily. Patients in the adjustable maintenance dose (AMD) group received 1 month of double-blind treatment with Symbicort FD followed by Symbicort AMD (1–4 inhalations twice daily) during the 6-month open-label extension.[50]

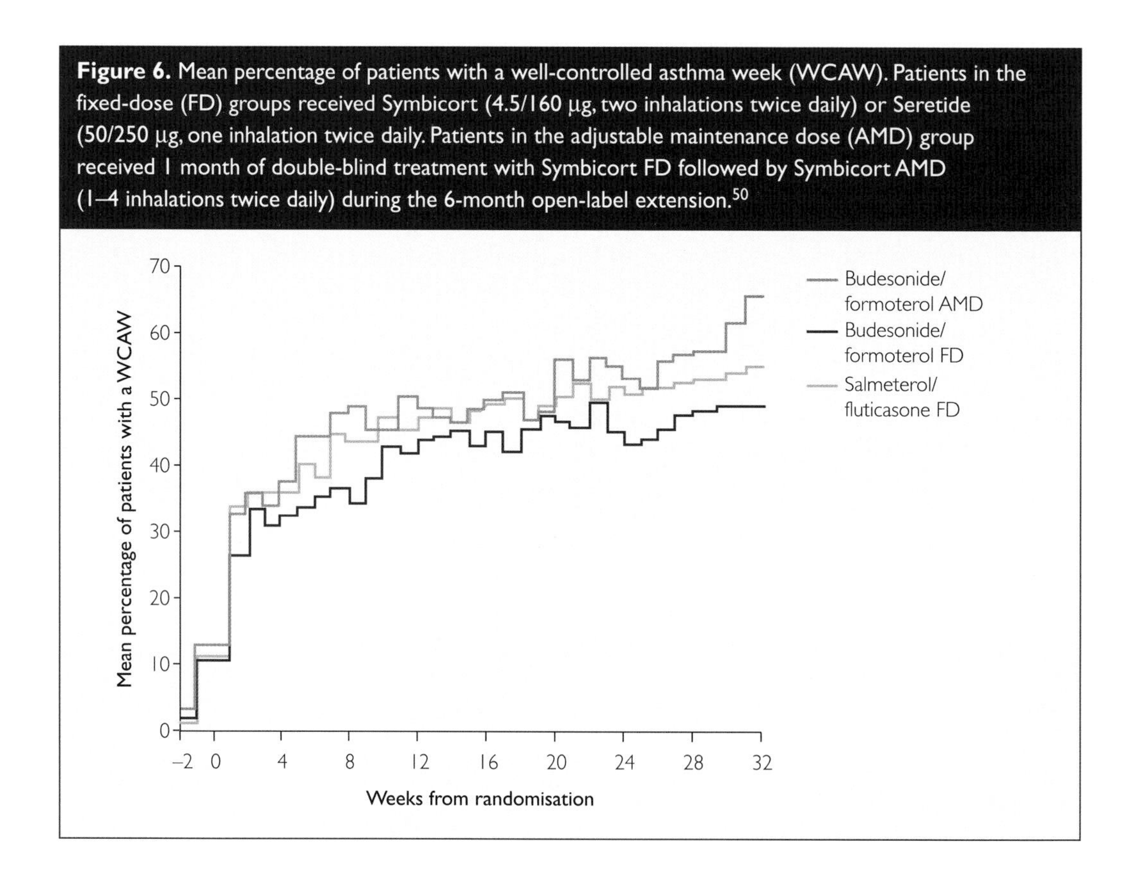

Seretide group. The improvement in FEV_1 induced by the fixed-dose Symbicort regimen was significantly greater than that in the Seretide group ($p<0.05$), both at the end of the double-blind phase and after the open-label extension. However, the mean changes from baseline in morning PEF, evening PEF, use of rescue medication and daytime symptom scores were all statistically equivalent between the fixed-dose Symbicort and Seretide groups during the double-blind phase and the open-label extension.

The incidence of adverse events was similar in the fixed-dose Symbicort and Seretide groups, though there was a trend for increased prevalence in the latter (58 and 66%). This trend was also seen in terms of the most commonly reported events (candidiasis in 2 *vs* 3%, dysphonia in 1 *vs* 7% and headache in 2 *vs* 4%, in each group, respectively). No serious events were reported in any group which were considered by the investigator to be related to the study drugs. One patient treated with fixed-dose Symbicort experienced an adverse event related to asthma, whereas none were reported in the fixed-dose Seretide group.

On the basis of the available data, Seretide and Symbicort appear broadly comparable in their efficacy and tolerability when used in fixed regimens. The benefits observed in the Aalbers study resulting from the adoption of an adjustable dosing regimen for Symbicort may extend to Seretide, and may represent the way forward for maintenance therapy for asthma.[50]

Efficacy in children

Almost all of the studies described previously have included patients under the age of 18 years, though the youngest patients enrolled into these studies were older than 12 years. US data indicate that up to 80% of children with asthma exhibit symptoms by 5 years of age.[51] Indeed, the incidence of asthma is higher in children under the age of 5 years than in any other segment of the population.[52] Thus, it is important to establish the efficacy and safety of asthma therapies in this paediatric patient population. Guidelines for the treatment of childhood asthma advise that in children under the age of 5 years with chronic or daily wheezing, inhaled corticosteroids are an appropriate choice of treatment.[3,53] Given the heightened concerns associated with the use of high doses of inhaled corticosteroids in children, the high potency and lipophilicity (which ensures retention in the lung tissue) of fluticasone means that it can be used at relatively lower doses than other corticosteroids, thereby making it an appropriate choice in this population. It is also associated with a lower risk of impaired growth velocity than beclometasone dipropionate.[54] Concern over increasing the dosage of corticosteroids in paediatric patients also indicates that add-on therapy with a long-acting β_2-agonist is a more preferable treatment strategy than an increase in the dose of corticosteroids in those patients whose asthma is inadequately controlled on monotherapy.[53] It is questionable, however, whether regular use of long-acting β_2-agonists as add-on therapy is effective in this patient population. Rather, it appears that in children, more effective bronchodilation and bronchoprotection is obtained with long-acting β_2-agonists when they are administered according to an intermittent, as-needed regimen.[55]

A retrospective, multicentre analysis has been conducted to evaluate the efficacy and safety of the fluticasone/salmeterol combination in patients between the ages of 5 months and 5 years.[e,52] Each patient (n=50) had a history of wheezing and was treated with concurrent fluticasone (88–440 µg/day) and salmeterol (doses not reported), administered by two separate MDIs fitted with chambers and face masks. Patients were required to have been treated with this combination for at least 3 months, though the mean duration of treatment was 19.1 months.

The number of emergency room visits in the year after fluticasone/salmeterol treatment was significantly lower than that in the year before (visits reduced from 78 to 5; $p<0.001$). The same was true of the number of hospitalisations (reduced 43 to 2; $p<0.001$). Combination treatment was also associated with a significant reduction in the frequency of wheezing ($p<0.001$). Of the 45 patients included in this part of the analysis, 24 were wheezing daily prior to treatment. After treatment, 22 of these patients were wheezing no more than monthly.

One of the major safety concerns in paediatric patients treated with inhaled corticosteroids is the potential for retarded growth velocity. However, in the 21 patients included in the safety analysis in this study, there was no significant difference in the mean height percentile before (46.2%) and after (42.8%) treatment with fluticasone/salmeterol. When male and female subjects were analysed separately, there was a trend for a reduction in mean growth percentile in males (–5.6 *vs* +1.3%). This reduction was not statistically significant, though a failure to detect a difference between these groups may reflect the limited sample size (n=13).

The use of Seretide specifically in a paediatric patient population has been evaluated in a double-blind, double-dummy trial, which compared its relative efficacy and safety profile with the salmeterol/fluticasone combination administered concurrently via separate devices.[56] Patients included in this trial (n=257) had reversible airways obstruction, were aged between 4 and 11 years, and remained symptomatic on beclometasone dipropionate (400–500 µg/day or equivalent inhaled corticosteroid dose[f]) for at least 4 weeks prior to the study. Patients entered a 2-week run-in phase, during which time they continued to use their regular inhaled corticosteroid therapy. Patients subsequently randomised to active treatment had symptom scores of at least 1 on at least 4 of the last 7 consecutive days prior to the run-in phase. They also had a mean morning PEF of 50–85% of that measured 15 minutes after an inhaled dose of salbutamol (400 µg). Patients were randomised to active treatment with Seretide (50/100 µg twice daily, administered via a DPI) or the equivalent doses of salmeterol and fluticasone given by two separate DPIs.

---

[e]Seretide is not licensed in the UK for children under the age of 4 years

[f]Budesonide or flunisolide, 400–500 µg/day, or fluticasone, 200–250 µg/day.

In both treatment groups, the mean morning PEF increased significantly. The mean change from baseline was greater in the Seretide group (33 *vs* 28 L/minute), though this difference was not statistically significant. However, at week 2 the benefit of Seretide in terms of PEF was significantly superior compared with the concurrently administered agents (p=0.017). The same pattern emerged for the mean change in evening PEF, which again was not significantly different between the Seretide and concurrent groups at the end of the study (29 *vs* 25 L/minute), but favoured Seretide at week 2 (p=0.027). Both Seretide and concurrent therapy improved FEV_1, symptom scores, the percentage of symptom-free days and nights, and the percentage of days and nights without any need for rescue medication, by a statistically equivalent extent.

Both active treatments were well tolerated. Adverse events considered to be drug-related by the study investigators occurred in 10% of those receiving Seretide and 5% of those receiving concurrent therapy. No serious adverse events were reported that were considered to be related to study treatment. Two patients in each group withdrew due as a result of these adverse events. However, neither treatment generated any significant increase in mean morning cortisol concentrations or any changes to vital signs or laboratory values.

The fluticasone/salmeterol combination appears, therefore, to be effective and well tolerated in young children. Data are not available, however, regarding the relative efficacy and safety of Seretide in comparison with an increased dose of fluticasone, or compared with placebo, fluticasone or salmeterol administered individually. Given that dosing complexity, and its impact on compliance, is an issue particularly pertinent amongst the paediatric population, the combination of fluticasone and salmeterol in a single inhalation device may prove to be particularly beneficial for these patients.

The fluticasone/ salmeterol combination appears to be effective and well tolerated in young children.

Safety and tolerability

The safety of maintenance treatment for persistent asthma is essentially the raison d'être of Seretide, as combination therapy was developed as an alternative strategy to increasing the dose of inhaled corticosteroids and incurring the associated risks of systemic side effects. Furthermore, the addition of salmeterol to low-to-moderate doses of fluticasone treatment does not appear to be associated with any significant impact upon tolerability.[15] The side-effect profile of Seretide reported in the clinical trial programme appears to be comparable with that reported for fluticasone alone. Adverse events include candidiasis of the mouth and throat, headache, tremor, palpitations, throat irritation, hoarseness/dysphonia and muscle cramps.[18]

One of the major underlying safety concerns associated with Seretide arises not from its corticosteroid component, but from salmeterol. This concern arose from the Salmeterol Multicenter Asthma Research Trial (SMART), which was halted early due to a routine interim analysis that highlighted a non-significant trend towards an increase in asthma-related life-threatening events with salmeterol than with placebo.[23] The primary endpoint of this trial was the number of respiratory-related deaths and life-threatening events, with secondary outcomes including asthma-related events, including deaths. Although the overall trend for asthma-related life-threatening events was non-significant, amongst the black population (who comprised 17% of the study population of nearly 26,000), salmeterol treatment was associated with significantly more primary and secondary outcomes than placebo. However, a subgroup analysis revealed that amongst the 50% of Caucasian and 38% of black patients who were receiving concurrent inhaled corticosteroid therapy within the SMART trial, no significant effect of salmeterol treatment on the number of primary or secondary outcomes was reported. In addition to raising queries regarding a possible association between ethnicity and asthma-related death, data from the SMART study have further reinforced management guidelines which recommend that salmeterol should not be used in isolation, either for immediate relief of acute asthma or as a substitute for inhaled corticosteroids in maintenance therapy for persistent asthma.[3] From these preliminary data, however, it would appear that the initial concerns over the association of salmeterol treatment with life-threatening asthma episodes and asthma-related deaths do not appear to apply when salmeterol is administered concurrently with corticosteroids, as is the case with Seretide. This issue was addressed in an analysis of data from a comparative double-blind, double-dummy trial.[43] There were no deaths among black patients treated with either fluticasone/montelukast or fluticasone/salmeterol, and the small increase in the number of asthma attacks, which occurred in both treatment groups, did not reach statistical significance.

Initial concerns over the association of salmeterol treatment with life-threatening asthma episodes and asthma-related deaths do not appear to apply when salmeterol is administered concurrently with corticosteroids.

Further concerns over the safety of Seretide relate to the uncertainty over whether salmeterol exerts any anti-inflammatory effects. As discussed previously, indications that salmeterol may promote the translocation of the corticosteroid–receptor complex to the cell nucleus and enhance apoptosis of inflammatory cells have not translated to any consistently detectable anti-inflammatory effect in patients. As a result of this uncertainty, concern has been expressed over whether add-on therapy with long-acting β_2-agonists may mask deteriorating or persistent airway inflammation, by relieving asthma symptoms without affecting the underlying disease process. Indeed, it has been reported that add-on salmeterol therapy in patients already receiving inhaled corticosteroids can control symptoms and improve lung function despite inflammation becomes significantly more advanced.[57] This observation underlies the importance of establishing a suitable maintenance dose of inhaled corticosteroid before supplemental treatment is added.

Concern has been expressed over whether add-on therapy with long-acting β_2-agonists may mask deteriorating or persistent airway inflammation.

Cautions and contra-indications

No adjustment of dose is required in patients with renal impairment or in the elderly.[15] Children under the age of 12 years should only receive the lowest dose formulation (50/100 µg), and Seretide is not licensed in the UK for children under the age of 4 years.[58] No data are yet available on the use of Seretide in patients with hepatic impairment, though given the involvement of the CYP 3A4 isoenzyme in the metabolism of both fluticasone and salmeterol, caution is advised when using Seretide in these patients.[15] Caution is also advised in patients with cardiovascular disorders (e.g. coronary insufficiency, heart rhythm abnormalities or hypertension), diabetes mellitus, untreated hypokalaemia or thyrotoxicosis.

The use of Seretide during pregnancy has not been formally studied in humans. In studies in rodents, salmeterol has been reported to increase the rate of benign smooth muscle tumours, but there is strong evidence that these effects are species-specific.[16] Sparse data on the safety of Seretide in human pregnancy have been obtained from a study that compared Seretide with concurrent budesonide and formoterol treatment.[49] During the course of this study, two pregnancies occurred. Both patients were receiving Seretide, and neither pregnancy was associated with any birth defects.

Pharmacoeconomics

Persistent asthma is associated with significant direct costs as a consequence of medical care, such as physician visits, hospitalisations and drug costs, but also with indirect costs, relating to absenteeism from work or school, and reduced productivity at work. Generally, the improved asthma control offered by combination treatment is associated with higher direct costs than monotherapy.[59] Although monotherapy is clearly a less costly option in an appropriate patient population, poorly controlled asthma leads to indirect cost implications, and therefore adoption of combination therapy may prove to be a more cost-effective strategy in those with more severe asthma. Compared with other available combination treatments, asthma-related costs with Seretide are low, as demonstrated in a 6-month US-based pharmacoeconomic study (Table 2).[59] When focusing on the comparisons which are most relevant for clinical practice in the UK, the fluticasone/salmeterol combination has consistently been shown to be more cost-effective than inhaled corticosteroids administered together with leukotriene receptor antagonists.[60,61] Furthermore, in trials comparing Seretide with Symbicort, Seretide was shown to be more cost-effective.[49,50]

Compared with other available combination treatments, asthma-related costs with Seretide are low.

Table 2. Total asthma-related costs of various drug combinations for maintenance treatment of asthma over a 6-month period.[59]

Combination	Total cost (US$)
Corticosteroid + mast cell-stabilising agents	359.72
Fluticasone + salmeterol	408.63
Corticosteroid + xanthines	455.24
Corticosteroid (excluding fluticasone) + salmeterol	460.30
Salmeterol + leukotriene receptor antagonist	537.08
Corticosteroid + leukotriene receptor antagonist	560.84

Key points

- Fluticasone and salmeterol have complementary mechanisms of action and target two major components of asthma – airway inflammation and bronchoconstriction. Seretide is a single inhaled combination product containing both agents, which offers the potential for increased compliance due to simplified dosing.
- Seretide offers superior efficacy in terms of pulmonary function, symptom control and the need for rescue medication, in comparison with placebo, the individual monotherapies administered at equivalent doses or at least double the dose of fluticasone.
- Seretide is at least as effective as the equivalent doses of fluticasone and salmeterol administered concurrently via separate inhalers.
- The CFC-free HFA-formulation of Seretide is more effective than concurrent treatment with CFC-based fluticasone and salmeterol. Head-to-head comparisons of HFA– and CFC–Seretide are needed to confirm their relative efficacy.
- Seretide is considerably more effective than montelukast administered alone, whilst there is some evidence to indicate superiority over a fluticasone/montelukast combination.
- Seretide (50/250 μg) and Symbicort (4.5 μg/160 μg) are broadly equivalent in clinical efficacy. However, an adjustable maintenance dosing regimen has been shown to improve efficacy with Symbicort treatment, which may also apply to Seretide.
- Seretide is well tolerated, with a side-effect profile similar to that reported for fluticasone monotherapy. Concerns regarding the incidence of asthma-related life-threatening events in patients treated with salmeterol, particularly amongst black patients, do not appear to apply when the drug is used concurrently with fluticasone.
- The combination of fluticasone and salmeterol is effective and well tolerated in a paediatric patient population.
- In patients whose asthma is inadequately controlled by inhaled corticosteroids alone, Seretide appears to be a cost-effective option.

References

A list of the published evidence which has been reviewed in compiling the preceding section of *BESTMEDICINE*.

1 MacKenzie C. Effects of inhaled corticosteroids on growth. *J Allergy Clin Immunol* 1998; **101**: S451–5.
2 Wallin A, Sue-Chu M, Bjermer L *et al.* Effect of inhaled fluticasone with and without salmeterol on airway inflammation in asthma. *J Allergy Clin Immunol* 2003; **112**: 72–8.
3 British Thoracic Society and Scottish Intercollegiate Guidelines Network. British Guideline on the Management of Asthma. 2004. *www.sign.ac.uk*
4 Ringdal N. Long-acting beta2-agonists or leukotriene receptor antagonists as add-on therapy to inhaled corticosteroids for the treatment of persistent asthma. *Drugs* 2003; **63(Suppl 2)**: 21–33.
5 Greening AP, Ind PW, Northfield M, Shaw G. Added salmeterol versus higher-dose corticosteroid in asthma patients with symptoms on existing inhaled corticosteroid. Allen & Hanburys Limited UK Study Group. *Lancet* 1994; **344**: 219–24.
6 Woolcock A, Lundback B, Ringdal N, Jacques LA. Comparison of addition of salmeterol to inhaled steroids with doubling of the dose of inhaled steroids. *Am J Respir Crit Care Med* 1996; **153**: 1481–8.
7 Nelson HS, Wolfe JD, Gross G *et al.* Efficacy and safety of fluticasone propionate 44 microg/salmeterol 21 microg administered in a hydrofluoroalkane metered-dose inhaler as an initial asthma maintenance treatment. *Ann Allergy Asthma Immunol* 2003; **91**: 263–9.
8 D'Souza S. The Montreal Protocol and essential use exemptions. *J Aerosol Med* 1995; **8(Suppl 1)**: S13–7.
9 Nelson HS, Chapman KR, Pyke SD, Johnson M, Pritchard JN. Enhanced synergy between fluticasone propionate and salmeterol inhaled from a single inhaler versus separate inhalers. *J Allergy Clin Immunol* 2003; **112**: 29–36.
10 Baumgarten C, Geldszus R, Behre U, Peslis N, Trautmann M. Initial treatment of symptomatic mild to moderate bronchial asthma with the salmeterol/fluticasone propionate (50/250 microg) combination product (SAS 40023). *Eur J Med Res* 2002; **7**: 1–7.
11 Walters EH, Bjermer L, Faurschou P, Sandstrom T. The anti-inflammatory profile of inhaled corticosteroids combined with salmeterol in asthmatic patients. *Respir Med* 2000; **94(Suppl F)**: S26–31.
12 Stoloff S, Poinsett-Holmes K, Dorinsky PM. Combination therapy with inhaled long-acting beta2-agonists and inhaled corticosteroids: a paradigm shift in asthma management. *Pharmacotherapy* 2002; **22**: 212–26.
13 Lee DK, Jackson CM, Currie GP, Cockburn WJ, Lipworth BJ. Comparison of combination inhalers *vs* inhaled corticosteroids alone in moderate persistent asthma. *Br J Clin Pharmacol* 2003; **56**: 494–500.
14 Currie GP, Stenback S, Lipworth BJ. Effects of fluticasone vs. fluticasone/salmeterol on airway calibre and airway hyperresponsiveness in mild persistent asthma. *Br J Clin Pharmacol* 2003; **56**: 11–7.
15 Markham A, Jarvis B. Inhaled salmeterol/fluticasone propionate combination: a review of its use in persistent asthma. *Drugs* 2000; **60**: 1207–33.
16 Allen and Hanburys Ltd. Serevent® (salmeterol) *Summary of product characteristics.* Uxbridge, Middlesex, 2004.
17 Allen and Hanburys Ltd. Flixotide® (fluticasone) *Summary of product characteristics.* Uxbridge, Middlesex, 2004.
18 Allen and Hanburys Ltd. Seretide®. *Summary of product characteristics.* Uxbridge, Middlesex, 2004.
19 Cazzola M, Testi R, Matera MG. Clinical pharmacokinetics of salmeterol. *Clin Pharmacokinet* 2002; **41**: 19–30.
20 Kirby S, Falcoz C, Daniel MJ *et al.* Salmeterol and fluticasone propionate given as a combination. Lack of systemic pharmacodynamic and pharmacokinetic interactions. *Eur J Clin Pharmacol* 2001; **56**: 781–91.
21 Kavuru M, Melamed J, Gross G *et al.* Salmeterol and fluticasone propionate combined in a new powder inhalation device for the treatment of asthma: a randomized, double-blind, placebo-controlled trial. *J Allergy Clin Immunol* 2000; **105**: 1108–16.
22 Shapiro G, Lumry W, Wolfe J *et al.* Combined salmeterol 50 microg and fluticasone propionate 250 microg in the diskus device for the treatment of asthma. *Am J Respir Crit Care Med* 2000; **161**: 527–34.
23 Wooltorton E. Salmeterol (Serevent) asthma trial halted early. *CMAJ* 2003; **168**: 738.
24 Condemi JJ, Goldstein S, Kalberg C *et al.* The addition of salmeterol to fluticasone propionate versus increasing the dose of fluticasone propionate in patients with persistent asthma. Salmeterol Study Group. *Ann Allergy Asthma Immunol* 1999; **82**: 383–9.
25 Busse W, Koenig SM, Oppenheimer J *et al.* Steroid-sparing effects of fluticasone propionate 100 microg and salmeterol 50 microg administered twice daily in a single product in patients previously controlled with fluticasone propionate 250 microg administered twice daily. *J Allergy Clin Immunol* 2003; **111**: 57–65.
26 Bergmann KC, Lindemann L, Braun R, Steinkamp G. Salmeterol/fluticasone propionate (50/250 microg) combination is superior to double dose fluticasone (500 microg) for the treatment of symptomatic moderate asthma. *Swiss Med Wkly* 2004; **134**: 50–8.
27 Ind PW, Dal Negro R, Colman NC *et al.* Addition of salmeterol to fluticasone propionate treatment in moderate-to-severe asthma. *Respir Med* 2003; **97**: 555–62.

28 Bateman ED, Boushey HA, Bousquet J *et al.* Can guideline-defined asthma control be achieved? The Gaining Optimal Asthma ControL study. *Am J Respir Crit Care Med* 2004; **170**: 836–44.

29 Rabe KF, Vermeire PA, Soriano JB, Maier WC. Clinical management of asthma in 1999: the Asthma Insights and Reality in Europe (AIRE) study. *Eur Respir J* 2000; **16**: 802–7.

30 Bateman E, Britton M, Carrillo Jea. Salmeterol/fluticasone combination inhaler: a new effective and well tolerated treatment for asthma. *Clin Drug Invest* 1998; **16**: 193–201.

31 Chapman KR, Ringdal N, Backer V *et al.* Salmeterol and fluticasone propionate (50/250 microg) administered via combination Diskus inhaler: as effective as when given via separate Diskus inhalers. *Can Respir J* 1999; **6**: 45–51.

32 Aubier M, Pieters WR, Schlosser NJ, Steinmetz KO. Salmeterol/fluticasone propionate (50/500 microg) in combination in a Diskus inhaler (Seretide) is effective and safe in the treatment of steroid-dependent asthma. *Respir Med* 1999; **93**: 876–84.

33 Nelson HS. Advair: combination treatment with fluticasone propionate/salmeterol in the treatment of asthma. *J Allergy Clin Immunol* 2001; **107**: 398–416.

34 Stoloff SW, Stempel DA, Meyer J, Stanford RH, Carranza Rosenzweig JR. Improved refill persistence with fluticasone propionate and salmeterol in a single inhaler compared with other controller therapies. *J Allergy Clin Immunol* 2004; **113**: 245–51.

35 Carter ER, Ananthakrishnan M. Adherence to montelukast versus inhaled corticosteroids in children with asthma. *Pediatr Pulmonol* 2003; **36**: 301–4.

36 Jenkins C, Woolcock AJ, Saarelainen P, Lundback B, James MH. Salmeterol/fluticasone propionate combination therapy 50/250 microg twice daily is more effective than budesonide 800 microg twice daily in treating moderate to severe asthma. *Respir Med* 2000; **94**: 715–23.

37 Juniper EF, Jenkins C, Price MJ, James MH. Impact of inhaled salmeterol/fluticasone propionate combination product versus budesonide on the health-related quality of life of patients with asthma. *Am J Respir Med* 2002; **1**: 435–40.

38 Pearlman DS, White MV, Lieberman AK *et al.* Fluticasone propionate/salmeterol combination compared with montelukast for the treatment of persistent asthma. *Ann Allergy Asthma Immunol* 2002; **88**: 227–35.

39 Busse W, Raphael GD, Galant S *et al.* Low-dose fluticasone propionate compared with montelukast for first-line treatment of persistent asthma: a randomized clinical trial. *J Allergy Clin Immunol* 2001; **107**: 461–8.

40 Meltzer EO, Lockey RF, Friedman BF *et al.* Efficacy and safety of low-dose fluticasone propionate compared with montelukast for maintenance treatment of persistent asthma. *Mayo Clin Proc* 2002; **77**: 437–45.

41 Nelson HS, Busse WW, Kerwin E *et al.* Fluticasone propionate/salmeterol combination provides more effective asthma control than low-dose inhaled corticosteroid plus montelukast. *J Allergy Clin Immunol* 2000; **106**: 1088–95.

42 Ringdal N, Eliraz A, Pruzinec R *et al.* The salmeterol/fluticasone combination is more effective than fluticasone plus oral montelukast in asthma. *Respir Med* 2003; **97**: 234–41.

43 Ilowite J, Webb R, Friedman B *et al.* Addition of montelukast or salmeterol to fluticasone for protection against asthma attacks: a randomized, double-blind, multicenter study. *Ann Allergy Asthma Immunol* 2004; **92**: 641–8.

44 Bjermer L, Bisgaard H, Bousquet J *et al.* Montelukast and fluticasone compared with salmeterol and fluticasone in protecting against asthma exacerbation in adults: one year, double blind, randomised, comparative trial. *BMJ* 2003; **327**: 891.

45 Zetterstrom O, Buhl R, Mellem H *et al.* Improved asthma control with budesonide/formoterol in a single inhaler, compared with budesonide alone. *Eur Respir J* 2001; **18**: 262–8.

46 Rosenhall L, Heinig JH, Lindqvist A *et al.* Budesonide/formoterol (Symbicort) is well tolerated and effective in patients with moderate persistent asthma. *Int J Clin Pract* 2002; **56**: 427–33.

47 Pauwels RA, Lofdahl CG, Postma DS *et al.* Effect of inhaled formoterol and budesonide on exacerbations of asthma. Formoterol and Corticosteroids Establishing Therapy (FACET) International Study Group. *N Engl J Med* 1997; **337**: 1405–11.

48 O'Byrne PM, Barnes PJ, Rodriguez-Roisin R *et al.* Low dose inhaled budesonide and formoterol in mild persistent asthma: the OPTIMA randomized trial. *Am J Respir Crit Care Med* 2001; **164**: 1392–7.

49 Ringdal N, Chuchalin A, Chovan L *et al.* Evaluation of different inhaled combination therapies (EDICT): a randomised, double-blind comparison of Seretide (50/250 microg bd Diskus vs. formoterol (12 microg bd) and budesonide (800 microg bd) given concurrently (both via Turbuhaler) in patients with moderate-to-severe asthma. *Respir Med* 2002; **96**: 851–61.

50 Aalbers R, Backer V, Kava TT *et al.* Adjustable maintenance dosing with budesonide/formoterol compared with fixed-dose salmeterol/fluticasone in moderate to severe asthma. *Curr Med Res Opin* 2004; **20**: 225–40.

51 Kemp JP, Skoner DP, Szefler SJ *et al.* Once-daily budesonide inhalation suspension for the treatment of persistent asthma in infants and young children. *Ann Allergy Asthma Immunol* 1999; **83**: 231–9.

52 Sekhsaria S, Alam M, Sait T, Starr B, Parekh M. Efficacy and safety of inhaled corticosteroids in combination with a long-acting beta2-agonist in asthmatic children under age 5. *J Asthma* 2004; **41**: 575–82.

53 British Asthma Guidelines Coordinating Committee. Asthma in children under five years of age. The General Practitioner in Asthma Group, the British Association of Accident and Emergency Medicine, the British Paediatric Respiratory Society and the Royal College of Paediatrics and Child Health. *Thorax* 1997; **52(Suppl 1)**: S9–10, S18–21.

54 Wolthers OD, Pedersen S. Short-term growth during treatment with inhaled fluticasone propionate and beclomethasone dipropionate. *Arch Dis Child* 1993; **68**: 673–6.

55 Bisgaard H. Long-acting beta(2)-agonists in management of childhood asthma: A critical review of the literature. *Pediatr Pulmonol* 2000; **29**: 221–34.

56 Van den Berg NJ, Ossip MS, Hederos CA *et al.* Salmeterol/fluticasone propionate (50/100 microg) in combination in a Diskus inhaler (Seretide) is effective and safe in children with asthma. *Pediatr Pulmonol* 2000; **30**: 97–105.

57 McIvor RA, Pizzichini E, Turner MO *et al.* Potential masking effects of salmeterol on airway inflammation in asthma. *Am J Respir Crit Care Med* 1998; **158**: 924–30.

58 *British National Formulary (BNF) 48.* London: British Medical Association and Royal Pharmaceutical Society of Great Britian. September 2004.

59 Wang SW, Liu X, Wiener DJ *et al.* Comparison of prevalence, cost, and outcomes of a combination of salmeterol and fluticasone therapy to common asthma treatments. *Am J Manag Care* 2001; **7**: 913–22.

60 O'Connor RD, O'Donnell JC, Pinto LA, Wiener DJ, Legorreta AP. Two-year retrospective economic evaluation of three dual-controller therapies used in the treatment of asthma. *Chest* 2002; **121**: 1028–35.

61 O'Connor RD, Nelson H, Borker R *et al.* Cost effectiveness of fluticasone propionate plus salmeterol versus fluticasone propionate plus montelukast in the treatment of persistent asthma. *Pharmacoeconomics* 2004; **22**: 815–25.

Acknowledgements

Figure 2 is adapted from Shapiro *et al.*, 2000.[22]
Figure 3 is adapted from Ind *et al.*, 2003.[27]
Figure 4 is adapted from Ringdal *et al.*, 2003.[42]
Figure 5 is adapted from Aalbers *et al.*, 2004.[50]

11. Drug review – Symbicort®

Dr Eleanor Bull
CSF Medical Communications Ltd

Summary

Symbicort® is a single combined formulation of the inhaled corticosteroid, budesonide, and the long-acting β_2-adrenoceptor agonist (β_2-agonist), formoterol. The combined administration of these agents is currently recommended in asthma patients in whom moderate doses of inhaled corticosteroids are failing to provide adequate control. Whether the optimised asthma control that results from co-administration of both agents is a result of synergistic drug–drug interactions or simply the improved convenience of a single inhaler regimen remains unclear. Clinical studies have shown that Symbicort is as effective as budesonide and formoterol administered via separate inhalers and more effective than higher doses of budesonide monotherapy. By limiting the dose of inhaled corticosteroid, Symbicort may help to minimise long-term systemic safety concerns related to the prolonged use of inhaled corticosteroids. Patient-controlled adjustable Symbicort maintenance dosing regimens are associated with at least the same level of asthma control as fixed-dose regimens, but at a lower overall dose. Comparative studies with Seretide® – the single inhaler formulation of fluticasone propionate and salmeterol – have been largely inconclusive to date, though both combinations provide significant improvements compared with their respective monotherapies.

The addition of a long-acting β_2-agonist to an inhaled corticosteroid gives optimal control of asthma in most patients and is more effective than increasing the dose of the inhaled corticosteroid.

Introduction

Current asthma management includes corticosteroids as prophylactic therapy in all but the mildest cases of asthma with persistent symptoms, and advocates the use of long-acting β_2-agonists as the preferred second-line controller therapy in addition to inhaled corticosteroids. The addition of a long-acting β_2-agonist to an inhaled corticosteroid gives optimal control of asthma in most patients and is more effective than increasing the dose of the inhaled corticosteroid.[1]

Guidelines issued in 2004 jointly by the Scottish Intercollegiate Guidelines Network (SIGN) and the British Thoracic Society (BTS), recommend the use of long-acting β_2-agonists as add-on therapy if moderate doses of inhaled steroids (usual maintenance dose of 400 μg/day for adults and 200 μg/day for children aged 5–12 years of beclometasone dipropionate or equivalent) are failing to adequately control asthma.[2] The Global Initiative for Asthma (GINA) guidelines echo these recommendations and add that control should be established initially with a high level of therapy (i.e. a high dose of inhaled corticosteroid plus a long-acting β_2-agonist that corresponds to the severity of the patient's asthma), which should then be stepped down after control is sustained for at least 3 months.[3]

Corticosteroids and β_2-agonists have complementary mechanisms of action; corticosteroids suppress the chronic inflammation of the airways associated with asthma and also reduce airway hyper-responsiveness, whereas β_2-agonists have predominantly bronchodilatory effects.[1] The combined effects of these drugs are superior to the actions of either drug when given as monotherapy and in general, their low systemic activities do not result in an increase in the frequency or severity of adverse events when used together.[1]

Aside from the mechanistic benefits of combining these drugs, administering two drugs simultaneously may also serve to improve patient adherence to therapy. The success of any asthma treatment regimen is highly dependent on the compliance of the individual patient and in general, adherence declines as the regimen becomes more complex.[4] A multiple inhaler approach is potentially confusing to the patient. Adherence is compromised further if the effects of a drug are not immediately apparent to the patient. Therefore, it is speculated that the addition of budesonide, for which there is no immediate perceived effect on breathing, to formoterol, a drug with a rapid onset of action, may also improve adherence and ultimately asthma control.

Symbicort is indicated for the regular treatment of asthma where the use of a combination of an inhaled corticosteroid and a long-acting β_2-agonist is appropriate.

Symbicort is a combined formulation of the second-generation inhaled corticosteroid, budesonide, and the long-acting β_2-adrenoceptor selective agonist, formoterol, administered via the Turbohaler®, a dry powder, inspiratory flow driven inhaler.[5] Each metered inhalation of Symbicort delivers the same quantity of budesonide and formoterol as the respective metered doses when administered as separate inhalations.[6] Symbicort is indicated for the regular treatment of asthma where the use of a combination of an inhaled corticosteroid and a long-acting β_2-agonist is appropriate.[5] This includes patients not adequately controlled with inhaled corticosteroids and as-needed inhaled short-acting β_2-agonists and patients already adequately controlled on both inhaled corticosteroids and long-acting β_2-agonists.[5]

The current review discusses the pharmacological properties of Symbicort and its efficacy in controlled clinical trials in adults and children with asthma. In line with other reviews of anti-asthma drugs previously published in the journal *Drugs in Context*, clinical trials of Symbicort in patients with Chronic Obstructive Pulmonary Disease (COPD) are beyond the scope of the review and are not discussed herein. Symbicort is currently available in three formulations, the metered doses of which are 100/6, 200/6 and 400/12 μg, of budesonide and formoterol, respectively. In this article, we have reviewed data specific to the combined administration of budesonide and formoterol, either from single or separate inhaler devices. Clinical data pertaining to budesonide and formoterol as individual formulations are discussed in detail in the other chapters of this edition of *BESTMEDICINE*.

Pharmacology

Chemistry

The chemical structures of budesonide and formoterol (or eformoterol) are illustrated in Figure 1. The formulation of budesonide in clinical use is a racemic mixture of two epimers, 22R and 22S, that do not interconvert.[7] Budesonide is non-halogenated, in contrast to many other inhaled corticosteroids (e.g. beclometasone dipropionate, triamcinolone acetonide), which may contribute to its high topical-to-systemic activity ratio.[8]

The clinical formulation of formoterol is a pure diastereomer of the RR and SS enantiomers of the fumarate dihydrate salt. The unique pharmacological profile of formoterol can be attributed to its intermediate physiochemical properties.[9] Formoterol is less hydrophilic than salbutamol and less lipophilic than salmeterol, which consequently produces a hybrid compound that shares the most therapeutically valuable attributes of these short- and long-acting β_2-compounds.[9]

The chemistry of Symbicort® is of essentially academic interest and most healthcare professionals will, like you, skip this section.

Mechanism of action

Budesonide

Budesonide is a potent anti-inflammatory drug that acts by inhibiting the production and release of inflammatory mediators (e.g. cytokines, histamine, eicosanoids, leukotrienes), enhancing the synthesis of anti-inflammatory proteins and accelerating the apoptosis of inflammatory cells (lymphocytes, eosinophils, neutrophils, macrophages and mast

Figure 1. The chemical structures of budesonide and formoterol.

Budesonide

Formamide moiety

Aralkyl group

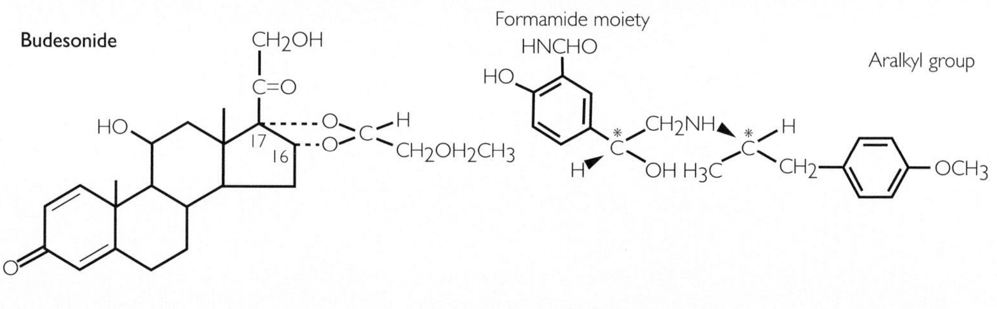

Budesonide is retained in airways tissue for longer than other inhaled corticosteroids as a result of a unique esterification process.

cells).[8,10,11] Budesonide has also been shown to improve airway hyper-responsiveness, manifested as a reduction in airway reactivity to histamine and methacholine in susceptible patients.[12]

Budesonide is retained in airways tissue for longer than other inhaled corticosteroids (e.g. fluticasone propionate or mometasone furoate), as a result of a unique esterification process.[8,13] Following administration and passage into the lungs, excess budesonide is esterified to budesonide oleate in a rapid, reversible process to form an essentially inactive intracellular ester pool.[14] As the intracellular concentration of budesonide decreases, the esterified budesonide is hydrolysed and active budesonide is released from the depot in a continuous manner, thus prolonging its duration of effect and sustaining its local anti-inflammatory activity.[14]

Formoterol

In humans, bronchodilation occurs within 1–3 minutes of inhalation of formoterol and is maintained for a mean duration of 12 hours.

Formoterol is a potent and selective β_2-adrenoceptor agonist that relieves bronchoconstriction by relaxing airway smooth muscle.[15] In humans, bronchodilation occurs within 1–3 minutes of inhalation of formoterol and is maintained for a mean duration of 12 hours.[16] Formoterol displays very high binding affinity and selectivity for the β_2-adrenoceptor in lung preparations (dissociation constant [KD] 8.12 *vs* 6.44 and 7.10 for formoterol, salbutamol and the non-selective β_2-agonist, isoprenaline, respectively).[15] Both short- and long-acting β_2-agonists also afford protection against bronchoconstrictive stimuli such as methacholine and adenosine monophosphate, and the bronchoprotective efficacy of formoterol was approximately three-times greater than that of the short-acting β_2-agonist, terbutaline, in a double-blind placebo-controlled study of 72 patients with stable mild-to-moderate asthma.[17]

Rationale for budesonide/formoterol combination therapy

Budesonide and formoterol treat two different components of asthma; chronic inflammation of the airways and airways obstruction, respectively.[11] The proposed complementary actions of the two drug types are illustrated schematically in Figure 2.[1] Corticosteroids increase the expression of β_2-adrenoceptors by increasing gene transcription.[1] This counteracts the downregulation of pulmonary β_2-adrenoceptors that is associated with the long-term use of β-agonists.[1] In turn, β_2-agonists increase the nuclear localisation of glucocorticoid receptors (GC), the cytoplasmic receptors through which corticosteroids exert their effects, and ultimately, may increase corticosteroid-induced gene transcription of inflammatory mediators.[1,18] Currently, although the clinical benefits of combining the two drugs are undisputed, the exact pharmacological mechanisms through which corticosteroids and β_2-agonists may interact remain unconfirmed.

Figure 2. The complementary actions of inhaled corticosteroids and long-acting β_2-agonists (LABA) on the pathophysiology of asthma (top) and the interaction of corticosteroids and β_2-agonists (bottom).[1]

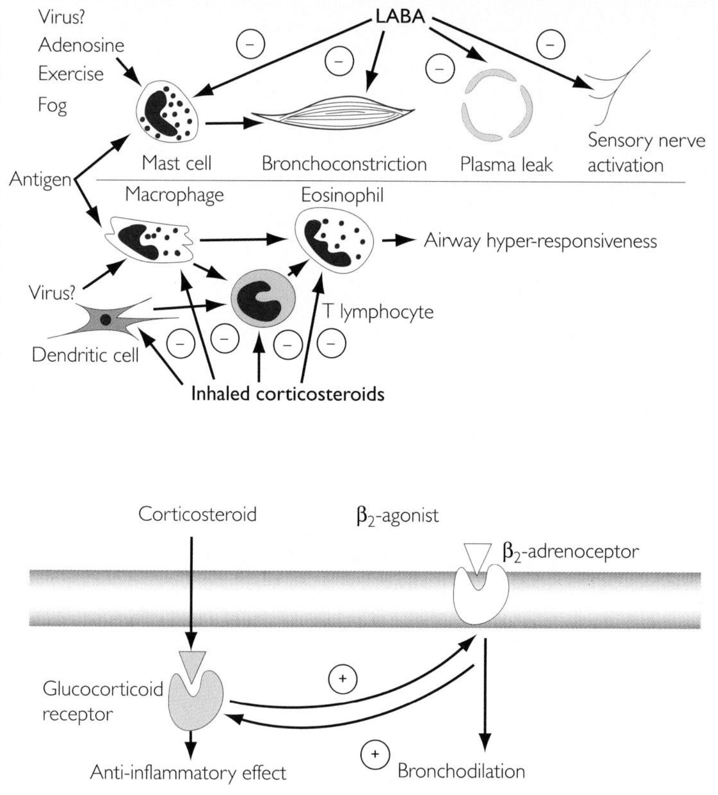

Effects on inflammatory cells

A double-blind study in 60 patients with moderate asthma, analysed the composition of sputum following 1 year of treatment with either low-dose budesonide and formoterol in combination, or a higher dose of budesonide alone.[19] Following a 4-week run-in period during which all participants received high-dose budesonide, 800 µg twice daily, patients were randomised to receive a twice-daily dose of either budesonide, 400 µg plus placebo, or budesonide, 100 µg plus formoterol, 12 µg. At baseline, mean forced expiratory volume in 1 second (FEV_1) was 83.3% of the predicted normal value. During the run-in phase, high-dose budesonide significantly reduced median sputum eosinophils from 4.5 to 0.68% (p<0.0005). There were no significant changes in the number of eosinophils, other inflammatory cells or levels of eosinophil cationic protein (ECP), over the subsequent year of treatment. The proportion of eosinophils in sputum collected from patients in the budesonide plus formoterol treatment group was slightly higher than in sputum derived from the budesonide only group, but this did not reach significance (3.41 *vs* 1.74%; $p>0.05$). These data show that the anti-inflammatory properties of budesonide that arise from a reduction in the number of eosinophils, are not compromised when formoterol is added to a regimen in which the dose of budesonide is dramatically reduced.

Onset of bronchodilation

A study conducted in 30 patients with a mean FEV_1 of 2.54 L, compared the onset of action of Symbicort with that of a fixed combination of Seretide (fluticasone and salmeterol).[20] Patients were randomised to receive either one or two inhalations of Symbicort, 160/4.5 µg, one inhalation of Seretide, 250/50 µg, or placebo, and serial measurements of FEV_1 were performed over a 3-hour period. Both doses of Symbicort showed a faster onset of action, in terms of improvement of FEV_1, than Seretide (mean FEV_1 at 3 minutes: 2.74, 2.75, 2.56 and 2.46 L for Symbicort one and two inhalations, Seretide and placebo, respectively; $p<0.001$ *vs* Seretide).

The pharmacokinetics of a drug are of interest to healthcare professionals because it is important for them to understand the action of a drug on the body over a period of time.

Pharmacokinetics

The pharmacokinetic properties of budesonide and formoterol are presented in Table 1.[5,21] Symbicort is bioequivalent to the corresponding constituent parts with regard to systemic exposure.[5] There is no evidence for clinically relevant pharmacokinetic interactions between the two drugs, although the rate of absorption and maximal plasma concentration of budesonide may increase slightly following co-administration with formoterol.[5] Each metered inhalation of

Table 1. The pharmacokinetic properties of budesonide and formoterol.[5,21]

Pharmacokinetic parameter	Budesonide	Formoterol
Systemic availability (%)	49	61
C_{max} (nmol/L)	3.5 (following dose of 1 mg)	NA
t_{max} (minutes)	15–45	15
Volume of distribution (L/kg)	3	4
Mean lung deposition	32–44	28–49% of delivered dose
Plasma protein binding (%)	90	50
Total clearance (L/minute)	1.2	1.4
$t_{1/2}$ (hours)	4	17
Excretion (% delivered dose)	41 (mouth or inhaler) 32 (urine) 15 (faeces)	8–13 (urine)

t_{max}, time to reach maximum drug plasma concentration (C_{max}); $t_{1/2}$, elimination half-life; NA, not available.

Symbicort from the dry powder Turbohaler delivers the same quantity of budesonide and formoterol as the respective metered doses when administered separately.[6] The recommended doses of budesonide and formoterol when given in combination are presented in Table 2.[5,6,22,23]

Symbicort is bioequivalent to the corresponding constituent parts with regard to systemic exposure.

Budesonide

Following inhalation, budesonide is rapidly and extensively absorbed through the lung, reaching peak plasma concentrations within 30 minutes of inhalation, although there is considerable inter-individual variability in lung absorption.[7,12] Budesonide reaches the systemic circulation either through the lungs or via gastrointestinal absorption of the negligible amount of drug that is inadvertently swallowed. Ninety per cent of budesonide undergoes biotransformation in the liver.[12] The major metabolites of budesonide – 6β-hydroxybudesonide and 16α-hydroxyprednisolone – are relatively inactive, demonstrating less than 1% of the anti-inflammatory activity of budesonide. The metabolism of budesonide is primarily mediated by cytochrome P450 (CYP) 3A4.[12]

Formoterol

Formoterol is absorbed rapidly following inhalation, and reaches peak plasma concentration approximately 15 minutes after administration.[16] The total plasma clearance and volume of distribution of formoterol has

Table 2. The recommended doses of budesonide and formoterol when given in combination.[5,6,22,23]

Formulation	Metered dose (μg)		Recommended dosage regimen
	Budesonide	Formoterol	
Symbicort® 100/6	80	4.5	**Adults:** 1–2 inhalations twice daily (maximum of 4 inhalations twice daily, reduced to 1 inhalation once daily if control is maintained) **Adolescents 12–17 years:** 1–2 inhalations twice daily (reduce to 1 inhalation once daily if control is maintained) **Children over 6 years:** 2 inhalations twice daily
Symbicort® 200/6	160	4.5	As for Symbicort® 100/6 but not recommended in children under 12 years
Symbicort® 400/12	320	9	**Adults:** 1 inhalation twice daily (maximum of 2 inhalations twice daily, reduce to 1 inhalation once daily if control is maintained) **Adolescents** 12–17 years: 1 inhalation twice daily (reduce to 1 inhalation once daily if control is maintained) Not recommended in children under 12 years

not been determined in pharmacokinetic studies.[16] Formoterol is extensively metabolised via direct glucuronidation and O-demethylation followed by further glucuronidation. Although the precise enzyme responsible for O-demethylation has not been identified, it is likely that the CYP isoenzymes 2D6, 2C19, 2C9 and 2A6 are involved.[16]

Special patient groups

There is no need for dosage adjustment when administering Symbicort to elderly patients.

Formoterol is not indicated for use in children aged under 6 years and to date, there are no pharmacokinetic data available that relate specifically to children in this age category.[16] There is no need for dosage adjustment when administering Symbicort to elderly patients and there are no data in patients with hepatic or renal impairment.[5] Since both budesonide and formoterol are primarily eliminated via metabolism, increased exposure can be expected in patients with severe liver cirrhosis and appropriate caution should therefore be observed.[5]

Clinical efficacy

Single vs *separate inhalers*

The increase in morning PEF was significantly greater following budesonide/ formoterol administered via single and separate inhalers than with budesonide alone.

The overall efficacy of concurrent budesonide and formoterol, administered using either single or separate inhalers, was examined in a placebo-controlled, double-blind study in 362 adult patients with asthma not fully controlled with inhaled corticosteroids alone.[24] Patients were randomised to receive either Symbicort, 160/4.5 µg two inhalations twice daily, or equivalent doses of each of the components from separate inhalers, or budesonide alone, for a period of 12 weeks. At baseline, mean FEV_1 was 73.8% of the predicted normal value and the mean daily dose of inhaled corticosteroid was 960 µg. The rate of premature treatment withdrawals was similar in the different treatment groups (16, 14 and 13% for single, separate and budesonide alone groups, respectively; *p*-value not reported). The increase in morning peak expiratory flow (PEF) was significantly greater following budesonide/ formoterol administered via single and separate inhalers than with budesonide alone (35.7 and 32.0 *vs* 0.2 L/minute for single, separate and budesonide alone groups, respectively; $p<0.001$ for both comparisons). A similar pattern emerged in terms of evening PEF measurements (i.e. corresponding increases: 24.8 and 22.3 *vs* –3.7 L/minute; $p<0.001$ for both comparisons). The onset of action following both single and separate inhaler therapy, was apparent from day 1 ($p<0.0001$ *vs* budesonide alone for both comparisons). The changes in asthma symptom scores are presented in Figure 3. The percentages of symptom-free and asthma control days were increased significantly in both the single and separate inhaler groups compared with budesonide alone (increases of 25 and 22.3 *vs* 8.0% for symptom-free and 28.5 and 26.9 *vs* 12.1% for asthma control days, respectively; $p<0.0001$ for all comparisons *vs* budesonide). All treatments were well tolerated and showed comparable adverse event profiles.

Figure 3. The change in total asthma symptom score during 12 weeks' treatment with Symbicort, budesonide plus formoterol given by separate inhalers or budesonide alone.[24]

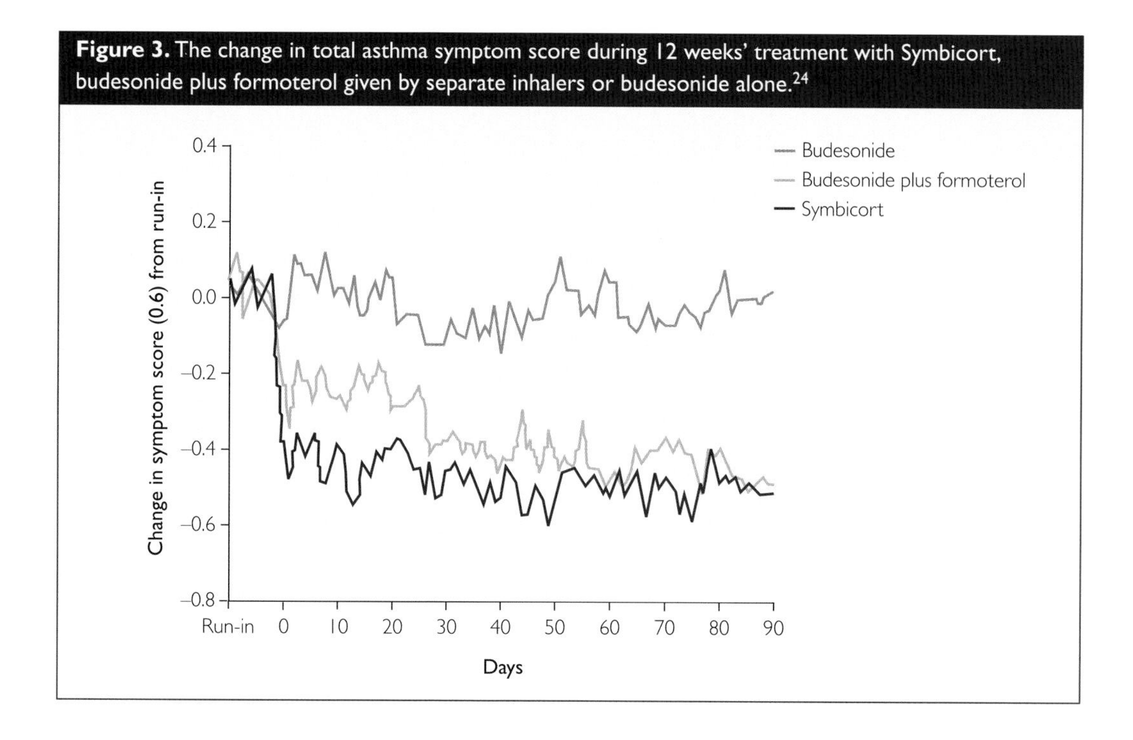

A longer-term, open-label study compared the safety and efficacy of Symbicort with identical doses of the mono-products administered separately, over 6 months in 585 adult patients with moderate persistent asthma.[25] Patients received budesonide, 160 µg, and formoterol, 4.5 µg, as two inhalations twice daily, and treatment allocation was 2:1 biased in favour of single inhaler therapy. At baseline, mean FEV_1 was 94.5% of the predicted normal value. The study completion rate was higher in the single inhaler group, though this did not reach significance (93.6 *vs* 89.3% for Symbicort and separate inhaler groups, respectively; p=0.085). Improvements in lung function, measured as the change in mean FEV_1 values from baseline, were comparable between the treatment groups (increases of 5–6% for both groups; *p*-value not reported). The proportion of patients requiring treatment with oral corticosteroids was also similar between treatment groups (15 *vs* 14% for Symbicort and separate inhaler groups, respectively; *p*-value not reported). Changes in health-related quality of life, determined by the Asthma Quality of Life Questionnaire (AQLQ) were similarly improved from baseline in both treatment groups (–0.50 *vs* –0.46 points, respectively; *p*-value not reported).

A 6-month extension of this study, conducted in 321 patients and using identical treatment regimens, examined the relationship between the method of inhalation and study completion rate further.[26] Following a total of 1 year of treatment, the percentage of patients who withdrew prematurely from the study – either as a result of asthma deterioration or adverse events – was significantly higher in the separate inhaler groups (19 *vs* 9% for separate inhaler and Symbicort groups, respectively;

The percentage of patients who withdrew prematurely from the study was significantly higher in the separate inhaler groups.

Administering budesonide and formoterol via a single inhaler is as effective as using separate inhalers.

p=0.008). Thus, this finding confirmed the trend identified in the original 6-month study. Moroever, the improvements in lung function and AQLQ scores reported in the original study at 6 months were maintained over 12 months of treatment.

Taken together, these data demonstrate that administering budesonide and formoterol via a single inhaler is as effective as using separate inhalers, and both single and separate inhalers are more clinically effective than budesonide when given alone. The lower rate of treatment discontinuation associated with the Symbicort may reflect the improved convenience of such a regimen.

Adding formoterol to budesonide vs increasing dose of budesonide

A number of large-scale clinical studies have investigated the merits of adding formoterol to a budesonide treatment regimen in comparison with an increase in the total dose of budesonide, with respect to asthma control.[27–31] These investigations have included patients with moderate-to-severe and mild-to-moderate asthma, and are described in detail below.

Moderate-to-severe asthma

The Formoterol and Corticosteroid Establishing Therapy (FACET) study examined the effects of adding formoterol to low- or high-dose budesonide treatment regimens in adult patients with moderate-to-severe asthma who were already receiving inhaled corticosteroids.[27] Following a 4-week run-in phase, during which time all participants received high-dose budesonide, 800 μg twice daily, patients who became controlled (n=852) were randomised to the following twice-daily dosing regimens for a 1-year period:

- budesonide, 100 μg, plus placebo
- budesonide, 100 μg, plus formoterol, 12 μg
- budesonide, 400 μg, plus placebo
- budesonide, 400 μg, plus formoterol, 12 μg.

The greatest reductions in the rates of severe and mild exacerbations were observed when formoterol was added to high-dose budesonide.

At baseline, mean FEV_1 was 75.8% of the predicted normal value. The main outcomes from the study, including the primary outcome variables – the rates of severe and mild asthma exacerbations – are presented in Table 3. The greatest reductions in the rates of severe and mild exacerbations were observed when formoterol was added to high-dose budesonide (63 and 62% reductions for severe and mild exacerbations, respectively). Symptoms of asthma and lung function improved with both formoterol and the higher dose of budesonide, but the improvements were most pronounced following the addition of formoterol.

Further analysis of the 425 severe asthma exacerbations reported over the course of the FACET study revealed that the time-course and severity of exacerbations were similar across all treatment groups.[32] All

Table 3. Clinical outcomes from the Formoterol and Corticosteroid Establishing Therapy (FACET) study.[27] Low-dose budesonide, 100 μg twice daily; high-dose budesonide, 400 μg twice daily; formoterol, 12 μg twice daily.

Efficacy variable	Low-dose budesonide plus placebo	Low-dose budesonide plus formoterol	High-dose budesonide plus placebo	High-dose budesonide plus formoterol	*p*-value	
					Formoterol *vs* placebo	Low- *vs* high-dose budesonide
Exacerbations (n)						
Severe	153	125	90	57		
Mild	5953	3980	4289	2241		
Withdrawals due to severe exacerbations (n)	10	7	4	0		
Estimated yearly rate of exacerbations (n/patient/year)						
Severe	0.91	0.67	0.46	0.34	0.01	<0.001
Mild	35.4	21.3	22.3	13.4	<0.001	<0.001
Patients without severe exacerbations (%)	61.4	70.3	71.8	80.8		
Episode-free days (mean % of year)	41.7	51.1	45.7	54.8	0.001	0.16
Mean symptom score (night-time)	0.37	0.31	0.38	0.20	<0.001	0.08
Mean symptom score (daytime)	0.57	0.46	0.53	0.33	<0.001	0.01
Use of night-time rescue medication (number of inhalations)	0.29	0.18	0.20	0.11	<0.001	0.003
Use of daytime rescue medication (number of inhalations)	0.91	0.57	0.82	0.44	<0.001	0.08
Night-time awakenings (number each night)	0.14	0.11	0.10	0.05	0.03	0.003

exacerbations were characterised by a gradual decline in PEF over several days, followed by more rapid changes over 2–3 days, an increase in symptoms and the increased use of β_2-agonist rescue medication use. The major patient characteristic associated with an increased risk of having a severe exacerbation was female gender, with an odds ratio of 1.89. However, the pattern of severe exacerbations was not affected by the dose of inhaled corticosteroid administered or whether or nor the patient was taking formoterol.

A quality of life assessment of 470 patients enrolled in the FACET study examined whether patients' health-related quality of life improved following budesonide/formoterol treatment and whether any improvements were sustained when improvements in clinical indices reached a plateau.[33] Patients completed the AQLQ on seven occasions over the 12-month duration of the FACET study. During the high-dose budesonide run-in period, AQLQ scores improved significantly, averaging an overall score of ~0.50 (p<0.0001 *vs* baseline). Following randomisation, further significant improvements in quality of life were observed amongst patients who received the high-dose budesonide/formoterol combination (0.21 points; p=0.028). One month after treatment randomisation, improvements in all groups had stabilised and were then sustained over 12 months, such that the pattern mirrored that of the improvement in clinical parameters reported in the original study. The correlation between individual changes in clinical indices and changes in AQLQ score over 12 months was weak-to-moderate (r=0.51).

Significant improvements in quality of life were observed amongst patients who received the high-dose budesonide/ formoterol combination.

In summary, the FACET study has demonstrated that the addition of formoterol to a budesonide treatment regimen, leads to an improvement in lung function, asthma symptoms and health-related quality of life, without compromising asthma control. Since increasing the dose of budesonide also showed pronounced clinical benefits, in some patients it may be appropriate to increase the dose of budesonide, as well as adding formoterol to the treatment regimen.

Mild-to-moderate asthma

The OPTIMA study investigated the effects of adding formoterol to a low dose of budesonide in patients with mild asthma who had not previously received an inhaled corticosteroid or who had received only a low corticosteroid dose (≤400 µg budesonide or equivalent) for at least 3 months before entry into the study.[28] Corticosteroid-naïve patients (n=698) were randomised at baseline to receive budesonide, 100 µg twice daily, with or without formoterol, 4.5 µg twice daily, or placebo. The 1272 corticosteroid-experienced patients were assigned to twice-daily budesonide, 100 µg or 200 µg, with or without formoterol, 4.5 µg twice daily. The year-long study was completed by 81% of corticosteroid-naïve patients and 87% of corticosteroid-experienced patients (p-value not reported). In the corticosteroid-naïve patients, budesonide treatment significantly reduced the risk for the first severe asthma exacerbation by 60% and reduced the rate of poorly controlled asthma days by 48%, compared with placebo. The addition of formoterol to budesonide provided additional benefit over budesonide alone, with regard to both FEV_1 and morning PEF (FEV_1 5.87 *vs* 4.04%; PEF 31.81 *vs* 15.12 L/minute for budesonide plus formoterol *vs* budesonide alone, respectively; p=0.023 and p=0.0001). In contrast, in corticosteroid-experienced patients, adding formoterol to budesonide reduced the risk for a first severe asthma exacerbation by 43% and that for poorly controlled asthma days by 30%, compared with either dose of budesonide alone. This risk reduction was more effective than simply doubling the dose of budesonide, which elicited respective risk reductions of 19 and 13% compared with the lower dose of budesonide. The changes in morning PEF in both patient subsets over the course of the study are shown in Figure 4. All treatments were well tolerated throughout the study and the frequency of adverse events was similar in corticosteroid-naïve and corticosteroid-experienced patients.

In corticosteroid-experienced patients, adding formoterol to budesonide reduced the risk for a first severe asthma exacerbation by 43% and that for poorly controlled asthma days by 30%.

The FLOW study (Formoterol in the Management of Mild Asthma – Formoterol Turbohaler with Budesonide Turbohaler) examined the impact upon asthma control and exacerbations of adding formoterol to budesonide in 663 patients with mild-to-moderate asthma and whether the dose of corticosteroid could be tapered more successfully in the presence of formoterol.[29] Patients were randomly assigned to budesonide, 400 μg twice daily, together with either formoterol, 9 μg (delivered dose), or placebo, twice daily. All treatments were administered via separate inhalers. After 4 weeks of treatment, those patients whose asthma was well controlled (according to pre-defined criteria: <20% diurnal variation in PEF and less than four daily inhalations of rescue medication) were re-randomised to receive half the dose of steroid (budesonide, 400 μg once daily), and either formoterol, 9 μg or placebo, twice daily, for a further 6 months. At entry to the first part of the study, mean PEF was 385 L/minute, which was 74% of the predicted normal value. Of those patients receiving formoterol in the first part of the study, 52% achieved asthma control at 4 weeks, compared with 41% of those patients who originally received placebo (p=0.003). Furthermore, the time to the first mild asthma exacerbation was significantly prolonged amongst patients receiving formoterol and budesonide in combination compared with budesonide alone (35 *vs* 47% of patients, respectively, experiencing a mild exacerbation by 24 weeks; p=0.01). Both treatment groups had a significant reduction in the daytime use of β_2-agonist rescue medication after 4 weeks though this was more pronounced in the budesonide plus formoterol group (–1.18 *vs* –0.85 inhalations/day for budesonide plus formoterol *vs* budesonide plus placebo, respectively; p<0.001 between groups). The frequency of symptom-free days followed a similar trend (9.7 *vs* 7.5 days, respectively; p=0.004). The improvements in morning and evening PEF values over 4 weeks were more pronounced amongst patients treated with budesonide plus formoterol than those who received budesonide plus placebo (mean differences of 19.0 and 15.7 L/minute for morning and evening, respectively; p<0.001 for both comparisons). Following re-randomisation, the frequency of mild exacerbations over 6 months was significantly lower in the budesonide plus formoterol group than in those patients receiving budesonide alone (7.2 *vs* 10.5 per patient per

Figure 4. The mean change from baseline in morning peak expiratory flow (PEF) in corticosteroid-naïve (top) and corticosteroid-experienced (bottom) patients treated with budesonide and/or formoterol, or placebo, over a 1-year period.[28]

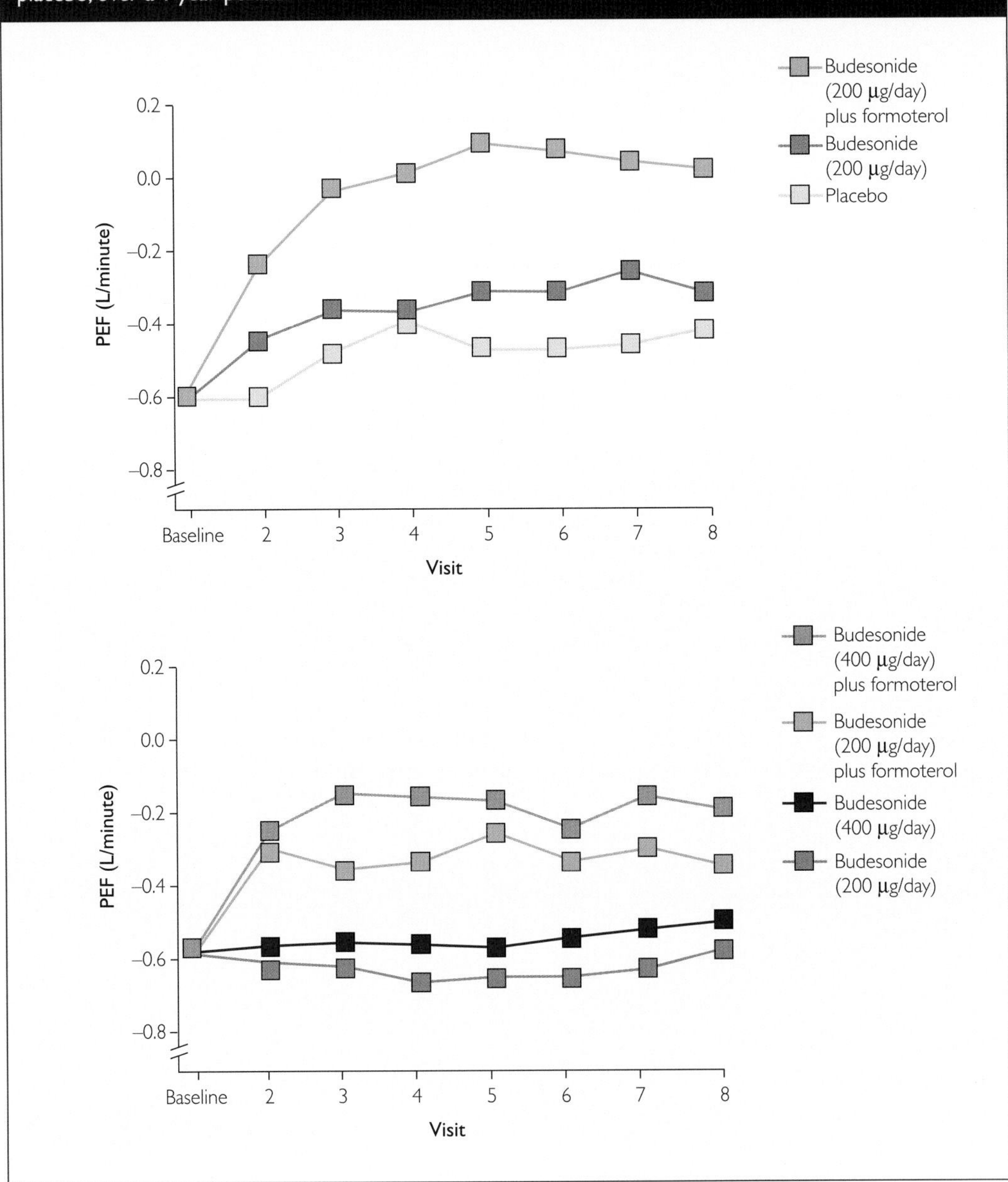

6 months; p=0.03). The median time to the first poorly controlled asthma day was more than doubled by the addition of formoterol to budesonide (97 *vs* 42 days, respectively; p=0.003). Again, the daytime use of β_2-agonist rescue medication (–0.17 *vs* +0.20 inhalations/day; p=0.0001), the frequency of symptom-free days (89.0 *vs* 71.6 days; p=0.002) and the changes in morning and evening PEF (differences of 17.1 and

17.3 L/minute, respectively; $p<0.0001$) were significantly improved in patients receiving budesonide plus formoterol compared with patients receiving budesonide alone. The safety profiles observed in both phases of the study were comparable between treatment groups. Thus, adding formoterol to low-to-moderate doses of budesonide resulted in faster and more effective asthma control than budesonide alone in patients with mild-to-moderate asthma. This treatment approach also allowed more patients to have their dose of budesonide tapered.

Adding formoterol to low-to-moderate doses of budesonide resulted in faster and more effective asthma control than budesonide alone in patients with mild-to-moderate asthma.

The efficacy of a low-dose combination of Symbicort (80/4.5 µg [delivered dose] twice daily) was compared with that of a higher dose of budesonide (200 µg twice daily) in a double-blind study of 467 patients with mild-to-moderate asthma.[30] Following a 2-week run-in phase during which time all patients received budesonide, 100 µg twice daily, participants were randomised to their respective treatment allocations for a further 12 weeks. Patient demographics were well balanced at baseline, and the mean FEV_1 was 82% of the predicted normal value, with 22% mean reversibility. The rates of premature treatment discontinuation over the course of the study were 6.5 and 9% for Symbicort and budesonide treatment groups, respectively (*p*-value not reported). Over the 12 weeks of the study, the mean increases in morning and evening PEF were significantly higher in patients receiving Symbicort than in those receiving budesonide alone (16.5 *vs* 7.3 and 13.7 *vs* 4.2 L/minute, for morning and evening, respectively; $p=0.002$ and $p<0.001$). The use of β_2-agonist rescue medication was also significantly lower in the Symbicort group (–0.33 *vs* –0.1 inhalations/day, respectively; $p=0.025$). The percentages of symptom-free and asthma control days were improved significantly in the Symbicort group compared with the budesonide monotherapy group (differences of 6 and 8%, respectively; $p=0.007$ and $p=0.002$). Furthermore, the relative risk of an asthma exacerbation was reduced by 26% following Symbicort compared with budesonide alone ($p=0.02$). In conclusion, this study demonstrates the superiority of low doses of Symbicort, compared with higher doses of budesonide, in patients with mild-to-moderate asthma that is not fully controlled with inhaled corticosteroids alone.

Dosage regimen

Having established the benefits of administering budesonide and formoterol together from the same inhaler, the effects of further simplification of the regimen to once-daily dosing was examined over a 12-week period in 523 patients with moderate persistent asthma.[31] Thus, the efficacy of once-daily Symbicort (160/4.5 µg [delivered dose], two inhalations) was compared with that of once-daily budesonide (400 µg) and twice-daily Symbicort (160/4.5 µg, one inhalation). All patients received budesonide 200 µg twice daily during the 2-week run-in period. At baseline, mean FEV_1 was 77.4% of the predicted normal value. Compared with budesonide alone, the changes in mean morning and evening PEF were significantly greater in both Symbicort treatment groups (differences: 27 and 17 L/minute for once daily; 23 and

Symbicort administered once daily was as effective clinically, as twice-daily administration of the equivalent dose.

24 L/minute for twice daily; both for morning and evening PEF respectively; $p<0.001$ for both comparisons). Similarly, the percentage of patients with an asthma-control day (no night-time awakening, no asthma symptoms and no use of rescue medication) was increased following both once- and twice-daily Symbicort compared with budesonide alone ($p\leq0.05$, Figure 5). The risk of experiencing a mild asthma exacerbation was significantly reduced in both once- and twice-daily Symbicort treatment groups (risk reductions of 38 and 35%, for once- and twice-daily doses, respectively; $p\leq0.002$). Thus, Symbicort administered once daily was as effective clinically, as twice-daily administration of the equivalent dose, and more effective than budesonide when given alone.

Adjustable- vs fixed-dosing regimens

Current guidelines recommend that patients are educated to adjust their controller medication according to the severity of their asthma, using physician-guided self-management plans.[2] Studies implemented under the Symbicort Adjustable Maintenance Dosing (SAMD) plan have shown that adjustable-maintenance dosing with Symbicort is associated with a lower overall dosage of drug and appears to maintain control as effectively or better than fixed dosing.[21] Table 4 summarises the major open-label studies, which have compared adjustable-maintenance dosing with fixed-dosage regimens of Symbicort, administered via a single inhaler.[34–39]

Figure 5. The percentage of patients with an asthma-control day (no night-time awakening, no asthma symptoms and no use of rescue medication) during treatment with once-daily Symbicort, twice-daily Symbicort or once-daily budesonide alone.[31]

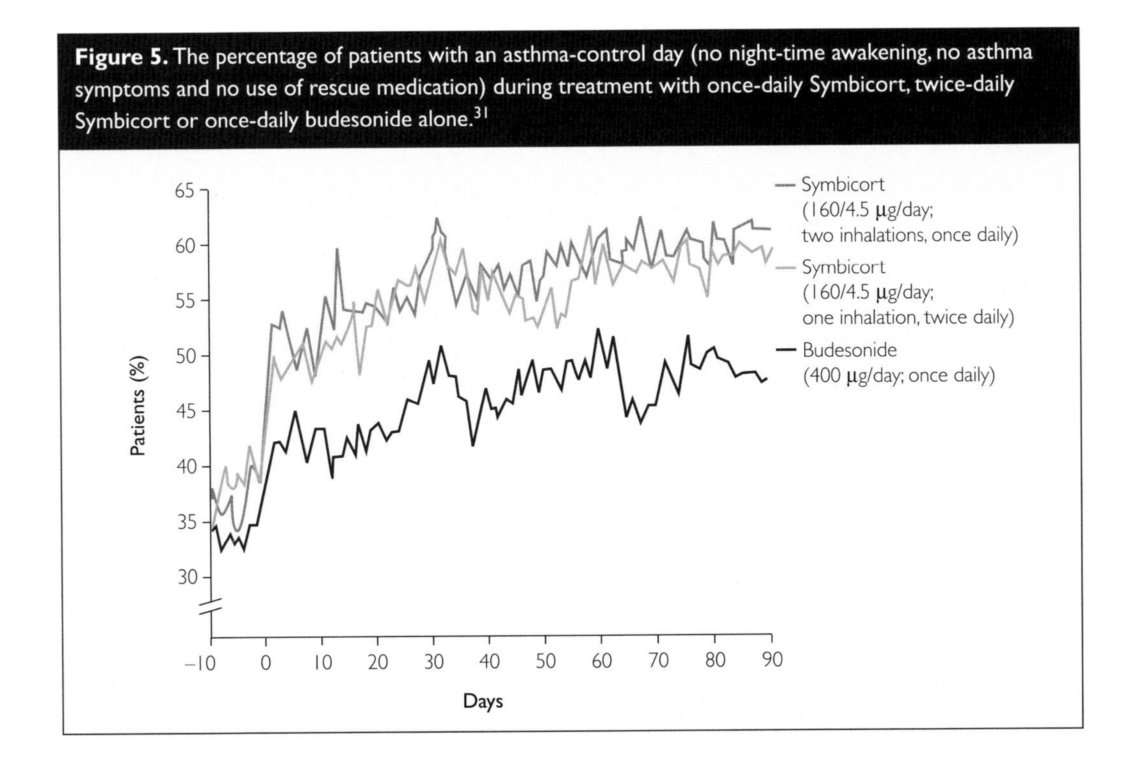

Table 4. Summary of the major open-label clinical trials examining adjustable[a] vs fixed Symbicort dosing regimens in patients with persistent asthma.[34–39]

Study	Dosage regimen	Main outcomes
Stallberg *et al.*, 2003[34] Open-label n=1034 7 months	Budesonide/formoterol, 80/4.5 µg, or 160/4.5 µg Two inhalations, twice daily for 4 weeks Fixed- or self-adjustable dose thereafter for 6 months	• Significantly fewer patients receiving the adjustable- than the fixed-dose regimen experienced an asthma exacerbation over the course of the study (6.2 *vs* 9.5%; $p<0.05$). • Patients in the adjustable group required significantly fewer daily inhalations of Symbicort (2.35 *vs* 3.95; $p<0.001$ [Figure 6]). • The economic costs of the adjustable regimen were significantly lower than those with the fixed regimen (6-month saving: €98; $p<0.001$)
Leuppi *et al.*, 2003[35] Open-label n=127 16 weeks	Budesonide/formoterol, 160/4.5 µg Two inhalations, twice daily for 4 weeks Fixed- or self-adjustable dose thereafter for 12 weeks	• 72% of patients on the adjustable regimen reduced their maintenance dose within 2 weeks. • The reduction in symptom severity (NHLBI) from baseline was only significant in the adjustable-dosing group (33.3 *vs* 25.9% patients shifted to lower severity status; $p=0.004$). • Nocturnal awakenings were significantly less frequent in adjustable-dosing group (0.057 *vs* 0.067 per night; $p=0.006$). • The use of rescue medication was significantly less frequent in adjustable-dosing group (0.15 *vs* 0.23 inhalations/day; $p<0.001$).
Fitzgerald et *al.*, 2003[36] Open-label n=995 5 months	Budesonide/formoterol, 100/6 µg or 200/6 µg (metered dose) Two inhalations, twice daily for 4 weeks Fixed- or self-adjustable dose thereafter for 5 months	• Significantly fewer patients on the adjustable- than the fixed-dose regimen experienced an asthma exacerbation over the course of the study (4.0 *vs* 8.9%; $p=0.002$). • Patients in the adjustable-dose group required 36% fewer overall inhalations of Symbicort (2.5 *vs* 3.9 inhalations/day; $p<0.001$). • The reduction in symptom severity (NHLBI) from baseline was maintained or improved in 97% or greater of patients in both groups. • The economic costs of the adjustable regimen were significantly lower than those of the fixed regimen (5-month saving: CAN$141).

[a]Patients on the adjustable regimen were able to step down their treatment to one inhalation twice daily if symptoms were controlled, with the option to step up to four inhalations twice daily for 7–14 days if symptoms worsened.
AQLQ, Asthma Quality of Life Questionnaire; CAN, Canadian; CAST, Control of Asthma by Symbicort® Turbohaler®; NHLBI, National Heart, Lung and Blood Institute; PEF, peak expiratory flow.

Table 4. Continued

Study	Dosage regimen	Main outcomes
Ind *et al.*, 2004[37] Open-label n=1539 16 weeks ASSURE study group	Budesonide/formoterol, 80/4.5 μg or 160/4.5 μg Two inhalations, twice daily for 4 weeks Fixed- or self-adjustable dose thereafter for 12 weeks	• During the run-in phase, the severity status of patients improved significantly (37 *vs* 52% of patients were categorised with severe- or moderate-persistent asthma; $p<0.001$). • Symptom severity in the adjustable- and fixed-dose groups was improved in 29 and 28% of patients, respectively ($p>0.05$). • Patients in the adjustable group required fewer inhalations of Symbicort (3.2 *vs* 3.8 inhalations/day; $p<0.05$). • 79% of patients in the adjustable group reduced the dosage of their medication. • Overall, 28 of patients in the adjustable group increased their dosage to eight inhalations/day at least once.
Buhl *et al.*, 2004[38] Open-label n=4025 16 weeks Single inhaler	Budesonide/formoterol, 160/4.5 μg Two inhalations, twice daily for 4 weeks Fixed- or self-adjustable dose thereafter for 12 weeks	• The mean improvements in AQLQ, morning and evening PEF and symptom-severity score were significant during the run-in period (0.73 points, 42.5 and 24.8 L/minute, and 0.36 points, respectively; $p\leq0.05$ for all comparisons). • These improvements were maintained in both groups over the 12-week randomisation period. • Patients on the adjustable-dosage regimen required 31% fewer daily inhalations of Symbicort than patients receiving the fixed-dose regimen (2.63 *vs* 3.82; $p<0.001$).
Canonica *et al.*, 2004[39] Open-label 16 weeks n=2358 Single inhaler CAST study group	Budesonide/formoterol, 160/4.5 μg or 80/4.5 μg Two inhalations, twice daily for 4 weeks Fixed- or self-adjustable dose thereafter for 12 weeks	• The proportion of patients who experienced an asthma exacerbation was similar in both the adjustable- and fixed-dose groups (5% for both groups; $p>0.05$). • Improvements in lung function were comparable between treatment groups. • Patients on the adjustable-dosage regimen required significantly fewer daily inhalations of Symbicort than those receiving the fixed-dose regimen (2.95 *vs* 3.86; $p<0.001$). • Patient and physician satisfaction scores were similar for both treatment groups (patients: 7.47 for both groups; physicians: 7.45 and 7.38 for adjustable- and fixed-dose groups, respectively).

[a]Patients on the adjustable regimen were able to step down their treatment to one inhalation twice daily if symptoms were controlled, with the option to step up to four inhalations twice daily for 7–14 days if symptoms worsened.
AQLQ, Asthma Quality of Life Questionnaire; CAN, Canadian; CAST, Control of Asthma by Symbicort® Turbohaler®; NHLBI, National Heart, Lung and Blood Institute; PEF, peak expiratory flow.

In general, adjustable Symbicort maintenance regimens resulted in lower overall drug use over test periods of up to 6 months. When patients were given the option of controlling their own asthma medication, the majority considered their asthma sufficiently controlled to merit a dosage reduction, as illustrated in Figure 6.[34] Patients on adjustable Symbicort maintenance regimens also showed lower asthma exacerbation rates, lower use of rescue medication and more pronounced reductions in asthma severity scores (Table 4). The economic benefits associated with adjustable dosing regimens are discussed in more detail in the Pharmacoeconomics section.

Adjustable Symbicort maintenance regimens resulted in lower overall drug use over test periods of up to 6 months.

Comparative studies

Budesonide/formoterol *vs* fluticasone propionate/salmeterol

The efficacy of adjustable-maintenance dosing with Symbicort was compared with fixed-dosing regimens of either Symbicort or Seretide in 658 patients with symptomatic asthma, over 7 months, in a double-blind study with an open-label extension.[40] Mean FEV_1 at baseline was 84% of the predicted normal value and the mean daily dosage of inhaled corticosteroid was 735 µg. For the first 4 weeks of double-blind treatment, patients assigned to fixed- and adjustable-dosing regimens received either Symbicort, 160/4.5 µg, two inhalations twice daily, or Seretide, 250/50 µg, one inhalation twice daily. At the end of the double-blind period, those patients whose asthma was well controlled stepped down to one inhalation twice daily. Those patients in the

Figure 6. Mean number of inhalations of Symbicort over 6 months of adjustable or fixed dosing.[34]

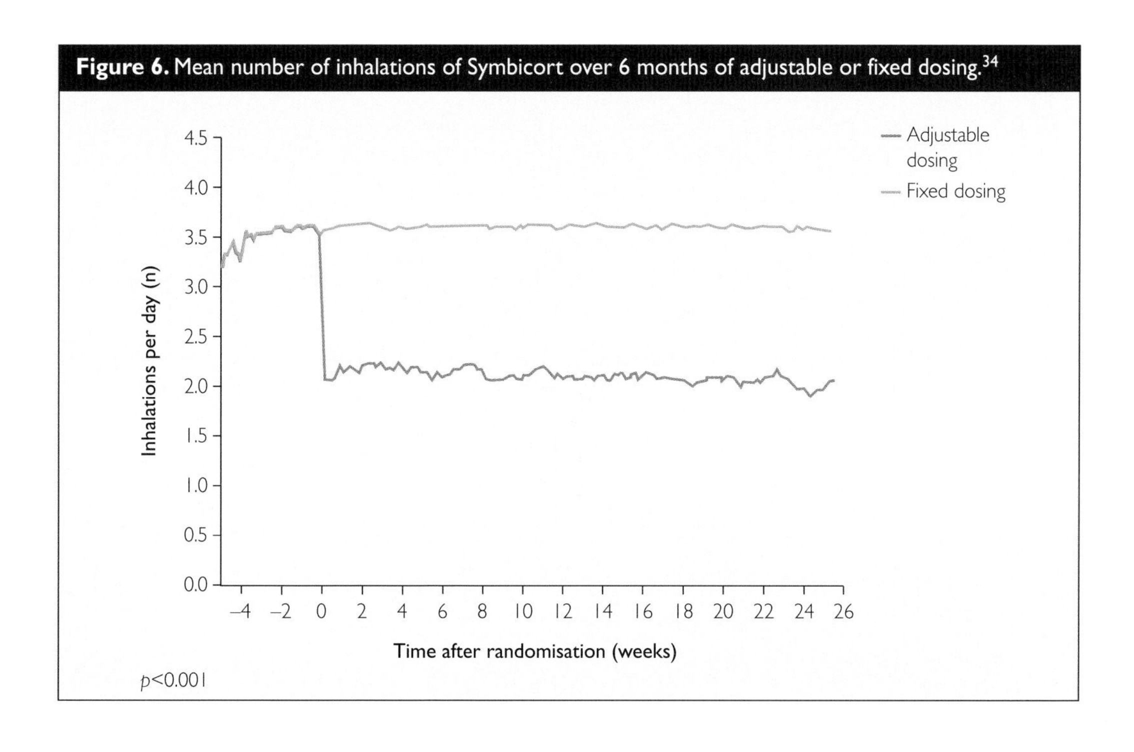

adjustable arm who did not meet the criteria for stepping down their dose, remained on two inhalations twice daily. Throughout the 6-month open-label period, if patients in the adjustable arm experienced worsening of symptoms (defined in study protocol), they stepped up their dose to four inhalations twice daily. Once these symptoms resolved, these patients then stepped down their dose to the level they were receiving previously. Over the whole treatment period, the odds ratios for achieving a well-controlled asthma week (WCAW) were comparable between the Symbicort and Seretide fixed-dose regimen groups. During the extension period, the likelihood of achieving a WCAW was significantly improved in patients receiving the adjustable-dosing regimen, compared with the fixed-dose Symbicort dosage regimen (ratio 1.335; p=0.049), despite a 15% reduction in mean study drug use. However, no improvement in terms of the likelihood of a WCAW was observed for adjustable Symbicort compared with fixed-dose Seretide formulations (ratio 1.048; p>0.05). Patients receiving adjustable Symbicort experienced a lower rate of exacerbations over the 7 months of the study, than patients receiving fixed-dose Symbicort (32% reduction; p>0.05) and those receiving fixed-dose Seretide (39.7% reduction; p=0.018). The daytime use of reliever medication and asthma symptom scores after asthma exacerbations are shown in Figure 7. Improvements from baseline in parameters of lung function during the double-blind treatment period were comparable between Symbicort and Seretide groups, with the notable exception of FEV_1, for which the improvement following Symbicort was significantly greater than that associated with Seretide (mean difference of –0.05 L; p<0.05).

Patients receiving adjustable Symbicort experienced a lower rate of exacerbations over the 7 months of the study, than patients receiving fixed-dose Symbicort and those receiving fixed-dose Seretide.

Figure 7. Mean daytime asthma symptom scores and daytime reliever medication use 30 days before and 30 days after asthma exacerbations following 7 months of treatment with fixed-dose (FD) Symbicort or Seretide, or 6 months of adjustable Symbicort maintenance dosing (AMD).[40]

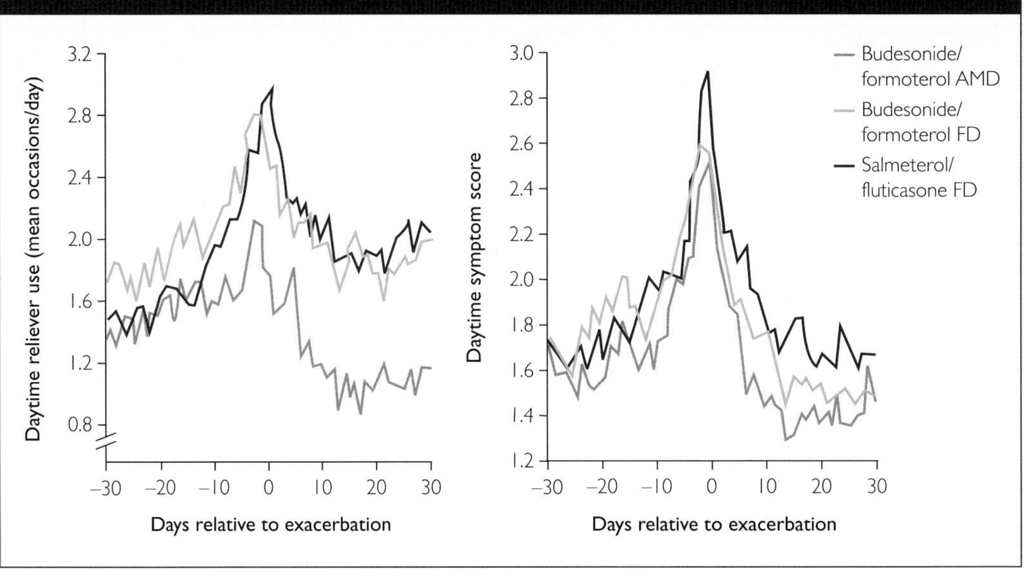

Overall, adjustable dosing with Symbicort provides more effective asthma control, in terms of the rate of asthma exacerbations, than a fixed-dose regimen of Seretide.

The Evaluation of Different Inhaled Combination Therapies (EDICT) study compared the relative efficacies of budesonide (800 µg, twice daily) and formoterol (12 µg, twice daily), given concurrently via separate inhalers, with a fixed dose of fluticasone/salmeterol (50/250 µg, twice daily), administered from a single inhaler.[41] The study included 428 patients with moderate-to-severe asthma that were uncontrolled on existing corticosteroid therapy and study treatments were administered over a 12-week double-blind treatment period. The mean improvements in morning PEF after 12 weeks were similar between the different treatment groups (increases of 41 and 43 L/minute for budesonide plus formoterol and fluticasone/salmeterol, respectively; p=0.59). The mean rate of asthma exacerbations over 12 weeks was significantly lower following fluticasone/salmeterol treatment (0.472 *vs* 0.735, respectively; p<0.001), corresponding to a 36% risk reduction. Similarly, the median percentage of symptom-free nights (difference 2.7%; p=0.04), and the percentage of nights without awakenings (difference 4.9%; p=0.02) were significantly improved amongst patients in the fluticasone/salmeterol treatment group compared with the budesonide plus formoterol group. Both treatments were well tolerated throughout the study. However, as budesonide and formoterol were administered via separate inhalers, it is not appropriate to extrapolate these data into a direct comparison of Symbicort and Seretide.

Symbicort *vs* salbutamol for the relief of acute asthma

A double-blind study of 104 patients admitted to hospital with acute asthma, examined the comparative efficacies of two doses of Symbicort (two inhalations of 320/9 µg [delivered dose]) and two doses of salbutamol (eight inhalations of 100 µg) for the relief of acute asthma symptoms.[a,42] Patients received the two doses of their respective study medications 5 minutes apart and were monitored for 3 hours after drug administration. All patients received a single dose of prednisolone, 60 mg, at 90 minutes. At treatment allocation, mean FEV_1 was 43% of the predicted normal value. After 90 minutes, mean FEV_1 had increased by a comparable extent in both treatment groups (30 and 32% for budesonide/fomoterol and salbutamol, respectively; p=0.66). The incidence of treatment-related adverse events was similar between treatment groups, though the mean increase in pulse rate over 3 hours, was significantly higher in the salbutamol treatment group (92 *vs* 88 beats/minute, respectively; p<0.001). Thus, the efficacy profile of the Symbicort combination for the treatment of acute asthma resembled that of salbutamol.

The efficacy profile of Symbicort for the treatment of acute asthma resembled that of salbutamol.

[a]Symbicort is not licensed for the relief of acute asthma.

Efficacy in children with asthma

The efficacy of Symbicort was compared with that of an equivalent dose of budesonide given alone in a double-blind, randomised study of 286 children (mean age 11 years) with moderate persistent asthma who had previously been treated with inhaled corticosteroids, at a mean daily dosage of 548 μg.[43] After a 2–4-week run-in period, patients were randomised to receive either Symbicort (80/4.5 μg, two inhalations twice daily) or budesonide (100 μg, two inhalations twice daily) for a period of 12 weeks. At baseline, the mean FEV_1 was 75% of the predicted normal value. The rate of premature treatment discontinuation was comparable between treatment groups (6 and 7% for Symbicort and budesonide, respectively; *p*-value not reported). Over the course of the study, morning PEF improved by a greater extent in patients receiving Symbicort than in those patients receiving only budesonide (increases of 7.22 *vs* 3.45%, respectively; $p<0.001$). Changes in evening PEF followed a similar trend (increases of 6.13 *vs* 2.72%, respectively; $p<0.001$). Serial measurements of FEV_1 carried out over 12 hours at 12 weeks in a subgroup of 81 children, showed a 6% improvement in mean FEV_1 during the first 10 minutes after inhalation of Symbicort, relative to budesonide ($p<0.05$). An improvement in mean FEV_1 over budesonide of approximately 5% was maintained for up to 12 hours after administration of Symbicort. Improvements in asthma symptoms and the use of rescue medication were similar between treatment groups whilst the adverse events profiles in both groups were also comparable.

Serial measurements of FEV_1 carried out in a subgroup of children, showed a 6% improvement in mean FEV_1 during the first 10 minutes after inhalation of Symbicort, relative to budesonide.

Safety and tolerability

The co-administration of budesonide and formoterol does not affect the individual adverse event profiles associated with each drug.[5] Thus, the side-effects, prescribing precautions and the drug-interaction profile for Symbicort are the same as those for each drug administered separately.

Controlled clinical studies conducted to date have confirmed the favourable tolerability profile of Symbicort. The most common adverse events associated with treatment include tremor in the extremities, palpitations, oral candidiasis, mild throat irritation, hoarseness and headache.[25,44] As with all inhaled medications, the potential for paradoxical bronchospasm should be considered when prescribing budesonide and formoterol in combination.[5]

The acute tolerability of high-dose Symbicort was examined in a double-blind, crossover, placebo-controlled study.[45] Fourteen patients with asthma who were already receiving Symbicort maintenance therapy (160/4.5 μg, twice daily) were also administered high-dose Symbicort (1600/45 μg, daily), formoterol (45 μg, daily) or placebo, on three separate study days. Serum potassium and blood glucose levels remained within their normal reference ranges throughout the study in all treatment groups. Pulse rate increased and small increases in systolic blood pressure and decreases in diastolic blood pressure were measured after dosing with both active treatments. Electrocardiogram (ECG) evaluations were normal for all patients, although the QT interval was slightly prolonged initially after dosing with both active treatments.

Moreover, the majority of adverse events reported were mild in intensity. These data would suggest that high-dose Symbicort is well tolerated when administered from a single inhaler.

Adverse events associated with budesonide

Although inhaled corticosteroids have considerably fewer systemic effects than oral corticosteroids, adverse events have been reported following regular use.[6] High doses in particular have been associated with an increased risk of adrenal suppression, reduced bone mineral density, glaucoma, cataracts and hoarseness and candidiasis of the mouth or throat.[6] The use of a dry powder inhaler may prevent or minimise oropharyngeal deposition.[6] In general, the linear growth retardation that is associated with oral corticosteroid therapy does not appear to be a significant issue as long as the dose of inhaled corticosteroid remains within the recommended dose range.[6]

Budesonide itself is generally well tolerated at therapeutic doses. Hoarseness, sore throat and local irritation causing cough are amongst the most common side-effects reported.[6,12,46] Furthermore, at therapeutic doses, budesonide produced little or no reduction in plasma cortisol levels in healthy individuals or in patients with persistent asthma, compared with other inhaled corticosteroids.[47] The lower incidence of systemic effects associated with budesonide than with other inhaled corticosteroids (e.g. fluticasone propionate and mometasone), may be due in part, to its short systemic half-life and limited volume of distribution.[48] In addition, budesonide's high rate of clearance and linear pharmacokinetics further enhances its tolerability profile.[48]

Although budesonide treatment has been associated with a slowing of initial growth velocity, there appears to be no effect on achieving normal adult height.[49] However, regular monitoring of height is advocated in children receiving prolonged exposure to inhaled corticosteroids.

Although budesonide treatment has been associated with a slowing of initial growth velocity, there appears to be no effect on achieving normal adult height.

Adverse events associated with formoterol

The β_2-agonists in general, are associated with fine tremor (particularly in the hands), nervous tension, headache, peripheral dilatation and palpitations.[6] Tachycardia and arrhythmias and disturbances of sleep and behaviour in children have also been reported following the regular use of β_2-agonists.[6] These side-effects are usually mild in severity and tend to resolve within the first few days of treatment.[6,16] Clinical experience drawn from large-scale trials of asthmatic adults and children have shown that whilst the use of formoterol may be accompanied by these adverse events, it is generally well tolerated.[9,50] Oropharyngeal irritation, taste disturbances, rash, insomnia, nausea and pruritus have been reported rarely following formoterol treatment.[6] It should also be noted that treatment with formoterol may cause prolongation of the corrected QT interval (QTc) of the ECG.[6,16] The risk of potentially serious hypokalaemia following treatment with formoterol, and β_2-agonists in general, merits the monitoring of serum potassium levels in some

The β_2-agonists in general, are associated with fine tremor, nervous tension, headache, peripheral dilatation and palpitations.

patients. Concomitant treatment with xanthine derivatives, steroids and diuretics may potentiate the risk of hypokalaemia.[16]

Precautions for use

Caution should be observed when administering formoterol to patients with:

- thyrotoxicosis
- phaeochromocytoma
- hypertrophic obstructive cardiomyopathy
- idiopathic subvalvular aortic stenosis
- severe hypertension
- aneurysm
- severe cardiovascular disorders (e.g. ischaemic heart disease, tachyarrhythmias, severe heart failure)
- prolongation of the QTc interval
- diabetes (additional blood glucose monitoring is recommended initially).[16,51]

Budesonide is contra-indicated in patients with active pulmonary tuberculosis or hypersensitivity to budesonide.[12] Caution should be also observed when administering budesonide to patients with quiescent lung tuberculosis or fungal or viral infections of the airways.[12] Those patients transferring from oral corticosteroid therapy to inhaled budesonide may experience unmasking of allergic or arthritic symptoms such as rhinitis, eczema, and muscle and joint pain. As mentioned previously, the routine monitoring of height in children receiving long-term budesonide treatment is advised.[12]

Asthma is one of the most common medical conditions that can complicate pregnancy and adequate control of asthma is vital to prevent maternal and foetal hypoxia. However, the benefits of Symbicort use during pregnancy should be weighed against the potential risk to the foetus, and doses should be kept to the absolute minimum.[5]

Drug interactions

Although to date, no specific drug interaction studies have been conducted, the co-administration of formoterol with the following substances merits caution:

- other sympathomimetic substances (may potentiate adverse events associated with formoterol)
- xanthine derivatives, steroids or diuretics (may potentiate the possible hypokalaemic effect of formoterol)
- L-dopa, L-thyroxine, oxytocin and alcohol (may impair cardiac tolerance towards β_2-agonists)
- monoamine oxidase inhibitors, including agents with similar properties, such as furazolidone and procarbazine (may cause hypertensive reactions)
- β-adrenoceptor antagonists (may weaken the effect of formoterol).[5,16]

No specific drug interaction data are available regarding inhaled budesonide, although in view of its metabolic pathway, drugs that markedly inhibit CYP 3A4 (e.g. ketoconazole) have the potential to increase systemic exposure to budesonide.[6,12] Thus, the concurrent use of these compounds with budesonide should be avoided where possible. The action of corticosteroids in general may be adversely affected by co-administration with amphotericin, barbiturates, carbamazepine, coumarins, methotrexate, phenytoin, primidone and rifamycins.[6] High doses of corticosteroids may also impair the immune response to live vaccines and concomitant use should therefore be avoided.

Pharmacoeconomics

The financial costs associated with asthma management are principally related to the cost of hospitalisation, emergency care and drug therapy. Indirectly, asthma also accounts for costs attributed to the absence from school or work. In theory, an effective anti-asthma drug would lower the number of hospitalisations and emergency pharmacological treatments, thereby reducing the total economic burden associated with the condition. One of the potential financial benefits of combining two anti-asthma medications, aside from the cost savings associated with improved asthma control, is the reduced cost of drug acquisition compared with the cost of obtaining each drug separately.

A number of pharmacoeconomic investigations have directly assessed the financial implications of combining budesonide and formoterol in a single inhaler. When compared with the cost of treating a patient with budesonide alone, budesonide/formoterol in combination is the more cost-effective option. Although prescribing costs were higher for the combination formulation, these were partially offset by reduced healthcare service utilisation as a result of fewer asthma exacerbations and a reduced need for other physician consultations and additional medications.[52,53]

Clinical data derived from the FACET study described previously, were combined with an expert survey on average resource use in connection with mild and severe asthma exacerbations in the UK, Sweden and Spain.[27,54] In general, the extra costs of adding formoterol to a budesonide treatment regimen were offset against the savings generated from a reduction in asthma exacerbations and the use of healthcare resources. Depending on the country, between 50 and 100% of the extra formoterol costs were recouped. If productivity losses resulting from work and school absences were included in this analysis, net savings were observed for all countries and ranged from €267 to €1183 per patient per year.

> The extra costs of adding formoterol to a budesonide treatment regimen were offset against the savings generated from a reduction in asthma exacerbations and the use of healthcare resources.

In addition to its clinical advantages, an adjustable Symbicort maintenance regimen is also associated with cost savings, as demonstrated by an economic evaluation of the ASSURE study.[55] From the perspective of the NHS in the UK, the mean daily cost per patient receiving adjustable Symbicort was £1.13, compared with £1.31 in patients receiving a fixed-dose of the combination ($p<0.001$). This difference in mean daily cost led to an annual per patient cost difference of £65.70, further testament to the benefits of adjustable dosing.

Key points

- Symbicort – the single inhaler formulation of the corticosteroid, budesonide, and the long-acting β_2-adrenoceptor agonist, formoterol – is recommended for the treatment of asthma in patients for whom moderate doses of inhaled corticosteroids alone are failing to provide adequate control.
- The improved asthma control associated with the combined administration of budesonide and formoterol may be attributed to their complementary mechanisms of action (anti-inflammatory and bronchodilatory, respectively).
- Combining these drugs in a single inhaler may also promote patient adherence through the simplification of the asthma treatment regimen.
- The pharmacokinetic and drug interaction profiles of budesonide and formoterol are largely unaffected by co-administration.
- Clinical studies have shown that Symbicort provides asthma control similar to that achieved by administering the drugs through separate inhalers.
- Large controlled studies in patients with mild-to-moderate and moderate-to-severe asthma have demonstrated that adding formoterol to a budesonide treatment regimen is at least as effective as increasing the total dose of budesonide.
- Open-label studies of up to 7 months duration have highlighted the benefits associated with a patient-controlled adjustable Symbicort maintenance regimen.
- Symbicort is effective and well tolerated amongst children with persistent asthma.
- The adverse event profile of Symbicort closely resembles that of the component drugs when given individually. Tremor, palpitations, oral candidiasis, mild throat irritation, hoarseness and headache are amongst the most commonly reported side-effects.
- The combination of budesonide and formoterol is more cost-effective than budesonide alone. Cost savings have also been associated with the use of the adjustable-maintenance regimen over fixed dosing with Symbicort.

References

A list of the published evidence which has been reviewed in compiling the preceding section of *BESTMEDICINE.*

1 Barnes P. Scientific rationale for inhaled combination therapy with long-acting beta2-agonists and corticosteroids. *Eur Respir J* 2002; **19**: 182–91.

2 Scottish Intercollegiate Guidelines Network & the British Thoracic Society. British Guidelines on the Management of Asthma. SIGN, Edinburgh, 2004. *www.sign.ac.uk*

3 Global Initiative for Asthma. *Pocket Guide for Asthma Management and Prevention.* 2004: 1–30.

4 Tal A. Symbicort: controlling asthma in children. *Respir Med* 2002; **96**: S23–8.

5 AstraZeneca UK Limited. Symbicort 100-6 Turbohaler. *Summary of product characteristics.* Luton, Bedfordshire, 2004.

6 *British National Formulary (BNF) 48.* London: British Medical Association and Royal Pharmaceutical Society of Great Britain. September, 2004.

7 Donnelly R, Seale J. Clinical pharmacokinetics of inhaled budesonide. *Clin Pharmacokinet* 2001; **40**: 427–40.

8 O'Connell E. Review of the unique properties of budesonide. *Clin Ther* 2003; **25**: C61–74.

9 Bartow R, Brogden R. Formoterol. An update of its pharmacological properties and therapeutic efficacy in the management of asthma. *Drugs* 1998; **55**: 303–22.

10 Boobis A. Comparative physicochemical and pharmacokinetic profiles of inhaled beclomethasone dipropionate and budesonide. *Respir Med* 1998; **92**: B2–6.

11 Kuna P, Kuprys I. Symbicort Turbuhaler: a new concept in asthma management. *Int J Clin Pract* 2002; **56**: 797–803.

12 AstraZeneca UK Limited. Pulmicort Turbohaler 100. *Summary of product characteristics.* Luton, Bedfordshire, 2004.

13 Banov C. The role of budesonide in adults and children with mild-to-moderate persistent asthma. *J Asthma* 2004; **41**: 5–17.

14 Edsbacker S, Brattsand R. Budesonide fatty-acid esterification: a novel mechanism prolonging binding to airway tissue. Review of available data. *Ann Allergy Asthma Immunol* 2002; **88**: 609–16.

15 Anderson G. Formoterol: pharmacology, molecular basis of agonism, and mechanism of long duration of a highly potent and selective beta 2-adrenoceptor agonist bronchodilator. *Life Sci* 1993; **52**: 2145–60.

16 AstraZeneca UK Limited. Oxis Turbohaler 12. *Summary of product characteristics.* Luton, Bedfordshire, 2004.

17 Lipworth B, Tan S, Devlin M *et al.* Effects of treatment with formoterol on bronchoprotection against methacholine. *Am J Med* 1998; **104**: 431–8.

18 Spoelstra F, Postma D, Hovenga H, Noordhoek J, Kauffman H. Additive anti-inflammatory effect of formoterol and budesonide on human lung fibroblasts. *Thorax* 2002; **57**: 237–41.

19 Kips J, O'Connor B, Inman M *et al.* A long-term study of the antiinflammatory effect of low-dose budesonide plus formoterol versus high-dose budesonide in asthma. *Am J Respir Crit Care Med* 2000; **161**: 996–1001.

20 Palmqvist M, Arvidsson P, Beckman O, Peterson S, Lotvall J. Onset of bronchodilation of budesonide/formoterol vs. salmeterol/fluticasone in single inhalers. *Pulm Pharmacol Ther* 2001; **14**: 29–34.

21 Goldsmith D, Keating G. Budesonide/Formoterol: a review of its use in asthma. *Drugs* 2004; **64**: 1597–618.

22 AstraZeneca UK Limited. Symbicort 200-6 Turbohaler. *Summary of product characteristics.* Luton, Bedfordshire, 2004.

23 AstraZeneca UK Limited. Symbicort 400-12 Turbohaler. *Summary of product characteristics.* Luton, Bedfordshire, 2004.

24 Zetterstrom O, Buhl R, Mellem H *et al.* Improved asthma control with budesonide/formoterol in a single inhaler, compared with budesonide alone. *Eur Respir J* 2001; **18**: 262–8.

25 Rosenhall L, Heinig J, Lindqvist A *et al.* Budesonide/formoterol (Symbicort) is well tolerated and effective in patients with moderate persistent asthma. *Int J Clin Pract* 2002; **56**: 427–33.

26 Rosenhall L, Elvstrand A, Tilling B *et al.* One-year safety and efficacy of budesonide/formoterol in a single inhaler (Symbicort Turbuhaler) for the treatment of asthma. *Respir Med* 2003; **97**: 702–8.

27 Pauwels R, Lofdahl C, Postma D *et al.* Effect of inhaled formoterol and budesonide on exacerbations of asthma. Formoterol and Corticosteroids Establishing Therapy (FACET) International Study Group. *N Engl J Med* 1997; **337**: 1405–11.

28 O'Byrne P, Barnes P, Rodriguez-Roisin R *et al.* Low dose inhaled budesonide and formoterol in mild persistent asthma: the OPTIMA randomized trial. *Am J Respir Crit Care Med* 2001; **164**: 1392–7.

29 Price D, Dutchman D, Mawson A *et al.* Early asthma control and maintenance with eformoterol following reduction of inhaled corticosteroid dose. *Thorax* 2002; **57**: 791–8.

30 Lalloo U, Malolepszy J, Kozma D *et al.* Budesonide and formoterol in a single inhaler improves asthma control compared with increasing the dose of corticosteroid in adults with mild-to-moderate asthma. *Chest* 2003; **123**: 1480–7.

31 Buhl R, Creemers J, Vondra V *et al.* Once-daily budesonide/formoterol in a single inhaler in adults with moderate persistent asthma. *Respir Med* 2003; **97**: 323–30.

32 Tattersfield A, Postma D, Barnes P *et al.* Exacerbations of asthma: a descriptive study of 425 severe exacerbations. The FACET International Study Group. *Am J Respir Crit Care Med* 1999; **160**: 594–9.

33 Juniper E, Svensson K, O'Byrne P *et al.* Asthma quality of life during 1 year of treatment with budesonide with or without formoterol. *Eur Respir J* 1999; **14**: 1038–43.

34 Stallberg B, Olsson P, Jorgensen L, Lindarck N, Ekstrom T. Budesonide/formoterol adjustable maintenance dosing reduces asthma exacerbations versus fixed dosing. *Int J Clin Pract* 2003; **57**: 656–61.

35 Leuppi J, Salzberg M, Meyer L *et al.* An individualised, adjustable maintenance regimen of budesonide/formoterol provides effective asthma symptom control at a lower overall dose than fixed dosing. *Swiss Med Weekly* 2003; **133**: 302–9.

36 Fitzgerald J, Sears M, Boulet L *et al.* Adjustable maintenance dosing with budesonide/formoterol reduces asthma exacerbations compared with traditional fixed dosing: a five-month multicentre Canadian study. *Can Respir J* 2003; **10**: 427–34.

37 Ind P, Haughney J, Price D, Rosen J, Kennelly J. Adjustable and fixed dosing with budesonide/formoterol via a single inhaler in asthma patients: the ASSURE study. *Respir Med* 2004; **98**: 464–75.

38 Buhl R, Kardos P, Richter K *et al.* The effect of adjustable dosing with budesonide/formoterol on health-related quality of life and asthma control compared with fixed dosing. *Curr Res Med Opin* 2004; **20**: 1209–20.

39 Canonica G, Castellani P, Cazzola M *et al.* Adjustable maintenance dosing with budesonide/formoterol in a single inhaler provides effective asthma symptom control at a lower dose than fixed maintenance dosing. *Pulm Pharmacol Ther* 2004; **17**: 239–47.

40 Aalbers R, Backer V, Kava T *et al.* Adjustable maintenance dosing with budesonide/formoterol compared with fixed-dose salmeterol/fluticasone in moderate to severe asthma. *Curr Med Res Opin* 2004; **20**: 225–40.

41 Ringdal N, Chuchalin A, Chovan L *et al.* Evaluation of different inhaled combination therapies (EDICT): a randomised, double-blind comparison of Seretide (50/250 microg bd Diskus vs. formoterol (12 microg bd) and budesonide (800 microg bd) given concurrently (both via Turbuhaler) in patients with moderate-to-severe asthma. *Respir Med* 2002; **96**: 851–61.

42 Balanag V, Yunas F, Yang P, Jorup C. Budesonide/formoterol in a single inhaler is as effective and well tolerated as salbutamol in relieving acute asthma in adults and adolescents. *Eur Respir J* 2003; **22**: S445.

43 Tal A, Simon G, Vermeulen J *et al.* Budesonide/formoterol in a single inhaler versus inhaled corticosteroids alone in the treatment of asthma. *Pediatr Pulmonol.* 2002; **34**: 342–50.

44 Remington T, Heaberlin A, DiGiovine B. Combined budesonide/formoterol turbuhaler treatment of asthma. *Ann Pharmacother* 2002; **36**: 1918–28.

45 Ankerst J, Persson G, Weibull E. Tolerability of a high dose of budesonide/formoterol in a single inhaler in patients with asthma. *Pulm Pharmacol Ther* 2003; **16**: 147–51.

46 Brogden R, McTavish D. Budesonide. An updated review of its pharmacological properties, and therapeutic efficacy in asthma and rhinitis. *Drugs* 1992; **44**: 375–407.

47 Skoner D. Therapeutic margin of budesonide in patients with mild to severe asthma. *Clin Ther* 2003; **25**: C61–74.

48 Pearlman D. Preclinical properties of budesonide: translation to the clinical setting. *Clin Ther* 2003; **25**: C75–91.

49 Agertoft L, Pedersen S. Effect of long-term treatment with inhaled budesonide on adult height in children with asthma. *N Engl J Med* 2000; **343**: 1064–9.

50 Cheer S, Warner G, Easthope S. Formoterol delivered by Turbuhaler: in pediatric asthma. *Paediatr Drugs* 2003; **5**: 63–8.

51 AstraZeneca UK Limited. Oxis Turbohaler 6. *Summary of product characteristics.* Luton, Bedfordshire, 2004.

52 Zetterstrom O, Buhl R, Mellem H, Andersson F. The whole story: treatment outcomes with Symbicort. *Respir Med* 2002; **96**: S29–35.

53 Rosenhall L, Borg S, Andersson F, Ericsson K. Budesonide/formoterol in a single inhaler (Symbicort) reduces healthcare costs compared with separate inhalers in the treatment of asthma over 12 months. *Int J Clin Pract* 2003; **57**: 662–7.

54 Andersson F, Stahl E, Barnes P *et al.* Adding formoterol to budesonide in moderate asthma–health economic results from the FACET study. *Respir Med* 2001; **95**: 505–12.

55 Price D, Haughney J, Lloyd A, Hutchinson J, Plumb J. An economic evaluation of adjustable and fixed dosing with budesonide/formoterol via a single inhaler in asthma patients: the ASSURE study. *Curr Med Res Opin* 2004; **20**: 1671–9.

Acknowledgements

Figure 2 is adapted from Barnes, 2002.[1]
Figure 3 is adapted from Zetterström *et al.*, 2001.[24]
Figure 4 is adapted from O'Byrne *et al.*, 2001.[28]
Figure 5 is adapted from Buhl *et al.*, 2003.[31]
Figure 6 is adapted from Ställberg *et al.*, 2003.[34]
Figure 7 is adapted from Aalbers *et al.*, 2004.[40]

PATIENT NOTES

Dr Mike Thomas and Professor David Price

Introduction

Asthma is a disease characterised by persistent inflammation in the airways (or the tubes that transfer air from the mouth to the air-sacs in the lungs). Inflammation leads to over-reactive airways that can become temporarily constricted (narrowed) in response to triggers, resulting in the characteristic symptoms of breathlessness, cough, chest tightness and wheeze. Although inflammation persists in asthma, symptoms and limitations in air flow are variable, either spontaneously (because of the presence/absence of trigger factors) or as a result of treatment.

Asthma treatment: preventative and symptom relief

The treatment of asthma is divided into two main categories:

- preventative treatment – principally with anti-inflammatory drugs such as inhaled corticosteroids
- reliever treatment – principally with drugs that reverse the narrowing of the airways, such as bronchodilators.

In the long term, preventer medication is considered to offer by far the best protection against asthma symptoms and severe attacks.

Although reliever medications act rapidly to relieve symptoms and dilate the constricted airways making their effects more noticeable to the sufferer, they do not affect the underlying inflammation and therefore are a more temporary treatment. In contrast, preventer medications, by relieving inflammation and the over-reactivity of the airways, provide better long-term control of the condition. Preventer medications, however, need to be taken regularly to be effective, and their slower onset of action means that their effects are often less apparent to people with asthma compared with the faster-onset relievers. In the long term, however, preventer medication is considered to offer by far the best protection against asthma symptoms and severe attacks, including those which result in hospital admission or death.

Preventative treatment: anti-inflammatory medications

Inhaled corticosteroids

The principal anti-inflammatory class of medication used for the treatment of asthma is inhaled corticosteroids. Corticosteroids are naturally occurring substances made in the human body by the adrenal glands that have powerful actions in 'damping down' inflammation. Synthetic types of corticosteroids have been

After inhalation, the drug is deposited in the air tubes where it exerts a potent local anti-inflammatory effect.

developed and are used widely in medicine to control inflammation, either in tablet (oral) form or in local (topical) forms (such as skin creams, nose sprays or as inhaled medication). When given in tablet form, the drugs affect the whole body and may cause a number of well-known unwanted adverse events (side-effects). These include weight gain, high blood pressure, diabetes and weakened bones (osteoporosis). Although oral corticosteroids are very effective in asthma, and are sometimes given in short courses to treat asthma exacerbations (flare-ups), their associated side-effects mean that their potential risks are too great for them to be used regularly with the exception of the most severe and difficult-to-treat asthma.

On the other hand, inhaled corticosteroids are widely used to treat of asthma. The drugs are formulated either as a fine powder or as aerosolised droplets and are given by inhaler devices that deliver metered doses into the lungs of the patient. After inhalation, the drug is deposited in the air tubes (bronchi and bronchioli) where it exerts a potent local anti-inflammatory effect. Since the drug is delivered directly to the affected part of the body, a smaller dose can be given and side-effects are less likely to occur. Limited absorption of the active drug may occur with higher doses, either directly from the lungs or from the small amount of the drug that is deposited in the mouth and throat and which then reaches the stomach and is absorbed from the gut. At standard doses, the safety profile of inhaled corticosteroids is very good. Long-term surveillance studies, however, have indicated that some absorption and side-effects may occur in people receiving high doses of inhaled corticosteroids over long periods of time, with small increases in the risks of cataracts and fractures.

Inhaled corticosteroids may be formulated in gas-driven aerosols, in which a jet of gas containing dissolved droplets or fine suspensions of the drug is delivered, either when the patient presses a release mechanism (self-activated devices) or automatically when the patient starts to inspire (breath-activated devices). The propellant used to 'fire' the inhalers has traditionally been the inert 'CFC' (chlorofluorocarbon) gases, but due to concerns about the effect of these gases on the environment, these are currently being phased out and replaced with other 'non CFC' propellants. Alternatively, dry-powder inhaler devices may be used, in which a fine powder is sucked into the lungs by the patient.

A number of different inhaled steroids are now available. These include beclometasone dipropionate – the original inhaled corticosteroid used in Becotide® inhalers and still widely used today. Budesonide (Pulmicort®) is a more recently developed and widely used inhaled corticosteroid. Likewise, fluticasone propionate (Flixotide®) is a newer inhaled corticosteroid, and appears to be more potent than older-generation agents, and is not absorbed into the body from the gut. However, it may still be absorbed from the lung when used at higher doses. Mometasone, another potent inhaled corticosteroid, has recently been introduced in the UK and has the advantage of being able to be used once a day (rather than twice a day as is the case with most other inhaled corticosteroids). Newer, so-called 'soft' inhaled corticosteroids have recently been introduced (e.g. ciclesonide [Alvesco®]), which are designed to be broken down (metabolised) locally in the lungs and hence have less chance of being absorbed and reaching the rest of the body and causing side-effects.

Inhaled corticosteroids are considered to be very safe when used at standard doses. Local side-effects occasionally occur from deposition of the drug in the mouth and throat. These include candidiasis (or thrush [a minor fungal infection]), hoarseness and coughing, but they can be lessened by using 'spacer' devices (large plastic or metal bubbles that prevent the jet of gas hitting the back of the mouth) and by rinsing the mouth after use. These side-effects are reversible and can be treated if they do occur. When used in high doses, inhaled corticosteroids may be absorbed into the body and cause side-effects such as those described previously for the oral corticosteroids and may suppress the body's own steroid production – a potentially dangerous complication. As a consequence, guidelines recommend that the lowest effective dose of inhaled corticosteroids is used and that high-dose treatment should only be given after other options have been tried and failed.

Guidelines recommend that the lowest effective dose of inhaled corticosteroids is used and that high-dose treatment should only be given after other options have been tried and failed.

Leukotriene receptor antagonists

Leukotrienes are naturally occurring messenger molecules that promote inflammatory and allergic reactions. Importantly, the inflammation induced by leukotrienes is not suppressed by corticosteroids. Leukotrienes may be released in susceptible people by asthma triggers such as allergens, viral infections and allergens, which may then drive the asthma process. Drugs that block these effects have been developed (e.g. montelukast [Singulair®] and zafirulakast [Accolate®] and these can be used as 'add-on' therapy to standard doses of inhaled corticosteroids in patients who remain symptomatic. These drugs are available in oral (tablet) form, and can be given once or twice daily. They reduce inflammation and protect against constriction of the airways, thereby improving asthma symptoms and the flow of air into the lungs. They also reduce asthma exacerbations. As they are unrelated to corticosteroids they have none of the associated side-effects described previously and are generally well tolerated with few side-effects. Formulations of these drugs for children are

Leukotriene receptor antagonists appear to be particularly useful in patients who have asthma and allergic rhinitis as they improve both conditions.

also now available. They may be used, albeit in exceptional circumstances, as an alternative to inhaled corticosteroids, particularly in those with mild asthma triggered by exercise.

This class of therapy appears to be particularly useful in patients who have asthma and allergic rhinitis (nasal symptoms triggered by allergens such as pollen [e.g. 'hayfever') as it improves both conditions.

Theophyllines

These drugs are available in tablet form and have some degree of anti-inflammatory activity and some capacity to dilate constricted airways. They have been used as 'add-on' treatment in people whose asthma is uncontrolled on inhaled corticosteroids alone for many years. However, the use of this class of medication is limited by its tendency to cause nausea, and the use of these drugs is in decline.

Symptom relief: bronchodilators

Bronchodilators act by relaxing the muscle in the walls of the airways which become tightened when asthma is active, and their use results in opening up (dilatation) of the tightened (constricted) airway.

Short-acting β_2-agonists

This class of medication has been available for many years for the treatment of asthma. Drugs such as salbutamol (Ventolin®) and terbutaline (Bricanyl®) are usually given by the inhaled route by aerosol or dry powder inhalers. Patients are generally advised to use these reliever medicines on an 'as required' basis – i.e. to use them for the control of symptoms when needed but not in a regular manner. In well-controlled asthma, the need for such rescue medication is usually low, ideally used on less than two or three occasions each week, though everyone with asthma should have these inhalers available for occasional use. The effect of these drugs is rapid and people with constricted airways will usually notice a difference in their ability to breath and a reduction in their wheezing within minutes. A lack of an effect with the usual reliever medication can be a sign of a severe asthma attack and should prompt immediate medical attention. These drugs usually exert their effects for up to 6 hours, and the need for further doses of reliever medication within this time should again be a trigger for immediate medical attention.

Tablet and liquid formulations are available and have been used in the past, particularly in younger children, but the inhaled route is much safer and more effective and should be used wherever possible. In severe and life-threatening asthma these drugs are sometimes given by the 'nebulised' route, in which a jet of air (or oxygen) is bubbled through a solution of the drug and vaporised, with the patient breathing the enriched air/oxygen and bronchodilator mixture through a facemask.

Side-effects of short-acting β_2-agonists are usually mild, but include palpitations, trembling and a rapid pulse.

Long-acting β_2-agonists

Recently a number of drugs (e.g. salmeterol (Serevent®) and formoterol (Foradil® Oxis®) have been developed that act on the same receptors in the airways as the short-acting β_2-agonists but have a much longer duration of action. These drugs continue to act for 12 hours or longer to dilate constricted airways. They are used regularly, rather than on an 'as needed' basis (usually twice daily), and in addition to inhaled corticosteroids to prevent bronchoconstriction. When used in addition to standard doses of inhaled corticosteroids in patients whose asthma is not fully controlled, they have been shown to give very good results. The addition of a long-acting β_2-agonist is now recommended by guidelines as the first-choice therapy in adults and older children whose asthma is uncontrolled on inhaled corticosteroids alone.

Combining the different drugs in a single device is convenient for the patient and may result in better 'adherence'.

Long-acting β_2-agonists are available for use as inhalers alone or in combination with inhaled corticosteroids (see below), whilst longer acting 'once-daily' drugs are also under development.

Preventative and symptom relief: combination inhalers

As the combination of an inhaled corticosteroid and a long-acting β_2-agonist has proved to be very useful in providing excellent asthma control, and since both agents are used regularly (usually on a 'twice a day' basis), these drugs have now been combined in a single inhaled formulation. Several combination inhalers are now available (e.g. Seretide® and Symbicort®) and more are under development. Combining the different drugs in a single device is convenient for the patient, may result in better 'adherence' (use of medicine as recommended by the physician), whilst there are also some theoretical reasons why the delivery of the two active molecules in tandem may produce better results.

Future therapeutic developments

Although a number of effective treatments are available, a considerable burden of illness from asthma remains. New treatments are under development and may soon become available, which may in the long term reduce this burden.

As asthma is a variable disease over time and between individuals, no single treatment is right for all patients at all times. Medicines under development that may have a future role in asthma therapy include new, safer and longer-acting (once-daily) inhaled corticosteroids such as ciclesonide, and new types of oral anti-inflammatory agents, such as the 'phosphodiesterase 4' (PDE4) inhibitors. In addition, an injectable treatment given on a twice-weekly or once-monthly basis to 'mop up' the immunoglobulin E (IgE) antibodies involved in allergic asthma should soon be available as add-on treatment for those with the most severe asthma.

Although a number of effective treatments are available, a considerable burden of illness from asthma remains.

12. Improving practice

Kevin Gruffydd-Jones MA (Oxon) BM BCh MRCGP DRCOG Dip Sports Med Dip Occ Health
General Practitioner, Box, Wiltshire
Honorary Lecturer, University of Bath and University of Aberdeen
Member of the General Practice Airways Group

Remember that the author of the Improving Practice is addressing his healthcare professional colleagues rather than the 'lay' reader. This provides a fascinating insight into many of the challenges faced by doctors in the day-to-day practice of medicine (see Reader's Guide).

Summary

Despite recent improvements in structured care and the treatment of asthma within the primary-care sector, the condition remains a major burden on limited healthcare resources. Much remains to be done to address misconceptions amongst many clinicians that we have all but conquered this debilitating condition. With asthma not recognised as one of the main clinical priorities in the new NHS plan, making further improvements to its clinical management poses a significant challenge to GPs. There are also other significant barriers to its effective management, including confusion over appropriate diagnostic techniques and patient adherence to treatment. Here, practical solutions relating to improved education, diagnosis, patient communication and clinical audit are proposed to help overcome some of these barriers.

The burden of asthma in general practice

There have been huge improvements in the organisation of asthma care in general practice and in the treatment of asthma over the past two decades. In particular, there has been a significant reduction in asthma mortality – principally due to the widespread use of inhaled steroids – despite a significant rise in the prevalence of the disease during this period. However, asthma continues to represent a huge burden to primary care. For example, an average Primary Care Organisation (PCO) with a population of a third of a million patients can expect to include:

- 45,000 patients with diagnosed asthma
- more than 400 asthma-related emergency admissions to hospital per annum
- eight deaths from asthma per annum.

Asthma continues to represent a huge burden to primary care.

In addition, there is significant unmet need amongst asthmatics relating to successful treatment, with large surveys indicating that

20–40% of patients still have limitations in their everyday lives as a consequence of their condition, despite receiving active treatment.

What are the barriers to effective asthma management?

1. Professional complacency and lack of government prioritisation

There is a perception amongst health clinicians and administrators that asthma is essentially 'done and dusted'. However, the extent of the problem, as illustrated in the previous sections of this book, shows that this is far from true. The antipathy towards organised management of the condition is further reinforced by the fact that asthma is not one of the main priorities identified in the NHS plan. As a result, PCO and practice resources are inevitably diverted towards areas such as cardiovascular disease and diabetes which are the current government priorities.

2. Diagnostic confusion

A recent audit in our practice showed that fewer than 50% of adult asthmatics had objective evidence of asthma in their records.

Asthma continues to be misdiagnosed. In particular, there are significant diagnostic problems at both ends of the age spectrum. For example, the wheezing infant may too readily be given a diagnosis of asthma or inappropriately given antibiotics. Many of our 'asthmatics' over the age of 40 years in fact have Chronic Obstructive Pulmonary Disease (COPD). A recent audit in our practice, which has a strong interest in respiratory disease, showed that fewer than 50% of adult asthmatics had objective evidence of asthma in their records.

3. Poor patient compliance

Non-compliance to treatment is a significant problem in this area, and manifests in two distinct ways:

- poor compliance with preventative medication
- poor compliance with regular review in the surgery.

There is evidence that 50–60% of patients do not fully comply in either of these areas, and this in turn is linked to increased asthma morbidity. The common thread underlying this non-compliance appears to be patients' misperceptions about their asthma control. For example, it is common to hear statements from patients such as: "I'm not bad enough to need my preventer or to need a check-up". The reality may be quite different. For example, the Asthma Control and Expectations (ACE) study, which was published in 2002, showed that of the 1031 patients surveyed, 40% said that they felt well regarding their asthma, yet when questioned further one-third admitted to experiencing daily symptoms. Similarly, many patients accept restriction in their daily activities as a normal part of 'being an asthmatic'.

4. Lack of awareness of current management guidelines

It is perhaps inevitable that general health professionals who are faced with a multitude of disease entities, each with their own clinical guidelines, may not be up to date with all of them. To refresh the reader's memory, the management strategies described in this article are based on the 2003 British Guideline on the Management of Asthma (available via *www.brit-thoracic.org.uk*).

What should a practice do to overcome these barriers?

1. Overcoming complacency and improving compliance with review visits

Effective asthma management can be very rewarding for a GP! Asthma is a condition where effective treatment given within primary care can transform people's lives within just a few days. However, organising efficient asthma care within a practice requires more than enthusiasm, and demands time and resources. Achieving the quality standards for asthma outlined in the 2003 General Medical Services (GMS) GP contract can partially help this. These indicators are illustrated in Table 1.

Asthma is a condition where effective treatment can transform people's lives within just a few days.

Organised asthma care can be established either by dedicated asthma appointments or by an asthma clinic. Increasingly, nurses have taken over this role, and there is evidence that acquisition of a higher qualification such as an asthma diploma can further reduce asthma morbidity. However, it is equally important that a designated GP works in conjunction with the asthma nurse to reduce the chance of complacency ("we leave asthma management to the nurse") and to avoid 'de-skilling' the GP.

According to diagnostic criteria one of the most difficult quality markers is arranging regular review of our patients. This is perhaps best exemplified by surveys which estimate current non-attendance rates of 50–60% in asthma clinics. There are, however, a number of effective strategies that we can employ to encourage greater attendance. These include:

- reminders on repeat prescriptions
- written reminders (the GMS contract allows a non-attendee to be counted if three written reminders have been sent)
- telephone review – recent research has shown that more adult patients with asthma can be effectively reviewed by telephone consultation than traditional surgery or clinic review.

2. Improving diagnosis

Asthma diagnosis in older children and adults is largely based on a characteristic history and on objective lung function testing. Asthmatics usually present with one or more of cough, chest tightness, shortness of breath or wheeze. Characteristically these symptoms are variable and

Table 1. Indicators from the 2003 General Medical Services (GMS) GP contract for asthma management.

Indicator	Points	Maximum threshold
Records		
ASTHMA 1. The practice can produce a register of patients with asthma excluding patients with asthma who have been prescribed no asthma treatment in the last 12 months	7	N/A
Initial management		
ASTHMA 2. The percentage of patients aged 8 years and over diagnosed as having asthma from April 2003 where the diagnosis has been confirmed by spirometry or peak flow measurement	15	70%
Ongoing management		
ASTHMA 3. The percentage of patients with asthma between the ages of 14 and 19 years in whom there is a record of smoking status within the previous 15 months.	6	70%
ASTHMA 4. The percentage of patients aged 20 years and over with asthma whose notes record smoking status in the previous 15 months, except those who have never smoked where smoking status should be recorded at least once.	6	70%
ASTHMA 5. The percentage of patients with asthma who smoke and whose notes contain a record that smoking cessation advice has been offered within the last 15 months.	6	70%
ASTHMA 6. The percentage of patients with asthma who have had an asthma review in the last 15 months.	20	70%
ASTHMA 7. The percentage of patients aged 16 years and over with asthma who have had influenza immunisation in the preceding 1 September to 31 March.	12	70%

intermittent, being worse at night and provoked by trigger factors such as exercise or pollen. Although the results of the examination may be normal, it is important to exclude other causes of wheeze, for example, heart failure in the older patient.

Objective tests

The British Thoracic Society/Scottish Intercollegiate Guideline Network (BTS/SIGN) criteria for the objective diagnosis of asthma using peak flow or spirometry is illustrated in Table 2. In practice, it is often more convenient to carry out β_2-agonist reversibility testing when a patient first presents with asthma-like symptoms. This can provide a rapid diagnosis in addition to therapeutic relief for the patient. Peak flow charts are particularly useful in detecting occupational asthma and demonstrating 'before and after' benefits of preventative therapy. Exercise testing can be carried out by asking the patient to step up and down on an 18-inch high couch step for 6–8 minutes.

Table 2. Objective diagnosis of asthma using peak flow/spirometry.

- 20% or greater variability in peak flow (highest – lowest/highest × 100).
- Persists ideally for 3 days a week over 2 weeks.
- An increase in FEV_1/PEF following inhalation of a short-acting β_2-agonist such as 5 mg nebulised salbutamol or 400 μg salbutamol given via a metered-dose inhaler plus spacer.
- A decrease in FEV_1/PEF monitored every 10 minutes for 30 minutes after 6–8 minutes of exercise.
- An increase in FEV_1/PEF following a trial of oral prednisolone, 30 mg/day for 14 days.[a]
- With each of the above methods a change of ≥20% PEF and 60 L/minute or ≥15% FEV_1 and 200 mL provides objective evidence of asthma.

[a]Seldom used in primary care except in cases of uncertainty or where the presenting symptoms are in the form of acute asthma.
FEV_1, forced expiratory volume in 1 second; PEF, peak expiratory flow.

Other tests may be of help where doubt persists over the diagnosis. For example, a chest X-ray is advisable in patients presenting for the first time after the age of 45 years (especially in smokers) or in areas where there is a high prevalence of TB. Referral to a chest physician is indicated where significant diagnostic doubt persists (where histamine or methacholine challenge tests may be carried out) or where occupational asthma is present.

A chest X-ray is advisable in patients presenting for the first time after the age of 45 years (especially in smokers) or in areas where there is a high prevalence of TB.

Diagnosing asthma in young children

The diagnosis of asthma in young children is often problematic due to difficulties in performing objective testing in this patient population. Consequently, the diagnosis of asthma in pre-school children is principally based on:

- a suggestive history and high index of suspicion of alternative diagnoses
- assessment of the response to a trial of adequate asthma therapy.

The principal features of asthma in pre-school children are:

- recurrent and episodic cough and wheeze, which also occurs with respiratory tract infections, but also at other times (e.g. in response to exercise, or contact with pollen, animal antigens etc.)
- symptoms triggered by exercise or exposure to animal allergens etc.
- diurnal variation of symptoms – symptoms worse at night or early morning
- family history of allergic disease (especially maternal; e.g. asthma, allergic rhinitis or eczema)
- history of atopic eczema in the child.

A physical examination is absolutely vital in establishing a diagnosis in young children, as a child with bronchiolitis or pneumonia can often present with wheeze. An 'adequate trial of therapy' usually involves giving an anti-inflammatory agent for an appropriate length of time.

The response to inhaled β_2-agonists at this age can be highly variable and is therefore not used as a diagnostic test.

Inhaled steroids should be given via a large volume spacer with a mask for 4–8 weeks and the symptomatic response assessed. Relatively high doses of steroid (e.g. beclometasone, 200 μg twice daily, or equivalent) should be given intially, but if there is improvement the steroid dose can be reduced to an appropriate level to maintain control (usually 50 μg twice daily). An alternative is to give a 4-week course of montelukast, 4 mg/day. Oral steroids (prednisolone, 20 mg/day, for 3 days) can produce a dramatic improvement in symptoms, but have low specificity for asthma and should not be relied upon as a diagnostic test. It is vital that the child is closely followed up and a high index of suspicion held for alternative diagnoses. For example, at one end of the spectrum a child from a non-atopic background who wheezes only when a viral infection is present and is otherwise well is likely to have 'viral-induced wheeze' and thus requires symptomatic treatment only.

3. Improving management

Table 3 shows a scheme for the management of asthma in primary care, from initial presentation to regular review. Management of patients within this scheme occurs over several consultations and should involve both the doctor and the practice nurse.

In pre-school children, objective testing is unhelpful.

In pre-school children, as described above, objective testing is unhelpful. A therapeutic trial of inhaled steroids or montelukast should be given. It is likely that more frequent initial visits will be necessary to assess response than with an adult patient.

Pharmacological management

The classic SIGN/BTS step-up approach to asthma management in adults, children aged 5–12 years and pre-school children (under 5 years) has been presented in detail in the Disease Overview (see pages 11–14).

The initial pharmacological management of asthma in primary care depends very much on the nature of the initial presentation. All patients will require a short-acting β_2-agonist for the relief of symptoms. Inhaled steroids will be needed for patients with persistent night-time and daily symptoms. The majority of patients will show improvements in lung function and symptoms with beclometasone, 400 μg/day, or equivalent for adults, and 200 μg/day for children.[a] However, if there are problems with drug delivery, a 400 μg dose may be necessary in children under 5 years. Improvements are usually apparent within 48 hours, and then plateau after 4–6 weeks.

Oral steroids may be necessary to obtain control in patients who present with acute severe asthma.

[a]Mometasone is not currently recommended for use in children in the UK.

Table 3. Scheme for the management of asthma for adults and older children in primary care.

Visit 1	• Initial presentation • Provisional diagnosis of asthma on the basis of symptoms and examination • Explanation given with appropriate support materials • Patient issued with peak flow chart and/or reversibility testing carried out or arranged • Additional tests (e.g. chest X-ray if there is doubt over diagnosis) • Short-acting β_2-agonist prescribed (or for those with more severe asthma, oral steroids or inhaled steroids may need to be given to obtain control)
Visit 2 (allow 20–30 minutes)	• Confirmation of diagnosis by peak flow chart or reversibility testing • Establish severity of asthma and identify possible trigger factors (including smoking) • Reiterate explanation, deal with patient concerns and reinforce with self-help information • Establish control of asthma using appropriate pharmacotherapy (see text)
Visit 3	• Review asthma control and adjust medication • Check inhaler technique and compliance • Discuss non-pharmacological management (e.g. smoking cessation, influenza immunisation, avoidance of trigger factors) • Issue asthma action plan • Discuss outstanding patient concerns • Arrange regular review

Assessment of asthma control

Asthma control has traditionally been assessed in primary care by looking at changes in lung function or improvements in symptoms. Whilst these remain useful tools, it should be remembered that patients may present with few symptoms because they avoid activities which trigger their asthma. Similarly, patients may experience significant restrictions in their lives as a result of asthma, but have little change in lung function. One useful measure of asthma control is the Royal College of Physicians' Asthma Morbidity Index. At review patients are asked three questions relating to their symptoms in the last week or month.

- Have you had difficulty in sleeping because of your asthma symptoms (including cough)?
- Have you had your usual asthma symptoms in the day?
- Has your asthma interfered with your usual activities (e.g. work, school, housework)?

Asthma control has traditionally been assessed in primary care by looking at changes in lung function or improvements in symptoms.

If there is an affirmative response to any of these questions then the management of the patient should be adjusted. However, before medication is increased the following factors should also be checked:

- inhaler technique
- compliance with medication
- alteration in trigger factors.

The roles of various controller therapies are considered in the following sections.

Inhaled steroids

Inhaled steroid therapy is the cornerstone of asthma management and has been shown to improve lung function, symptoms and quality of life, and reduce exacerbations. For the majority of patients seen in general practice, inhaled steroids are generally safe and effective below the maximum daily dosage recommendations.

The choice of inhaled steroid largely depends on the choice of inhaler device and cost. There is some evidence that beclometasone may exhibit more short-term growth suppression in young children than low-dose budesonide or fluticasone.

Long-acting inhaled β_2-agonists/inhaled steroid combination therapy

The 2003 British Asthma Guidelines recommend that inhaled long-acting β_2-agonists (e.g. salmeterol and formoterol) should be added to the treatment of patients who are poorly controlled on low-dose inhaled corticosteroids, instead of increasing the inhaled corticosteroid dose. This is more conveniently given in the form of a combination inhaler (e.g. Seretide® or Symbicort®), which can improve compliance with treatment and give rapid improvement in asthma control.

Leukotriene receptor antagonists

Leukotriene receptor antagonists are considered as second-line controller therapy in the British Asthma Guidelines, but may be of particular help in the following groups:

- children under 5 years of age
- patients with exercise-induced asthma
- patients with allergen-induced asthma, especially when associated with allergic rhinitis
- patients with poor adherence with inhaled medication.

Referral to a specialist chest physician or paediatrician should be considered when a patient is still poorly controlled with inhaled steroids above 2000 μg per day in adults (800 μg in school-age children) and add-on therapy.

Once control has been obtained, step down of the dose of inhaled steroids to the lowest effective dose should be initiated in order to minimise the chance of side-effects. Bone densitometry should be performed in all patients on inhaled steroids above 800 μg/day for more than a few months. Growth should be checked regularly in all children with asthma.

Non-pharmacological management

Smoking cessation and influenza vaccination should be encouraged and are integral components of the quality markers for asthma in the GMS GP contract. Avoidance of trigger factors by the patient can be helpful, but radical avoidance measures (e.g. house dust eradication and pet avoidance) may be impractical and can cause huge distress. Exercise should be positively encouraged whilst breathing retraining may help patients with dysfunctional breathing.

Smoking cessation and influenza vaccination should be encouraged and are integral parts of the asthma quality markers in the GMS GP contract.

Personalised asthma action plans

Personalised action plans as part of structured asthma care have been shown to improve asthma morbidity, yet a recent survey showed that only 6% of asthma patients were given a written action plan. There is no evidence regarding the exact style of plan, but it is generally agreed that it should be individually tailored to the patient. An example of an appropriate asthma management plan is given in Table 4.

Clinical audit

Audit still fills many primary care professionals with dread. However, there is clear evidence to suggest that appropriately audited organised

Table 4. Example of an asthma action plan.

Good control	• No limits on daily activity • No night waking • Using reliever less than twice per week • Peak expiratory flow rate at highest recorded level
Worsening control	• If you wake at night because of asthma • Require reliever more than once per day • Daily activities restricted by asthma
	• **Increase preventer medication[a]** • **Increase reliever medication[a]**
Poor control	• If you need reliever more than four times in 24 hours • If peak flow is less than 60% of patients' best value
	• **See doctor or asthma nurse**
Danger signs	• If reliever only lasts 1 hour • Unable to speak in sentences because of breathing trouble
	• **Call doctor immediately**

[a]To be agreed between the individual patient and health professional.

asthma care markedly improves asthma morbidity. The new GMS GP contract has undoubtedly encouraged audit of certain 'process' markers. However, additional factors amenable to clinical audit could include the use of personalised action plans or the number of asthma exacerbations experienced by patients. The General Practice Airways Group website offers some further ideas and help for audit (*www.gpiag.org.uk*).

Conclusion

Asthma still provides a great challenge for primary care, with a large unmet need amongst asthmatics. However, treating asthma is rewarding for the physician and can produce huge improvements in sufferers' lives.

Key points

- Whilst significant advances have been made in the management and treatment of asthma in the past 20 years, it continues to represent a major clinical burden for primary care.
- Many of the practical issues that remain relate to complacency and a lack of government prioritisation towards the condition. In addition, diagnosis continues to be an issue, with a significant number of asthmatics misdiagnosed, and consequently not optimally managed.
- There are also significant issues relating to treatment adherence, and a lack of awareness of the latest clinical guidelines.
- Improving structured care should involve the whole primary healthcare team in the management of the condition. Practice nurses have a critical role to play, whilst establishing dedicated asthma clinics will also serve to improve care.
- The latest clinical guidelines offer useful advice in terms of diagnosis and treatment. Non-pharmacological interventions should be implemented to maximise the care of our patients. Personalised asthma plans are useful tools in improving care, and also open up lines of communication between doctors and their patients.

PATIENT NOTES

Dr Mike Thomas and Professor David Price

Most of the costs of asthma relate to poor asthma control, and it is likely that a better partnership between doctors and patients could significantly reduce this burden.

Introduction

For many people, asthma is a long-term 'chronic' condition and, despite effective treatment, outcomes of care are currently far from ideal. Asthma results in a large burden of ill health for sufferers and in a large economic burden on society at large. Most of the costs of asthma relate to poor asthma control, and it is likely that a better partnership between doctors and patients could significantly reduce this burden. There are a number of factors in the 'delivery of care' that could improve asthma outcomes.

Information provision

Many people with asthma feel that they have not been given enough information about their condition, and would like to feel better informed and more in control. This is particularly so when the illness is first diagnosed, as the news may come as a real shock and, as such, the patient may not ask or remember the answers to important questions they have about their condition. Providing sufficient time and the right environment of trust in which newly diagnosed patients (or their parents/carers) can ask important questions they have about asthma, can lead to greater confidence, understanding and 'empowerment', and consequently improved outcomes. The provision of written patient-orientated material (such as that provided by the UK charity, Asthma UK [see Useful Contacts, page 335]) can be very helpful.

Regular follow up

There is good evidence that regular asthma checks, in which there is a proper evaluation of asthma control, lead to better long-term outcomes than dealing with crises when they occur. Asthma check-ups should occur at least once a year and more often if asthma is not stable. Most GP surgeries now provide dedicated 'asthma clinics', where a full asthma assessment is made by a trained asthma nurse or GP. Factors covered in the 'annual review' should include the use of medication, concerns about medication (possibly leading to under use of recommended preventer treatment), a check of the inhaler technique and simple lung function tests such as measurement of the 'peak flow' (the fastest velocity of air exhaled from the lungs measured by a simple meter). The level of symptoms in the day and any night-time symptoms should also be assessed, whilst any restriction in activity caused by the condition should also be identified. The level of need for rescue medications should also be determined –

when asthma is well controlled there should be little need to use the blue rescue inhaler, and a regular need to use this more than twice a week may be an indication of the need for better preventative treatment. Any asthma attacks or need for additional medication or emergency contact with healthcare professionals should also be noted. Triggers should also be identified. Treatment should also be regularly assessed – in patients who are unstable it may need to be increased or changed, but equally in people who are very well controlled a 'step-down' of treatment can be attempted. Annual influenza vaccination is now offered to everyone with asthma in the UK and should be taken up where possible. A personal action plan should also be provided and checked during the follow up (see below). Finally, any concerns or worries that the patient has should be discussed and appropriate follow-up arranged.

There is good evidence that people undergoing regular checks have less asthma attacks, less time off work and a better quality of life. For people who are unable to get to the surgery for checks, telephone asthma checks have now been shown to be useful, and many surgeries now provide this facility.

Personal action plans

Everyone with asthma should know what to do when their condition deteriorates, and have a 'personal plan' of how to react to changes in their asthma.

Everyone with asthma should know what to do when their condition deteriorates, and have a 'personal plan' of how to react to changes in their asthma. Asthma is a variable condition, and even people who are well controlled can suffer exacerbations when they are exposed to a trigger (e.g. when they come into contact with an allergen or after a viral infection such as the 'flu). Such triggers can cause constriction of the airways leading to symptoms and even to full-blown asthma attacks, and therefore people with asthma need to know what to do when this occurs. Surveys consistently show that people with asthma want to be more independent of their doctors and nurses and wish to take control of their condition, but often they are not provided with the necessary skills to do so. Everyone with asthma should therefore sit down with their GP or asthma nurse to construct a personal plan that they feel comfortable with.

The contents of the plan will vary for each individual, but basically will include instructions on how to increase or decrease the levels of preventer and rescue medication in response to changes in their asthma, and when to call for medical help. This may be based on symptoms or on lung function. Some people find monitoring their 'peak flow' level with the use of a simple peak flow meter useful. People with asthma can blow hard into this device, and can measure their flow rate against their usual and best levels to see how they are doing. This can give an objective assessment of the level of constriction in the airways, and can be a guide to increasing treatment when needed. Simple peak flow meters can be provided on prescription by GPs. For other people an action plan based on changes in symptoms may be equally effective. It is important however that the information is written down and can be referred to when needed. Once again, Asthma UK provides excellent self-help and action-plan material on which to base such personal plans.

Patient–doctor partnerships

As with any long-term 'chronic' disease, a good partnership between the patient and the clinician lies at the heart of good quality care. Perhaps too often in the past, the doctor has 'told' the patient how to behave and what to do, but has failed to appreciate that person's understandings, aims and priorities in asthma care. In this situation it's not surprising that many people have chosen not to follow the recommended action, often without telling the doctor that this is the case. Best results are therefore achieved by a full and frank sharing of information, beliefs and objectives, and by shared decision making.

Best results are therefore achieved by a full and frank sharing of information, beliefs and objectives, and by shared decision making.

Glossary

α_1-adrenoceptors – Proteins on the surface of cells that mediate the biological effects of adrenaline and/or noradrenaline. Adrenoceptors are divided into α and β subtypes, with α receptors further subdivided into α_1 and α_2 receptors.

Absorption – The movement and uptake of a drug into cells or across tissues (such as the skin, intestine and kidney).

Acidic pH – A pH value of less than 7, indicating that a solution contains a high concentration of hydrogen ions (H^+). The pH value decreases as acidity increases.

Acute – A relatively short course of drug treatment lasting days or weeks rather than months. Can also refer to the duration of a disease or condition.

Adenylate cyclase pathway – A series of biochemical reactions catalysed by the adenylate cyclase enzyme. Adenylate cyclase promotes the conversion of adenosine triphosphate (ATP), the chemical form in which energy is stored in the body, into cyclic adenosine monophosphate (AMP). Cyclic AMP drives many important biochemical processes in the body, including the generation of signals within cells and the movement of calcium ions through cell membranes.

Adhesion molecule expression – The production of adhesion molecules on the surface of a cell. Adhesion molecules (e.g. integrins, cadherins and selectins) are protein–sugar complexes, which play an important role in many cellular processes, including cell growth and development, the migration of immune cells into and out of the circulatory system, and the growth of cancerous cells. In essence, adhesion molecules mediate interactions between cells.

Adrenal cortical reserve – The amount of the hormone, cortisol. Provides an indication of how well the adrenal cortex is functioning. Low plasma cortisol levels suggest that the adrenal cortical reserve is low and that the adrenal cortex is not functioning properly.

Adrenal glands – Two triangular-shaped glands located above the kidneys. The adrenal glands secrete the hormones aldosterone, hydrocortisone and corticosterone, which play an important role in the regulation of fat, protein and carbohydrate metabolism, and also in suppressing inflammatory reactions within the body. The adrenal glands also secrete adrenaline and noradrenaline, two chemicals involved in the transmission of nervous impulses in the sympathetic nervous system.

Adrenal suppression – The failure of the adrenal glands to secrete the corticosteroid hormones, aldosterone, hydrocortisone and cortisol.

Adrenocortical axis – See Hypothalamic–pituitary–adrenal (HPA) axis.

Adrenocorticotropic hormone (ACTH) – A hormone secreted by the pituitary gland that stimulates the adrenal glands to secrete corticosteroid hormones. These play an important role in the regulation of fat, protein and carbohydrate metabolism, and in suppressing inflammatory reactions in the body.

Adverse event – An unwanted reaction to a medical treatment.

Aetiology – The specific causes or origins of a disease, usually a result of both genetic and environmental factors.

Airway calibre – The width or diameter of the airways. The airways comprise the trachea (windpipe), the two bronchi and the smaller airways, or bronchioles, in the lungs.

Airway hyper-responsiveness – Increased sensitivity of the respiratory system to provocative stimuli, such as histamine and antigens (substances that stimulate an immune response [e.g. dust mites, pollen and animal fur]). Airway hyper-responsiveness is a characteristic feature of asthma.

Albuterol – See Salbutamol.

Allergen challenge – Controlled exposure to an allergen (a substance that causes an allergic reaction) in order to induce an inflammatory reaction in the airways. The patient inhales increasing doses of the allergen, and lung function (e.g. FEV_1) is measured before and after inhalation. The technique is commonly used to evaluate the anti-inflammatory effects of anti-asthma drugs.

Allergen inhalation challenge – A clinical test to determine which allergens are causing asthma or any other allergic respiratory disease in a person. The participant breathes in increasing amounts of a potential allergen as a fine mist. Lung function is measured before and after inhaling the substance using a technique known as spirometry.

Allergens – Substances that cause an allergic reaction in the body. Common allergens include dust, pet hair, pollen and peanuts.

Alveolus – Thin walled, air-filled pockets of the lungs in which gas exchange takes places (plural alveoli).

Amelioration – Improvement or moderation in the severity of a disease or the intensity of its symptoms.

Amphotericin – A drug used to treat severe fungal infections. It is available in liquid and injectable forms. The injectable form can cause serious side-effects, such as kidney damage, headache, vomiting and convulsions.

Aneurysm – Abnormal dilation (bulging) of a blood vessel wall. The condition most commonly affects the arteries at the base of the brain and the aorta. Can be fatal if the blood vessel wall ruptures.

Angioedema – Swelling under the skin and in the mucus membranes (the soft, pink lining of the body passages and cavities that connect with the exterior) as a result of an allergic reaction. Characterised by the development of wheals (flat, burning patches of skin).

Antibodies – Proteins present in the blood that target and destroy particular antigens.

Antigen – Any foreign substance within the body that stimulates an immune response.

Aorta – The large artery that carries oxygenated blood from the left ventricle of the heart to the other arteries of the body.

Arachidonic acid metabolism – The breakdown of arachidonic acid, a polyunsaturated fatty acid. Arachidonic acid, the building block of eicosanoids, is present in cell membranes and can be converted into prostaglandins and leukotrienes.

Area under curve (AUC) – A graphical plot of the concentration of a drug against the time since initial administration. It is a means of analysing the bioavailability of a drug. AUC_{24} describes the drug concentration over a 24-hour period (see Reader's Guide).

Arginine-16 polymorphism – The substitution of the arginine amino acid at position 16 of the protein chain that makes up the β_2-adrenoceptor in humans. Some individuals have arginine at this position, whilst others have glycine. The natural occurrence of different forms of the β_2-adrenoceptor is thought to account for the different responses of individuals to β_2-adrenoceptor agonists (e.g. salbutamol, salmeterol).

Ascaris aerosol – An aerosol containing antigens from the parasitic worm, Ascaris. The inhalation of ascaris protein stimulates an allergic reaction in animals and provides an animal model of asthma for medical research purposes.

Atopic – Suffering from atopy.

Atopic dermatitis – A type of immune-mediated (allergic) inflammatory skin disorder that results in an itchy, flaky rash and tends to affect the face, elbows, knees and arms. More commonly called atopic eczema.

Atopy – The tendency to suffer from allergies, such as asthma, eczema and hay fever. Atopy is commonly inherited.

Atrophy – Wasting away of a cell, tissue, organ or part of the body due to a lack of nourishment, disuse or the loss of its nerve supply.

β_2-adrenoceptor – Proteins on the surface of cells that mediate the biological effects of adrenaline and noradrenaline. β-adrenoceptors are subdivided into β_1, β_2 and β_3 receptors. The activation of β_2-adrenoceptors leads to relaxation of bronchial and vascular smooth muscle.

β_2-agonist – An agent that activates β_2-adrenoceptors, thereby mimicking the effects of adrenaline or noradrenaline. β_2-agonists (e.g. formoterol, salbutamol, salmeterol and terbutaline) are therefore effective bronchodilators (widen the airways) and are used in the treatment of asthma and other inflammatory diseases of the respiratory system.

17β-carboxylic acid metabolite – A substance formed from the breakdown (metabolism) of the corticosteroid drug, fluticasone propionate, in the liver.

Barbiturates – A group of drugs that work by depressing brain activity, thereby causing sedation and reducing anxiety. Owing to their danger in overdose (particularly when combined with alcohol) and abuse potential, barbiturates are currently used only in anaesthesia and the treatment of epilepsy.

Basal – Resting level.

Basal airway tone – The resting level of airway constriction. The width/flexibility of the airways under normal conditions.

Baseline – The starting point to which all subsequent measurements are compared. Used as a means of assessing improvement or deterioration during the course of a clinical trial.

Basement membrane thickening – Thickening or proliferation of the basement membrane, the thin layer of tissue beneath epithelial cells to which the epithelial cells are anchored.

Basophils – White blood cells that contain large granules in their cytoplasm and defend against large parasites. Basophils also play an important role in allergic reactions in that when activated, they secrete histamine and cytokines.

Binding affinity – An attractive force between substances that causes them to enter into and remain in chemical combination (see Reader's Guide).

Bronchi – Branched tubes of the respiratory system, located between the trachea (windpipe) and the bronchioles of the lungs.

Bronchial epithelium – The thin layer of cells lining the bronchi.

Bronchiectasis – A disease of the lungs in which the lining of the bronchi is damaged, and the bronchi become distorted and stretched. The disease used to be common in children, but the introduction of antibiotics has virtually wiped it out. The main symptom is a cough that produces green or yellow phlegm.

Bronchioles – Small tubules leading from the bronchi to the alveoli of the lungs. Less than 1 mm in diameter.

Bronchiolitis – Inflammation of the smaller airways in the lungs (the bronchioles) due to a viral infection. The condition mainly affects babies and young children and the main symptoms are a cough, rapid breathing, a temperature and, in severe cases, a blue complexion due to insufficient oxygen uptake.

Bronchoalveolar lavage – A procedure in which the bronchioles of the lungs are washed out with sterile saline solution delivered via a bronchoscope (a long, thin tube with a light at the end). The solution is then sucked back up the bronchoscope and is examined for the presence of various cells. The technique is useful for diagnosing and monitoring inflammatory diseases of the airways, including asthma.

Bronchoconstriction – Reduction of the diameter of the smaller airways in the lungs, which impedes the flow of air through the lungs.

Bronchodilation – Widening of the smaller airways in the lungs, which allows more air to flow in and out of the lungs.

Bronchodilators – A group of drugs used to treat asthma and other respiratory diseases that relax the smooth muscle in the walls of the airways, thereby widening the airways and allowing more air to flow in and out of the lungs. The major bronchodilators currently in clinical use include the short-acting β_2-agonists (e.g. salbutamol and terbutaline), the longer-acting β_2-agonists (e.g. formoterol and salmeterol) and the xanthines (e.g. theophylline).

Bronchoprovocation – Controlled exposure to agents that have the potential to cause an inflammatory reaction in the airways, such as histamine or methacholine. The patient inhales increasing doses of bronchoprovocator and lung function (e.g. FEV_1) is measured before and after inhalation. The technique is used to diagnose asthma, to identify factors that trigger the disease and to assess the response to anti-asthma treatment.

Calcitonin gene-related peptide (CGRP) – A small protein produced by the gene for calcitonin (a hormone produced by the thyroid gland that helps to control levels of calcium and phosphate in the blood) in nerve tissue. CGRP acts as a neurotransmitter and also inhibits the release of insulin (the hormone involved in controlling blood sugar levels) from the pancreas.

Candidiasis – Commonly known as thrush, this is an infection caused by the fungus *Candida albicans.* It most commonly affects the vagina, but may also affect the inside of the mouth. Oral candidiasis is characterised by sore, cream-coloured, raised patches in the mouth, and has been linked with the regular inhalation of corticosteroids for the treatment of asthma and other respiratory diseases. The risk of developing candidiasis may be reduced by gargling with water between corticosteroid applications.

Carbamazepine – An anticonvulsant drug used to treat epilepsy and to prevent seizures.

Catalysis – The acceleration of a chemical reaction by a catalyst, a substance that speeds up chemical reactions but is itself not used up in the process.

Catecholamines – A group of structurally related compounds occurring naturally in the body that act as hormones and/or neurotransmitters. Examples include dopamine, adrenaline and noradrenaline.

Cationic protein – A protein with a positive electrical charge due to the loss of negatively charged electrons. Eosinophilic cationic protein (ECP) is released from eosinophils and can be used clinically as a marker of airways inflammation in patients with asthma.

Chemokines – Inflammatory cytokines that have the ability to attract and activate white blood cells.

Chemotaxis – The movement of cells in a specific direction in response to a chemical stimulus. For example, white blood cells are attracted to a site of infection by chemokines produced by other cells of the immune system.

Chiral drugs – Drugs with a molecular structure that is not symmetrical. In other words, the structure cannot be superimposed on its mirror image. Thus, the drug exists in two forms: a 'right-handed' form (R) and a 'left-handed' (L) form, or enantiomer.

Chronic – A prolonged course of drug treatment lasting months rather than weeks. Can also refer to the duration of a disease or condition.

Chronic Obstructive Pulmonary Disease (COPD) – A potentially fatal, slowly progressive disease of the airways that is characterised by airflow obstruction that is not fully reversible. This is in contrast to asthma, in which the airflow obstruction is reversible. Tobacco smoking is a major cause of COPD, and leads to chronic inflammation of the small airways and lung tissue, and the destruction of lung tissue by certain enzymes. The main symptoms of COPD include chronic cough and/or wheezing, a tight chest, shortness of breath, difficulty in breathing, increased sputum production and frequent clearing of the throat. There is no cure, and treatment is aimed at controlling symptoms and preventing further progression of the disease through the use of bronchodilators.

Circadian rhythm – A biological pattern that occurs in approximately 24-hour cycles.

Cleavage – The splitting of a molecule by the breaking of a chemical bond (the attachment between two atoms in a molecule).

Co-administration – The simultaneous administration of more than one type of medication.

Comorbid – A co-existing medical condition.

Contra-indication – Specific circumstances under which a drug should not be prescribed, for example, certain drugs should not be given simultaneously.

Corticosteroids – A steroid produced by the adrenal cortex or a drug that resembles one. Corticosteroids (e.g. beclometasone, budesonide, fluticasone, mometasone and prednisolone) are potent anti-inflammatory agents, and are therefore used to treat a variety of inflammatory conditions, including asthma, rheumatoid arthritis, eczema, hay fever and Crohn's disease (inflammation of the digestive tract). Available in tablet, injectable and inhaled forms.

Cosynotropin – A synthetic form of corticotropin – the hormone that stimulates the adrenal glands to produce cortisol.

Cotton pellet model – An animal model of inflammation that is used to test the anti-inflammatory properties of drugs. Sterile cotton pellets are implanted into the 'armpit' of the animal (commonly rats). Inflammatory granuloma tissue (comprised of macrophages and lymphocytes) then develops around the cotton pellets, which are removed and weighed to determine how much granuloma tissue has formed.

Coumarins – A group of substances that occur naturally in plants (e.g. clover and grass) and inhibit the actions of vitamin K, which is necessary for the clotting of blood. Coumarin-like drugs (e.g. warfarin) are therefore used as anticlotting agents to prevent thrombosis (blockage of a blood vessel by a blood clot).

Cromones – A group of anti-inflammatory compounds that are used in the prophylactic (preventative) treatment of asthma and other allergic respiratory diseases. Cromones work by preventing inflammatory cells in the lungs (mast cells) from releasing histamine and other substances that cause constriction of the airways. Examples of cromones include sodium cromoglycate and nedocromil sodium.

Cromone therapy – Treatment with a chromone (e.g. sodium cromoglycate and nedocromil sodium). Chromones are a group of non-steroidal compounds with anti-inflammatory effects that are used in the prophylactic (preventative) treatment of asthma and other allergic respiratory diseases. They work by preventing inflammatory cells in the lungs (mast cells) from releasing histamine and other substances that cause constriction of the airways.

Cysteinyl leukotriene (cysLT$_1$) – A leukotriene containing the amino acid cysteine (e.g. leukotrienes C4, D4 and E4).

Cysteinyl leukotriene (cysLT$_1$) receptor – One of two membrane receptors for the cysteinyl leukotrienes. CysLT$_1$ receptors are found on airway smooth muscle, macrophages and other inflammatory cells and are targeted by the leukotriene receptor antagonists (e.g. montelukast, zafirlukast).

Cystic fibrosis – A disease characterised by the production of thick, sticky mucus in the nose, throat, airways, lungs and intestines. As a result, the patient is prone to lung infections, has difficulty in absorbing fats and other nutrients from food, and tends to show stunted growth. The condition is present at birth and is caused by a defective gene inherited from both parents. It is a serious condition and potentially fatal, but can be controlled to some extent with antibiotics and dietary supplements.

Cytochrome P450 (CYP) enzymes – A family of enzymes found in the liver that play an important role in the metabolism and detoxification of various compounds, including many drugs.

Cytokine receptors – Proteins on the surface of cells that have particular affinity for cytokines and mediate the biological effects of these proteins.

Cytokines – Small protein messengers secreted by immune cells (e.g. macrophages, monocytes, lymphocytes and neutrophils) in response to a stimulus, that affect the behaviour of other nearby cells. Examples of cytokines include histamine, prostaglandins, tumour necrosis factor (TNF) and the interleukins (IL).

Cytoplasm – Everything inside a cell except the nucleus. The main site of cellular chemical activity.

Cytoplasmic – Pertaining to the cytoplasm.

Dendritic cell – A highly branched extension of a nerve cell that receives information from other nerve cells.

Deposition – The distribution of drugs within the airways and lungs following inhalation.

Diastereomer – A stereoisomer in which the molecules consist of the same atoms but are not mirror images of each other.

Dihydrate salt – A salt of a compound, that contains two water molecules (hence dihydrate). A salt is a chemical compound produced by combining an acid with an alkali.

Dimerisation – The joining together of two protein subunits to form a protein complex.

Direct steroid-membrane interaction – One of the two main ways in which steroids exert their effect on cells. In this case, the steroid binds to a receptor in the cell membrane, and this triggers a series of events within the cell that does not involve an alteration in gene expression. This is a 'fast' pathway. The other way in which steroids exert their effects is to bind to receptors inside cells, triggering a series of events that involve an alteration in gene expression. This is a 'slow' pathway.

Diuretics – A group of drugs that remove excess water from the body by increasing the production of urine. Diuretics are used to treat many conditions associated with water retention, including heart failure, certain kidney and liver disorders, high blood pressure, glaucoma and premenstrual syndrome.

Diurnal – A biological pattern that fluctuates according to the time of day (e.g. cortisol secretion).

Double-blind – A clinical trial in which neither the doctor nor the patient are aware of the treatment allocation.

Drug interactions – In which the action of one drug interferes with that of another, with potentially hazardous consequences. Interactions are particularly common when the patient is taking more than one form of medication for the treatment of multiple disease states or conditions.

Dual energy x-ray absorptiometry (DXA) scanning – A technique used to measure the density of bone, bone mineral content and body fat content. It is particularly useful for the diagnosis of osteoporosis and assessing the response to treatment for this condition. A scanner machine beams x-rays from two different sources at the part of the body being examined. Any x-rays not absorbed are picked up by a detector, which produces an image of the bone.

Dysphonia – Difficulty in speaking.

Efficacy – The effectiveness of a drug against the disease or condition it was designed to treat.

Eicosanoids – A general term for the modified fatty acids that are the products of arachidonic acid metabolism (e.g. prostaglandins, thromboxanes and leukotrienes).

Enantiomers – See chiral drugs. A pair of chiral isomers that are non-superimposable mirror images of each other.

Endothelium – The inner lining of blood vessels. It has a number of functions, including acting as a barrier between blood and other body tissues, attracting white blood cells to the site of an infection, regulating blood flow, regulating blood clotting and controlling the contraction and relaxation of blood vessels.

Endpoint – A recognised stage in the disease process, used to compare the outcome in the different treatment arms of clinical trials. Endpoints can mark improvement or deterioration of the patient and signify the end of the trial.

Enzymatically converted – The conversion of one molecule into a different molecule by the action of enzymes, proteins produced by cells in the body that catalyse (increase the rate of) specific biochemical reactions in the body but are not themselves used up in the process.

Eosinophilic cationic protein (ECP) – A protein produced by activated eosinophils (white blood cells that play a role in allergic reactions) that has a positive electrical charge. ECP helps to destroy invading organisms, stimulates the release of histamine from mast cells, inhibits the proliferation of T lymphocytes, inhibits antibody synthesis in B lymphocytes, affects the blood clotting process and stimulates mucus secretion in the airways. Used clinically as a marker of airways inflammation in patients with asthma.

Eosinophilic vasculitits – Inflammation of the blood vessels due to the presence of abnormal numbers of eosinophils in the blood.

Eosinophils – White blood cells that destroy foreign organisms in the body and play a major role in allergic reactions. Eosinophils also secrete chemical mediators (e.g. eosinophilic cationic protein [ECP]) that can cause bronchoconstriction in asthma. Characterised by the presence of coarse granules in their cytoplasm and found in large numbers in the mucosa (the lining of the body passages and cavities that connect with the exterior).

Epidemiology – The incidence or distribution of a disease within a population.

Epimers – A stereoisomer that differs from its reference molecule at only one of its central carbon atoms.

Epithelial – Pertaining to the epithelium.

Epithelial goblet cells – A mucus-secreting cell located in the epithelium of the airways. Mucus helps to protect the airways by trapping foreign particles that enter the nose during breathing and keeps the airways moist.

Epithelium – A thin layer of cells that covers all of the internal and external surfaces of the body, including cavities, ducts and organs.

Ester – Organic substances containing a carbon atom that is double-bonded to one oxygen atom and single-bonded to another. Fats, such as cholesterol, are natural esters.

Esterification – The production of an ester through the reaction between an acid and an alcohol. Esters can also be manufactured in the body by enzymatic processes.

Ester pool – A store of esters within the body.

Exacerbation – A period during which the symptoms of a disease recur or become worse. Commonly used to describe an asthma attack.

Excretion – The elimination of a drug or substance from the body as a waste product, for example, in the urine or faeces.

Fibroblasts – Cells involved in the production of connective tissue (the tissues in the body that provide support, such as bone, tendons, ligaments and fat tissue). Fibroblasts are also themselves capable of developing into connective tissue cells (e.g. bone, fat and smooth muscle cells), and can migrate to the site of an injury to repair the damaged connective tissue.

Fumarate – A compound related to fumaric acid that is involved in cell metabolism (the production of energy) and sugar synthesis. The β_2-adrenoceptor agonist, formoterol, has a fumarate group.

Gene regulation – The control of protein production by genes, the units of hereditary information. Each gene consists of an ordered sequence of nucleotides (the building blocks of DNA) on a chromosome (strands of DNA containing many genes) and controls the production of a specific protein.

Genetic predisposition – An individuals' susceptibility to developing a disease or condition as a result of their genetic or chromosomal make-up.

Genotype – The genetic information carried by each individual that acts as a 'blueprint' to build and maintain that individual.

Glucocorticoid receptors – Protein molecules located inside cells that bind to glucocorticoids and mediate the biological effects of these hormones.

Glucocorticoids – Also known as glucocorticosteroids, these are the steroid (fat-like) hormones produced by the adrenal glands that regulate energy metabolism and play a role in immune and inflammatory responses. Cortisol is the most important glucocorticosteroid produced by the adrenal glands. Synthetic glucocorticosteroids are used to suppress allergic and inflammatory diseases (such as asthma) and the rejection of transplanted organs.

Glucocorticosteroids – See Glucocorticoids.

Glycine-16 genotype – Possessing the amino acid glycine at position 16 of the protein chain that makes up the human β_2-adrenoceptor. Some individuals have glycine at this position, whilst others have arginine. The natural occurrence of different forms of the β_2-adrenoceptor is thought to account for the different responses of individuals to β_2-adrenoceptor agonists (e.g. salbutamol, salmeterol).

Glycogenolysis – The breakdown of glycogen (the main storage form of glucose in the body, found mainly in the liver and muscle) into glucose.

Granuloma – A small mass or nodule of inflammatory tissue that develops in response to injury, inflammation or infection. Each nodule consists of a group of macrophages (scavenging cells) surrounded by a layer of lymphocytes (white blood cells). Granuloma formation is characteristic of a number of diseases, including tuberculosis and Crohn's disease (inflammation of the digestive tract).

Haematology – The study of blood and blood formation.

Heterozygous – Having two different forms of a gene, one inherited from each parent.

High affinity – Describes a substance that binds (attaches) strongly to its target, such as a receptor.

Histamine – An inflammatory substance that is released from mast cells during an allergic reaction. Histamine is one of the substances responsible for the swelling and redness associated with inflammation. Other effects include narrowing of the airways, itching and the stimulation of acid production in the stomach. The effects of histamine can be counteracted with antihistamine drugs (e.g. cetirizine, desloratadine and loratadine).

Homodimer complex – A protein arrangement consisting of two identical subunits.

Hydrofluoroalkane pressurised metered dose inhaler (MDI) – A canister containing a pressurised solution of an anti-asthma drug and the propellant (the substance used to expel the drug from the container) hydrofluoroalkane. When the canister is pressed down, the pressure in it is released briefly, allowing a measured dose of the asthma drug and hydrofluoroalkane to be released as a mist. The hydrofluoroalkane evaporates leaving behind small particles of the asthma drug, which are inhaled into the lungs. Hydrofluoroalkane is a non-chlorofluorocarbon propellant, which means that it is relatively 'environmentally friendly'.

Hyperplasia – An abnormal increase in the number of cells in an organ or tissue.

Hypertrophic obstructive cardiomyopathy – The abnormal thickening of the heart muscle leading to obstruction in the flow of blood from the heart into the aorta. The cells that make up the heart muscle are in disarray rather than lying in parallel rows. The condition has no apparent cause, but can be inherited. Symptoms include breathlessness and fatigue on exercising, chest pain, palpitations and dizziness. Can lead to congestive heart failure (failure of the heart to pump an adequate amount of blood around the body) and sudden death.

Hypoglycaemia – Abnormally low blood glucose (sugar) levels.

Hypothalamic–pituitary–adrenal (HPA) axis – The interaction between the hypothalamus, the pituitary gland and the adrenal glands. The hypothalamus lies just above the pituitary gland in the brain. It releases corticotropin-releasing hormone (CRH), which stimulates the pituitary gland to release adrenocorticotropic hormone (ACTH). This, in turn, stimulates the adrenal glands to secrete corticosteroid hormones, which play an important role in the regulation of fat, protein and carbohydrate metabolism, and in suppressing inflammatory reactions in the body.

Hypothalamic–pituitary–adrenal inhibitory potency – The extent to which a substance inhibits the hypothalamic–pituitary–adrenal (HPA) axis.

Idiopathic subvalvular aortic stenosis – Narrowing of the aorta below the aortic valve, the valve that controls the flow of blood from the left ventricle (lower chamber) of the heart into the aorta. The cause of the condition is unknown, but it is usually associated with hypertrophic obstructive cardiomyopathy and shares the same symptoms.

IgE antibodies – Protein–sugar complexes known as immunoglobulins that are produced by the body in response to the presence of an antigen (a foreign substance such as a virus or bacterium) and combine with the foreign substance to make it harmless. Antibodies are produced by certain white blood cells (B cells), and circulate in the blood and tissue fluids. Antibodies are grouped into five classes: IgA, IgD, IgE, IgG and IgM. IgE antibodies are the major antibodies involved in allergic reactions.

Immunological – Pertaining to immunology, the study of the body's immune system and diseases affecting this system. The immune system is the body's natural defence mechanism against infection and disease. It involves the action of antibodies, which are proteins that neutralise foreign particles in the body, and white blood cells, which attack and destroy foreign particles.

Inflammatory neurotransmitters – Chemicals that act as neurotransmitters but also have inflammatory effects. One example is substance P, which is involved in the transmission of pain and is also important in many inflammatory diseases (e.g. arthritis, asthma, hay fever, inflammatory bowel disease and migraine).

Inspiratory flow driven – Regulated by the air breathed into the lungs. Many inhaler devices used to administer anti-asthma drugs are inspiratory flow driven.

Inspired air – Air that has been breathed in.

Interleukins (IL) – A family of cytokines produced by white blood cells that play an important role in the functioning of the body's immune system. Twelve different interleukins have been identified, all with differing roles. For example, interleukin-4 (IL-4) plays a role in allergic reactions, IL-1, -6 and -11 are involved in the production of certain proteins by the liver in response to inflammation, and IL-9 stimulates mast cells to release histamine.

Intracellular ester pool – The accumulation of esters within a cell. Esters are fat-like substances containing a carbon atom that is double-bonded to one oxygen atom and single-bonded to another.

Intratracheal – Within the trachea or windpipe, the vertical tube that extends from the throat to just above the heart. Here it divides into the two main bronchi, which extend to the lungs.

Intubation – The insertion of a tube into a hollow organ, such as the trachea or the intestines, to keep it open or to reopen it if it was blocked.

In vitro – 'In glass'. Used with reference to experiments performed outside the living system in a laboratory setting.

In vivo – Used with reference to experiments performed within the living cell or organism.

Isoenzyme – Enzymes that catalyse the same chemical reaction, but differ in terms of their amino acid structure.

Isomer – Molecules (or drugs) that have the same chemical formula but a different spatial arrangement of their atoms.

Isotonic contraction – Muscular contraction in which the muscle shortens as it contracts.

Lassitude – Feeling tired, weak or exhausted.

Leakage – The undesirable loss of substances from a structure.

Leukotriene receptor antagonists – Drugs used in the treatment of asthma (e.g. montelukast and zafirlukast) that inhibit the binding of leukotrienes to their receptors. Leukotrienes are lipid (fat) molecules produced by white blood cells that mediate the inflammation associated with allergic and asthmatic reactions.

Leukotrienes – Inflammatory mediators produced by white blood cells and macrophages that mediate the inflammation associated with allergic and asthmatic reactions. Drugs that antagonise (inhibit) the effects of leukotrienes (e.g. montelukast and zafirlukast) are used in the treatment of asthma.

Lipid mediators – Lipids (fats) that play a role in biological or biochemical processes.

Lipolysis – The break down of lipids (fats).

Lipoxygenase pathway – A series of biochemical reactions that occurs in certain types of white blood cell (leukocytes and macrophages), platelets (cells involved in blood clotting) and lung cells. Results in the conversion of arachidonic acid into leukotrienes (fat molecules that mediate the inflammation associated with allergic reactions) and involves the action of the enzyme 5-lipoxygenase.

Lymphocytes – Another name for white blood cells. Form part of the body's immune system and play an important role in defending the body against invading organisms. There are two types of white blood cell: B lymphocytes and T lymphocytes. B lymphocytes produce antibodies and T lymphocytes attach to abnormal cells in the body (e.g. cells invaded by a virus, tumour cells or cells in transplanted tissue) and release chemicals that destroy the abnormal cells.

Macrophages – Cells that filter and remove foreign particles from the body, secrete cytokines and activate lymphocytes.

Main bronchi – The two major airways connecting the trachea (windpipe) to the smaller airways (bronchioles) in the lungs.

Mast cell – A cell that releases histamine and other chemicals involved in inflammation. Mast cells are responsible for the immediate reddening of the skin after an allergic response.

Matrix metalloproteinases – Enzymes that break down the proteins found in the spaces between cells, known as extracellular matrix proteins (e.g. collagen). Involved in wound healing, the formation of new blood vessels and the growth of cancerous cells. Metalloproteinases require the presence of zinc or calcium ions in order to function properly.

Matrix protein deposition – The laying down of proteins, that make up the extracellular matrix (the supporting tissue between cells). Examples of such proteins include collagen, elastin, fibrillin, fibronectin and laminin.

Mechanism of action – The manner in which a drug exerts its therapeutic effects.

Mellitus – Pertaining to diabetes mellitus.

Membrane receptors – Molecules (usually proteins) located in the cell membrane that show a particular affinity for a chemical, such as a hormone or a drug, and mediate the biological effect of that chemical.

Metabolism – The process by which a drug is broken down within the body.

Metabolites – The products of metabolism.

Metalloproteinase – Enzymes that break down proteins, and require the presence of zinc or calcium ions in order to function properly.

Methacholine – A drug that mimics the effects of histamine and is used to trigger short-term asthma attacks to determine whether or not a person has asthma.

Methacholine PC_{20} – The concentration of methacholine that reduces lung function (specifically the forced expiratory volume in 1 second or FEV_1 – see Spirometry) by 20%. This is evaluated by allowing the person to inhale increasing doses of methacholine and measuring lung function (FEV_1) after the inhalation of each dose. If the PC_{20} value is less than 4 mg/mL, the person is considered to have asthma.

Methotrexate – A drug used in the treatment of cancer and autoimmune diseases (diseases where the immune system attacks itself), such as rheumatoid arthritis. Methotrexate works by inhibiting the synthesis of folic acid, which is necessary for cell growth and proliferation.

Methylxanthines – A group of compounds (e.g. theophylline, caffeine) that act as mild stimulants and widen the airways by relaxing the smooth muscle in the airway walls. Sometimes used in the treatment of asthma.

Micronised particles – Very small particles of a drug. The minute particles have a high surface area, which helps them to dissolve faster in the body. Some of the drugs used to treat asthma are formulated as micronised particles, which are administered via an inhaler. The small size of the particles improves drug accessibility to the small airways of the lung.

Microvasculature – The smallest blood vessels in the body. Blood vessels less than 0.3 mm in diameter, such as venules and capillaries, are considered to be part of the microvasculature.

Mifepristone – A drug that antagonises (inhibits) the effects of progesterone (a hormone that helps to maintain pregnancy) and is used to terminate pregnancy or to induce labour when the foetus has died.

Monocytes – A type of white blood cell. These cells enlarge and develop into macrophages.

Morbidity – A diseased condition or state or the incidence of a disease within a population.

Mortality – The death rate of a population. The ratio of the total number of deaths to the total population.

Mucociliary – Pertaining to the movement of mucus in the airways due to the continual beating of finger-like projections known as cilia on the surface of the epithelial cells that line the airways. The cilia beat constantly in the same direction to clear mucus and foreign particles away from the airways.

Mucosa – The soft, pink lining of the body passages and hollow cavities that connect with the exterior, such as the respiratory and digestive tracts. The main functions of the mucosa are to give protection and support to the underlying structures, to absorb nutrients, and to secrete mucus, enzymes and salts.

Mucosal oedema – The abnormal accumulation of fluid in the mucosa, causing mucosal swelling.

Mucus gland – A collection of cells in the lining of the airways that secrete mucus. The mucus helps to protect the airways by trapping foreign particles that enter the nose during breathing, and keeps the airways moist.

Mucus gland proliferation – An increase in the number of mucus glands in the walls of the airways.

Mucus hypersecretion – The excessive production of mucus by the mucosa.

Multicentre – A clinical trial conducted across a number of treatment centres, either abroad or in the same country.

Multifactorial – A disease or state arising from more than one causative element.

Murine – Pertaining to mice.

Nebulisers – Devices used to administer bronchodilatory drugs (drugs that widen the airways) in the emergency treatment of asthma.

Necrotic epithelial cells – Epithelial cells having undergone cell death (necrosis). Epithelial cells line the internal and external surfaces of the body, including cavities, ducts and organs, and form the epithelium.

Negative exponential model – A statistical model used to determine the rate of decline of a particular population or the probability of survival in a particular population.

Neuropeptides – A family of small proteins that act as neurotransmitters (e.g. substance P, tachykinins, calcitonin gene-related peptide [CGRP]). Contribute to inflammatory reactions, for example, substance P and the tachykinins produce smooth muscle contraction and mucus secretion.

Neurotransmitter – A chemical that transmits nervous impulses from one nerve cell to another, or from nerve cells to muscles.

Neutrophil – A type of white blood cell that defends the body against invading organisms, such as bacteria or viruses. Neutrophils move to the site of infection or inflammation where they ingest and destroy the invading organism.

Neutrophil adhesion – The ability of neutrophils to adhere to endothelial cells (the cells that line blood vessels) at a site of inflammation or infection in the body. The neutrophils then migrate through the walls of the blood vessels to the site of infection and destroy the invading organism.

Neutrophil apoptosis – The deliberate and programmed death of a neutrophil. Death occurs after a neutrophil has ingested and destroyed an invading organism at the site of infection, and the dead neutrophil is then ingested by macrophages (scavenging cells). A number of diseases are associated with alterations in neutrophil apoptosis, including cancer.

Non-halogenated – A chemical compound in which the hydrogen atoms have not been substituted with a halogen (the chemicals chlorine, fluorine, bromine and iodine). Corticosteroids can be halogenated or non-halogenated.

Ocular – Pertaining to the eyes.

O-demethylation – A chemical reaction involving the removal of a methyl group (one carbon atom and three hydrogen atoms) from the O terminal (the end of the molecule containing an oxygen atom) of the molecule or compound in question.

Oleate – A salt of oleic acid, a naturally occurring fatty acid found in olive oil.

Open-label – A clinical trial in which all participants (i.e. the doctor and the patient) are aware of the treatment allocation.

Oropharyngeal – Pertaining to the oropharynx, the middle part of the passage that connects the back of the nose and mouth to the entrance of the trachea (windpipe) and oesophagus (the tube that conveys food from the mouth to the stomach).

Oropharyngeal deposition – The distribution of an inhaled drug in the oropharynx.

Osteocalcin – A protein produced by bone cells or osteoblasts that plays a role in bone formation. Serum levels of osteocalcin provide an indication of bone turnover.

Osteoporosis – A disease of skeletal fragility in which bone strength is compromised through the progressive deterioration of bone density and quality. Common in postmenopausal women, osteoporosis is also associated with other conditions, including rheumatoid arthritis, hyperthyroidism (the overproduction of thyroid hormones), use of corticosteroids and acromegaly (the excessive production of growth hormone resulting in an enlarged head, hands and feet).

Otitis media – Inflammation of the middle ear (the cavity between the ear drum and the inner ear, the latter containing the hearing structures) due to a bacterial or viral infection in the nose or throat passing up the eustachian tube (the tube that connects the middle ear to the back of the nose). Typical symptoms include severe earache, a feeling of fullness in the ear, deafness, ringing or buzzing in the ear and a temperature. Can be treated with antibiotics.

Ovalbumin-sensitised – Having increased the sensitivity of the airways to ovalbumin (a protein found in the white of an egg) through exposure to the protein. Future contact with this protein will then stimulate an asthma-like immune response. Ovalbumin-sensitised animals are used in medical research to study the pathogenesis of asthma.

Oxidative metabolism – A chemical process which uses oxygen to break down a substance.

Oxygen-derived free radicals – The splitting of oxygen within the body to produce free radicals; unstable atoms or molecules that contain an unpaired electron. Free radicals are highly reactive with other cellular structures because they take electrons from other molecules to become more stable. This process, known as oxidation, is toxic to many cells and can result in cellular damage.

***p*-value** – In statistical analysis, a measure of the probability that a given result occurred by chance. If the *p*-value is less than or equal to 0.05 then the result is usually considered to be statistically significant, and not due to chance.

Paradoxical bronchospasm – The apparently contradictory narrowing of the airways following the inhalation of a drug that is intended to relax the airways (e.g. β_2-agonists).

Pathogenesis – The processes involved in the development of a particular disease.

Pathogens – Agents (particularly micro-organisms) that cause disease, such as bacteria, viruses and fungi.

Pathophysiology – The functional changes that accompany a particular syndrome or disease.

Patient demographics – Patient characteristics, such as age, weight and height. Usually measured at the start of a clinical trial.

Perinatal – Pertaining to the period just before and just after birth (from week 28 of pregnancy to the end of the first week after birth).

Peripheral blood mononuclear cell proliferation – An increase in the number of peripheral blood mononuclear cells, a collective term to describe a number of different white blood cells including B and T lymphocytes, and granulocytes (eosinophils, basophils and neutrophils).

Peripheral dilatation – Widening of the blood vessels in the periphery (away from the central core) of the body (e.g. the arms and legs).

Phaeochromocytoma – A tumour of the adrenal glands, leading to the oversecretion of adrenaline and noradrenaline, which in turn, causes hypertension. Symptoms can include headaches, palpitations, flushing, nausea and vomiting.

Pharmacodynamics – The physiological and biological effects of a drug, including its mechanism of action – the process by which it exerts its therapeutic effects.

Pharmacokinetics – The activity of the drug within the body over a period of time.

Pharmacology – The branch of science that deals with the origin, nature, chemistry, effects and uses of drugs.

Pharynx – The passageway that connects the back of the nose and throat to the larynx (voice box) and the oesophagus (gullet).

Phenylethanolamine – A substance found in the brain that regulates the activity of the sympathetic nervous system.

Phenytoin – A non-sedating anticonvulsant drug used in the treatment of epilepsy, seizures due to head injury or neurosurgery, and cardiac arrhythmias (abnormal heart rhythms).

Phosphoinositide signalling cascade – A series of biochemical reactions within a cell. The pathway starts with the production of phosphoinositide (a type of fat molecule) which generates signals within the cell. The signalling pathways mediate many cellular activities, including growth, development, chemotaxis (cell movement in response to a certain chemical), glucose (sugar) metabolism and survival. Diseases associated with abnormal phosphoinositide signalling include cancer, diabetes and autoimmune inflammation (inflammation caused by the immune system attacking itself).

Pituitary gland – A pea-sized structure at the base of the brain. The pituitary is the most important endocrine (hormone-producing) gland and controls the activity of other endocrine glands and regulates many bodily processes.

Placebo – An inert substance with no specific pharmacological activity.

Placebo-controlled – A clinical trial in which a proportion of patients are given placebo in place of the active drug.

Platelet-activating factor (PAF) – A substance produced in response to specific stimuli by activated platelets, neutrophils and basophils in the blood. PAF stimulates platelets to clump together and form blood clots and also induces bronchoconstriction.

Polymyalgia – Pain in several muscles.

Pooled analysis – The amalgamation and processing of data derived from multiple clinical trials.

Post-bronchodilator FEV_1 – The volume of air that can be exhaled from fully inflated lungs during the first second of exhalation (the forced expiratory volume in 1 second or FEV_1) measured after inhaling a bronchodilator (a drug that widens the airways). Comparing this parameter with the pre-bronchodilator FEV_1 (see below) provides a measure of how well the airways have responded to the bronchodilator.

Posterior subcapsular cataracts – Cataracts (clouding of the lens of the eye) that develop towards the back of the cellophane-like capsule that surrounds the lens. People who take steroids for an inflammatory condition, such as asthma, are at increased risk of developing this type of cataract.

Pre-bronchodilator FEV_1 – The volume of air that can be exhaled from fully inflated lungs during the first second of exhalation (the forced expiratory volume in 1 second or FEV_1) measured before inhaling a bronchodilator (a drug that widens the airways). It gives an indication of whether or not a person has asthma. By measuring the pre- and post-bronchodilator FEV_1, it is possible to determine how well the airways respond to a particular bronchodilator.

Prednisolone – A synthetic corticosteroid used in the treatment of inflammatory conditions and to prevent the rejection of a transplanted organ.

Primidone – An anticonvulsant drug used to treat epilepsy, seizures and tremors.

Prophylaxis – Preventative treatment. Steps taken to prevent a disease before it occurs.

Prostaglandins – Naturally occurring chemicals in the body that act as hormones. Prostaglandins are found in many different tissues and have a wide range of effects in the body, including causing pain and inflammation in damaged tissues and the development of fever.

Pruritus – Itching.

Pulmonary disease – Lung disease or dysfunction.

Pulmonary tuberculosis – Infection of the lungs with the bacterium *Mycobacterium tuberculosis.* The lungs are usually the first organs to be infected since the bacterium is transmitted by inhalation. Once in the lungs, it can spread to other parts of the body in the bloodstream. Symptoms of tuberculosis include a general feeling of malaise, tiredness, loss of appetite, fever, sweating and a cough with blood-stained sputum.

Quiescent tuberculosis – Dormant tuberculosis. Once in the body, the *Mycobacterium tuberculosis* bacterium may remain inactive for many years. The bacterium may become activated at a later date, causing serious disease.

Racemic – Containing equal quantities of two enantiomers.

Radioactively labelled – Tagged with a radioactive substance. Commonly used to visualise biological processes *in vivo.*

Refill persistence – The compliance of patients in taking their medication as determined by counting the number of prescription refills (repeat prescriptions) for the medication over a certain amount of time.

Rescue medication – Medication that is taken to relieve an asthma attack (exacerbation) when it occurs. The most commonly used drugs are β_2-agonists (e.g. salbutamol, terbutaline). They are inhaled directly into the lungs, where they widen the airways and relieve the symptoms of asthma within minutes. Although rescue medication is fast acting, it does not have a long-term effect.

Resorption – The breakdown of a substance and the absorption of the breakdown products into the tissues of the body. Commonly used to describe the breakdown of bone in the bone remodelling process.

Reversible airflow limitation – Obstructed airflow in the airways, caused by narrowing or inflammation, that can be reversed with appropriate treatment. Asthma is a disease characterised by reversible airways obstruction.

Rhinovirus-induced – Caused by a rhinovirus, a group of viruses that are responsible for many infections of the respiratory tract, including the common cold.

Rifamycins – A group of antibiotics that are particularly effective against mycobacteria. Such antibiotics are used in the treatment of tuberculosis and leprosy.

RR enantiomers – The 'right-handed' form of a chiral compound.

Safety and tolerability – The side-effects associated with a particular drug and the likelihood that patients will tolerate a drug treatment regimen.

Salbutamol – Also known as albuterol, salbutamol is an inhaled drug used in the treatment of asthma and chronic obstructive pulmonary disease (COPD). It widens the airways by stimulating β_2 adrenoceptors, leading to relaxation of the smooth muscle in the walls of the airways. This allows more air to flow in and out of the lungs during breathing.

Secretory leucocyte protease inhibitor – A protein found in large quantities in the fluid secreted by mucosa cells that inhibits the serine proteases (a family of enzymes that break certain bonds in proteins) produced by mast cells and leucocytes (a collective term for white blood cells). Serine proteases have been implicated in the pathogenesis of asthma, and secretory leucocyte protease inhibitors are thought to provide protection against airway inflammation.

Serum cortisol – The concentration of the hormone, cortisol, in serum (the fluid component of blood after clotting agents have been removed). Cortisol is produced by the adrenal glands in response to the secretion of adrenocorticotropic hormone (ACTH) from the pituitary gland and plays a role in carbohydrate, fat and protein metabolism, functioning of the immune system and bone formation. Serum levels of cortisol are measured to determine how well the pituitary and adrenal glands are functioning.

Single-blind – A clinical trial in which only the patient is unaware of the treatment allocation.

Sinusitis – Inflammation of the membrane lining the facial sinuses (hollow cavities behind the forehead and cheekbones) due to a bacterial or viral infection, or an allergic reaction. Symptoms include pain in the face, headache, a blocked or runny nose, sensitive teeth and swelling around the eyes. The condition may be treated with decongestants (drugs that reduce nasal congestion) and, in the case of a bacterial infection, antibiotics.

Smooth muscle hypertrophy – An increase in the size of smooth muscle due to an increase in the size of its constituent cells. Smooth muscle is found in the walls of internal organs, such as the bladder, blood vessels and the digestive tract.

Socioeconomic impact – Social and economic factors that characterise the influence of a disease. Incorporates the financial cost incurred by the healthcare provider, patient and/or their employer.

Soft steroid – A synthetic corticosteroid that has a 'built-in' metabolic deactivator. When the drug reaches the bloodstream after it has exerted its effects on the respiratory system, it is rapidly deactivated. Thus, such drugs are active in the respiratory system without causing untoward effects in the rest of the body.

Spacer device – A large, plastic container with a mouthpiece at one end and a hole for inserting a metered dose inhaler (MDI) at the other end. Designed to make it easier to breathe in asthma medication from an MDI and to ensure that the asthma medication reaches the lungs. Young children may benefit from such a device.

Spasmogens – Substances that cause the contraction of smooth muscle, including that in the walls of the airways.

Spirometric – Pertaining to spirometry.

Spirometry – Techniques used to determine how well the lungs are functioning. The person breathes into a mouthpiece that is connected to a recording device known as a spirometer. This measures how quickly and how much air is moving in and out of the lungs.

SS enantiomers – The 'left-handed' form of a chiral compound.

Statistical significance – A measure of the probability that a given result derived from a clinical trial – be it an improvement or a decline in the health of the patient – is due to a specific effect of drug treatment, rather than a chance occurrence.

Status asthmaticus – A severe asthma attack that does not respond to conventional treatment and can therefore be fatal. It may require the injection of corticosteroids directly into the bloodstream or intubation (the passage of a tube down the trachea or windpipe to enable air to reach the lungs).

Stereoisomer – Molecules (or drugs) that have the same molecular formula, the same sequence of chemical bonds, but different spatial arrangements.

Steroidal agents – Compounds that act like steroids.

Subepithelial tissue – The tissue situated just underneath the epithelium (lining) of a cavity, duct or organ in the body.

Suboptimal – Below the 'best' or maximal level.

Surrogate markers – Laboratory or physical parameters that are used as a substitute for a direct biological measurement, such as how a patient feels, or how effective a particular treatment is.

Sustained-release theophylline – A formulation of theophylline that is released slowly into the body over a prolonged period of time. Theophylline is a drug used to treat diseases of the airways. Its main action is to relax the smooth muscle in the walls of the airways and blood vessels, thus widening these structures. This allows more air to flow in and out of the lungs during breathing.

Sympathetic nervous system – The part of the autonomic nervous system that controls the automatic functions of the body, such as breathing, digestion and the beating of the heart. Most sympathetic nerve cells, (but not all) use noradrenaline as a neurotransmitter.

Sympathomimetic – Produces effects similar to those of the sympathetic nervous system.

Terbutaline prodrug – An inactive form of terbutaline that becomes activated by a metabolic process once inside the body. Terbutaline is used in the treatment of asthma. It widens the airways by stimulating the β_2-receptors for adrenaline, leading to relaxation of the smooth muscle in the walls of the airways.

Th1 cells – A subset of helper T lymphocytes which manufacture and secrete interleukin-2, gamma-interferon, and interleukin-12. Involved in the destruction of invading organisms.

Th2 cells – A subset of helper T-lymphocytes which manufacture and secrete the interleukins (IL), Il-4, Il-5, Il-6 and Il-10. Involved in humoral immunity, which is the production of antibodies by B lymphocytes.

Th1 and Th2 phenotypes – Having the appearance of Th1 or Th2 cells, the two subsets of T helper cells.

T-helper cells – T lymphocytes, also known as $CD4^+$ cells, that co-ordinate the immune response. Destroyed by the human immunodeficiency virus (HIV).

Thymus involution – The shrinkage of the thymus gland, which occurs in most individuals after puberty. The thymus gland is located in the upper chest cavity between the neck and lungs and forms part of the body's immune system in early life.

Thyrotoxicosis – Overactivity of the thyroid gland, leading to the excessive production of thyroid hormones. This causes an increase in the body's metabolism, leading to weight loss, increased appetite, an increased heart rate, protruding eyes, sweating, shaking and hyperactivity. The condition may be treated with drugs that inhibit the production of thyroid hormones or by surgically removing part of the thyroid gland.

T lymphocytes – A type of white blood cell found in blood and the lymphatic system. T lymphocytes play a major role in the body's immune response, and are activated by the presence of an antigen (invading organism). Following activation, they migrate to the site of the antigen where they either destroy the invading organism or activate other immune cells (macrophages and natural killer cells) to do so. There are a number of different types of T lymphocyte, including cytotoxic T cells, helper T cells, suppressor T cells and regulatory T cells.

Topical-to-systemic activity – A comparison of the beneficial effects of an anti-asthma drug on the respiratory system and their unwanted effects elsewhere in the body. A drug with high topical-to-systemic activity is effective at reducing the symptoms of asthma without causing untoward effects in other body systems.

Trachea – Commonly known as the windpipe, the trachea is the tube that conveys air from the throat to the lungs.

Transmembrane helices – The parts of membrane proteins or receptors that span the membrane, forming links between the inside and the outside of the cell.

Trimester – A period of three months. One-third of the length of a pregnancy.

Tumour Necrosis Factor (TNF) – A cytokine that acts as a messenger between cells of the immune system. Produced by white blood cells in response to infection or the presence of cancer cells, and activates white blood cells seek and destroy foreign substances (e.g. bacteria and viruses) and cancer cells. However, TNF also causes certain types of inflammation, such as that occurring in rheumatoid arthritis (RA).

Tumour Necrosis Factor-α (TNF-α) – A member of the TNF family of cytokine proteins. TNF-α comprises 157 amino acids and has a wide range of proinflammatory actions. Two other types of TNF have been identified, β and γ. However, the term TNF (see previous entry) is often used synonymously with TNF-α.

Two-dimensional gamma scintigraphy – An imaging technique used to visualise different body systems. A chemical that emits gamma radiation is administered to the patient via injection, tablet or inhaler, depending on the body system to be examined. The gamma radiation is picked up by a detector, which produces a two-dimensional (flat) image. The technique is commonly used to study the distribution of inhaled drugs in the lungs.

Vascular permeability – The passage of water and small molecules (e.g. oxygen and carbon dioxide) through the walls of blood vessels.

Vasculitic rash – A rash characterised by small, red spots. The red spots are actually tiny blood blisters that are caused by the bursting of tiny blood vessels under the skin.

Wash-out – A period of time during a clinical trial when the participants do not receive any treatment so that the variables being evaluated (e.g. blood pressure) can return to their normal values.

Xanthine – A class of organic compounds (e.g. theophylline) with a ring structure containing nitrogen and oxygen atoms. In the human body, xanthines widen the airways by relaxing the smooth muscle in the airway walls. Thus, they are useful in the treatment of asthma.

Xinafoate – An acid salt of a compound.

Useful contacts

• Asthma UK

Providence House
Providence Place
London
N1 0NT
Asthma UK Adviceline: 08457 010203
Website: *http://www.asthma.org.uk/*
Registered charity
Formerly called the National Asthma Campaign

• Asthma UK Scotland

4 Queen's Street
Edinburgh
EH2 1JE
Asthma UK Advice line: 08457 010203
Website: *http://www.asthma.org.uk/*
Registered charity

• The British Thoracic Society

The British Thoracic Society
17 Doughty Street
London
WC1N 2PL
Email: *bts@brit-thoracic.org.uk*
Tel: 020 7831 8778
Website: *http://www.brit-thoracic.org.uk*
Registered charity

• The Lung and Asthma Information Agency

Community Health Sciences Department
St. George's Hospital Medical School
Cranmer Terrace
London
SW17 0RE
Website: *http://www.laia.ac.uk*
Academic resource unit sponsored by the asthma charities

• British Lung Foundation

73–75 Goswell Road
London
EC1V 7ER
Email: *enquiries@blf-uk.org*
Tel: 020 7688 5555
Website: *http://www.lunguk.org*
Registered charity

• Global Initiative for Asthma (GINA)

Website: *http://www.ginasthma.com*

• Best Treatments UK

Website:
http://www.besttreatments.co.uk/btuk/home.html
Produced by the British Medical Association

• NHS Direct

Website: *http://www.nhsdirect.nhs.uk/*

Index